Understanding Medical Professionalism

Understanding Medical Professionalism

Wendy Levinson, MD

Sir John and Lady Eaton Professor and Chair
Department of Medicine, University of Toronto
Toronto, Canada

Shiphra Ginsburg, MD, Med

Professor, Department of Medicine
Scientist, Wilson Centre for Research
   in Education
Staff Physician, Mount Sinai Hospital
Faculty of Medicine
University of Toronto
Toronto, Canada

Frederic W. Hafferty, PhD

Professor of Medical Education
Associate Dean of Professionalism,
College of Medicine
Associate Director, Program in
   Professionalism & Ethics
Mayo Clinic
Rochester, Minnesota

Catherine R. Lucey, MD

Professor of Medicine
Vice Dean for Education
School of Medicine
University of California, San Francisco
San Francisco, California

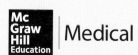 Medical

New York   Chicago   San Francisco   Athens   London   Madrid   Mexico City
Milan   New Delhi   Singapore   Sydney   Toronto

Understanding Medical Professionalism

1 2 3 4 5 6 7 8 9 0   CTP/CTP   19 18 17 16 15 14

ISBN 978-0-07-180743-2
MHID 0-07-180743-8

This book was set in Times LT Std by MPS Limited.
The editors were Jim Shanahan and Karen G. Edmonson.
The production supervisor was Catherine Saggese.
Project management was provided by Charu Khanna at MPS Limited.
The designer was Eve Siegel; the cover designer was Thomas De Pierro.
China Translation & Printing Services, Ltd. was printer and binder.

This book is printed on acid-free paper.

Library of Congress Cataloging-in-Publication Data

Levinson, Wendy, author.
Understanding medical professionalism/Wendy Levinson, Shiphra Ginsburg, Frederic W. Hafferty, Catherine R. Lucey.
    p. ; cm.
Includes bibliographical references and index.
ISBN 978-0-07-180743-2—ISBN 0-07-180743-8
I. Ginsburg, Shiphra, author. II. Hafferty, Frederic W., 1947- author.
III. Lucey, Catherine R., author. IV. Title.
[DNLM: 1. Clinical Competence. 2. Physician's Role.
3. Physician-Patient Relations. 4. Professional Practice. 5. Quality Assurance, Health Care. W 21]
R727.3
610.69'6—dc23

                                        2013043233

Contents

Chapter 1

A Practical Approach to "Professionalism" 1

Chapter 2

Resilience in Facing Professionalism Challenges 17

Chapter 3

A Brief History of Medicine's Modern-Day Professionalism Movement. 37

Chapter 4

Fostering Patient-Centered Care 55

Chapter 5

Integrity and Accountability 85

Chapter 10

Evaluating Professionalism 213

Chapter 11

When Things Go Wrong: The Challenge
of Self-Regulation 243

Chapter 12

Organizational Professionalism 277

Foreword

Spending the past decade as a dean for medical education charged with overseeing both undergraduate and graduate medical education at the University of Chicago, and for more than a decade before that serving as a residency program director, I have spent a considerable part of my career tackling modern-day issues of medical professionalism from the onset movement in the 1990s. In my various roles, I have sympathized with students who told me that being lectured to about professionalism is demeaning, discussed with residents the complexities of adhering to duty hours while ensuring that patients are well cared for, and brainstormed with faculty about elevating the ideals of professionalism across the entire medical enterprise.

Teaching professionalism is difficult. It can also be frustrating—how do you teach and impart core values? Influencing and creating a clinical learning environment can take years to bear fruit. This book's authors understand the profession's struggle and expertly reframe the issues by refocusing our attention on practical, specific behaviors, and coping techniques, while enlarging the discussion to focus on societal and systemic concerns. How can we thoughtfully design our healthcare system and our educational endeavors to help health professionals provide the best care for patients?

Implicit in nearly every discussion of professionalism up to this point is the hidden assumption that being professional is an immutable character trait, and one that the physician alone must carry. If a student, resident, or faculty member fails to act professionally, they have failed the profession. That is a heavy burden for anyone to carry and as educators we have asked our most inexperienced trainees to do just that. This book relieves us of the burden of this moral superiority.

Physicians are not, as Chapter 3 so aptly describes, superhuman. And being professional is not a superpower. It is a skill and competency which can be taught, and one that must be developed over our entire careers. Being professional, it turns out, is learning how to be completely human—learning how to manage challenging ethical situations, practicing telling patients "no" when they ask for unwarranted tests, and learning strategies for how to build up personal reserves so that we are better prepared to manage professional challenges. This requires practice. Throughout this book we are introduced to helpful tools. Communication training, faculty role modeling, the use of checklists and other rubrics focused on patient-centered care may all prove useful. The authors rightfully acknowledge that throughout the day, all health professionals struggle to act professionally. Occasional lapses in professional behavior are not character flaws, they are opportunities for learning. These opportunities appear at every level of practice, whether we are students, residents, or seasoned practitioners.

The message is clear: upholding the trust that our patients have placed in our hands is difficult. We all need guidance. Using challenge cases, checklists, and tables, this book provides the tools to help us bring the best version of ourselves to our daily interactions with patients. In today's world, being professional is synonymous with working in and leading team-based care. Physicians cannot and do not single-handedly treat patients. Professionalism is not an issue of *physician behavior*—it is an issue of the *team's behavior*—and fundamentally—an issue related to the *healthcare system*. Expanding the definition of professionalism beyond the physician does not abdicate the physician's responsibility for the patient; it simply expands the definition to acknowledge that all members of the healthcare system are equally responsible for providing the best possible care for patients. What does this mean for the nurses, assistants, and administrators who work with us to provide patient care? We are asking nurses and other healthcare professionals to help us by providing feedback when our behavior is not serving the patient. Fundamentally, this evolving definition means a willingness and openness to accept and learn from feedback—a fundamental acceptance of partnership.

Understanding Medical Professionalism places the issue of physician professionalism within the context of the healthcare system. Once we accept that professionalism is a competency that can be learned, we open up the possibility of focused interventions and systemic solutions. How can physicians influence the system and be advocates for change? Quite simply, get involved. This may take the form of participating in accreditation processes, quality task forces, or patient safety committees. Every day I work with medical students and residents who embrace civic professionalism and literally change the way our hospital does its business. The view from the trenches through the eyes of our students and residents provides a rarefied lens through which to see the world of healthcare. This view combined with their dedication and passion make a powerful impact for patients. The practical exercises in this book invite us all to reconnect with the thrill we experienced as students when we put on our white coat for the first time and believed that we could make a difference.

Understanding Medical Professionalism represents an important step forward in the ongoing discussion of medical professionalism. Hampered for decades with concerns that lapses in professional behavior were linked to deficits in character, this book reminds us to lay down our insecurities and defenses, acknowledge we all stumble in consistently being our best professional selves, and then invites us to roll up our sleeves, and get to work learning and relearning how to be professional in today's complex environment. Now is the time to create healthcare teams, institutions, and systems that foster an environment of respect, learning, and compassion to deliver the best possible care for patients. This book will help you do exactly that. Let's get started!

Holly J. Humphrey, MD
Chicago, Illinois
February 2014

Foreword

When I was 22 I was camping in the Pacific Northwest and broke my arm. I was a student with no health insurance and no money. I went to a couple of emergency rooms in the small towns in the area and all of them told me they couldn't treat me. Finally I found a physician—not an orthopedic surgeon—probably an internist—who would see me. We both scanned a book about fractures to see how to set my arm. When asked by his office staff how to code the bill, he said code it "H" for humanitarian.

This one example of medical professionalism was a defining moment for me. It led me to medical school. The combination of independence, intellectual curiosity and a higher purpose that this one physician exemplified was enough for me. It was why I became a physician. It was also one of the best examples of medical professionalism I've experienced in my decades' long career.

Often, the term physician professionalism is used to describe the motivations behind physician behavior—a physician's unique ability to see beyond personal self-interest or comfort—and do what is right for their patient and their community. Professionalism has at its heart a fundamental core—the idea that physicians are led by an intrinsic motivation to do their best for their patients.

On the flipside of the generous doctor noted above, all of us who practice medicine have seen the other side of the coin. Physicians who deride colleagues, who perform impaired, who lack the cognitive skills necessary to practice. These transgressions—or "unprofessional" behavior—undermine our ability to deliver on our promise to our patients and our communities. As a profession—have we done enough to address these shortcomings? Have we done enough to train physicians live up to the ideals embodied in the Hippocratic oath? Have we codified behaviors that are unacceptable?

What has characterized the definitions of professionalism in the past century was that it was defined, and controlled by the profession itself, primarily through its professional associations. Many outside the profession, however, have little understanding of the term. Some have dismissed the concept as a shield for physicians against criticism and action. They are concerned that professionalism equals "just trust us." In some ways, those worries are well-founded. We all know of shocking lapses in reporting and sanctioning of impaired colleagues—which get dismissed as "unprofessional behavior" and not remediated. These are the kinds of shortcomings that made even the term "professionalism" subject to suspicion from those outside the profession.

Attempts to codify the term—and bring into focus the core responsibilities of medical professionalism—were undertaken by a triumvirate of physician organizations in 2001: the ABIM Foundation, American College of Physicians Foundation, and the European Federation of Internal Medicine. *Medical Professionalism in the New Millennium: A Physician Charter* was written to provide affirmative expectations of professionalism—a definition if you will. While initiated by internists, the *Physician Charter* was endorsed by every specialty, and by medical organizations throughout the world.

The *Charter* remains alive more than a decade later and has spawned a rich and growing literature examining the meaning of this modern concept of professionalism. The *Charter's* impact in the contemporary practice of medicine is its usefulness for patients and for physicians in establishing a clear social contract needed in the twenty-first century. New realities in health care include expectations of transparency about errors and gaps in quality of care, expectations of patient experience as a key aspect to defining quality of care and of the patient voice as an essential one at every table. These new definitions of professionalism don't change the fundamental principle of devotion to the patient's well-being. But they reshape professionalism as embracing a full understanding of the patient's values, of the responsibility to make information available more broadly to consumers and purchasers, and the demand for continuous improvement.

In some ways the *Charter* is the proud father of this book. But this book takes the concept further than the *Charter* ever could.

There is growing awareness that institutions and organizations can create environments that foster professionalism, or they can create barriers to professional behavior. For organizations that want to improve quality of care, that want to create teams, that want to provide high value care, while reducing waste—professionalism can be an effectively lever for change. We have seen this with the national Choosing Wisely® campaign where leaders in medical specialties have called out tests and procedures that may be unnecessary—potentially undercutting reimbursements in the process. Their commitment to their patients and the health care system overrides their self-interest. Their professionalism drives this important effort.

With the growing emphasis on the value of systems in coordinating care, it is vitally important for health care organizations to consider their policies and their culture as key to advancing and supporting positive motivations of the professionals who work within their frameworks. This book is the first to place so firmly this responsibility with institutional leaders, and to include key practical considerations within every chapter.

In this past decade, scholarship on the topic of professionalism has expanded exponentially. But it is hard for the student, resident or fellow, or anyone in a busy practice to review this extensive literature and easily understand its implications for how they practice every day. In addition, health system leaders do not yet understand the link between physician leadership and professionalism and quality improvements.

Levinson and her colleagues have provided an extraordinary service to the profession, to health system leaders, to patients, and to society, in creating this important book. While built on the deep scholarship of philosophers and sociologists, and integrated with evidence on motivation, behavior, and learning it is accessible and actionable and focuses ultimately on what matters most to physicians—how to deliver the highest quality care possible.

Christine Cassel, MD
President and CEO, National Quality Forum
Immediate Past President and CEO,
American Board of Internal Medicine
and ABIM Foundation
February 2014

Preface

As medical students, residents, and practicing physicians, we all strive to be professional. We are dedicated to our work with patients and we strive to provide the highest level of excellence in all aspects of our work. We learn the codes of professionalism that govern medicine, starting from the Hippocratic oath that we all recite when we graduate from medical school to the modern day *Physician Charter*. Yet, despite our good intentions and the modern day charter, many of us think of professionalism as an abstract concept, a theoretical aspirational goal, or a set of written principles, rather than a set of core skills that we use in our daily clinical care, learning, and teaching.

This book will show that medical professionalism is part of our routine work and we do it best when we have specific skills. It is not just a theoretical concept or a set of principles distant from our clinical practice. This book is about medical professionalism in our work as students, residents, and practice physicians. It is also about professionalism in our medical institutions and hence, administrators and medical leaders are part of our target audience. We have designed this book to be highly practical and to help our readers develop or deepen their professionalism skills. Chapters include clinical scenarios all based on our personal experience in teaching and clinical care, learning exercises to stimulate active participation of readers, and "challenge cases." This is not a book about theory (although it includes some theoretical background); rather it is written to engage readers in reflection about professionalism in their own work.

There are several key premises of the book:

First, we define professionalism as a set of behaviors that can be demonstrated in our daily work. Defining professionalism as behaviors, enabled by specific skills that can be taught, and learned, makes "professionalism" practical and relevant.

Second, challenges to our professionalism occur every day in all clinical settings. Often physicians think of breaches of professionalism as something that most readers will never encounter; breaches where physicians commit serious offenses—like having sexual relations with patients. This is not our concept of every day professionalism challenges. Rather we think breaches in professionalism occur routinely in clinical care and teaching: the dilemma for a trainee of the need to adhere to work hour restrictions versus going to spend more time with a patient; observing or participating in a medical error that is undisclosed to the patient; disrespectful communication between physicians and nurses. These are all common examples of challenges to medical professionalism. We live with these challenges all the time. We need specific skills to handle them well.

Third, the responsibility to demonstrate professionalism is shared by individual physicians, the healthcare team, the medical institution, and medical professional organizations. Most physicians think that "being professional" is all their responsibility and often one that is a difficult burden to bear. Our premise is a novel one—medical professionalism is a system issue. All the stakeholders in the system can strive to enhance professionalism and can also create barriers to professionalism in a medical environment. Hence, the corollary is that all the stakeholders—trainees, physicians, healthcare team members, healthcare administrators, and leaders of professional organizations—have a key and important role to play.

Fourth, skills in medical professionalism need to be developed continuously over our lifetime. Just like we continuously learn new skills in diagnosis and treatment, we can and must keep learning how to demonstrate our professionalism in our daily work. The challenges we face are opportunities to learn new skills—just like seeing a rare presentation of a disease is an opportunity to deepen our knowledge and skills about diagnosis and treatment. Professionalism is a competency developed over time—that ca n result in mastery. We all need to develop "professional resiliency"—the ability to respond, based on skills, to challenging situations that inevitably arise.

The book presents professionalism in a *behavioral and systems approach*. This is done by a chapter that presents this core framework at the beginning (Chapter 1). The chapter presents our view that there are four key values that underlie medical professionalism—delivering patient-centered care; integrity and accountability; the pursuit of excellence; and the fair and ethical use of resources. For each of these values, there are specific behaviors that physicians, team members, healthcare administrators and leaders can demonstrate. Hence, the book has one chapter addressing each of these four values and presenting the specific behaviors and skills necessary to demonstrate that component of professionalism (Chapters 4, 5, 6, and 7).

Chapters on education and evaluation are relevant and practical for practicing physicians, medical students, residents, and faculty. These chapters are replete with learning and evaluation tools. Learning exercises are designed to allow readers to test their ability to handle professionalism challenges and to develop new approaches.

We are delighted to share this book with our readers who we hope will include students, residents in all specialties, faculty members, practicing physicians, healthcare administrators, and healthcare leaders. All of these healthcare professionals seek to achieve the highest level of professionalism in their care of individual patients, populations of patients, learning environments and care delivery systems. We hope this book will provide practical ways to make their efforts most effective. We think that readers will have fun working on the professionalism challenges presented in vignettes and learning exercises that are common situations we face in our daily work.

The Authors

Acknowledgments

We are incredibly grateful to several people who have helped us shape this book. The authors are very appreciative of the assistance of Karen McDonald from the University of Toronto for her help in preparation and review of all of the chapters. Also we wish to thank Amy Cunningham from the ABIM Foundation for her review of the manuscript and her contribution to the chapter on organizational professionalism. Daniel Wolfson, Executive Vice President and Chief Operating Officer, ABIM Foundation, encouraged us to write it in the first place. Our excellent chapter reviewers included Dr. Ayelet Kuper, Dr. Kaveh Shojania, Dr. Lynfa Stroud, Dr. Bob Wachter, Dr. Adina Weinerman, Dr. Brian Wong, and medical students, Marisa Leon, Sabrina Nurmohamed, and Raman Srivastava.

A PRACTICAL APPROACH TO "PROFESSIONALISM" | 1

Dr. Jackson is a 2nd-year medical resident doing a rotation on the wards of a teaching hospital. He was entering an order for an angiotensin-converting enzyme (ACE) inhibitor for Mrs. Shaw, an 80-year-old patient with congestive heart failure, when the chief resident interrupted him to discuss Mrs. Fraser, a patient with asthma who needed additional bronchodilator treatment. When Dr. Jackson returned to the computer, he incorrectly entered the order for salbutamol into the chart of Mrs. Shaw. The nurse noticed that this was a medication that had not previously been prescribed for Mrs. Shaw but did not question the order. The next day, the nurse sees Dr. Jackson during ward rounds and asks why the team started the salbutamol on Mrs. Shaw. When they realize there has been a medication error, the nurse and resident feel uncertain about whether they should tell the patient because she has not suffered any physical problems from the wrong drug. If they tell her, how should they do this and who should share the information with her? How might this be prevented in the hospital in the future? Dr. Jackson remembers he attended a lecture that mentioned that the hospital has an office that helps physicians with disclosing medical errors.

This case of a medication error illustrates a common occurrence and one in which multiple healthcare professionals play a role. Disclosing the error to the patient is a professional responsibility for the entire healthcare team. Dr. Jackson and the nurse will meet to plan how to tell Mrs. Shaw what occurred. The hospital has staff members who are experts in disclosing errors who will help Dr. Jackson and the nurse to prepare for this challenging disclosure conversation. Staff in the hospital's quality improvement department will conduct an analysis of the error to see how this error occurred and how they can prevent similar mistakes in the future. The hospital prides itself on compliance with the external standards set by the Joint Commission and the National Quality Forum Safe Practices regarding disclosing errors.

A medical error like this one is a challenge to our professionalism. Nobody working in healthcare intends to make a mistake, and yet, they occur routinely despite our best efforts to prevent them. Disclosing the error is a difficult task, but undertaking that conversation with the patient is an indication of the professionalism of each part of the system—the physician, the nurse, residents, medical students, and the hospital administration. Each player in the system, from an individual physician to the healthcare system itself, can demonstrate a high level of professionalism through behaviors that support the disclosure to the patient. Demonstrating professionalism is a team effort.

In this chapter, we describe a behavioral and systems approach to professionalism. Our basic tenets are the following:

1. Professionalism is demonstrated through a set of behaviors that can be observed;
2. The behaviors can be observed in four key domains:

    - the interaction between clinicians and patients/families;
    - the interaction among team members;
    - the practice settings (i.e., hospital, outpatient clinics, healthcare systems);
    - the professional organizations and external environment influencing care.

We have found this framework for describing professionalism to be a practical and useful approach for physicians, nurses, and healthcare administrators who seek to provide the highest quality of care (Lesser et al, 2010). We use examples of a variety of healthcare providers including practicing physicians, medical students, residents, nurse practitioners, physician assistants, and others, to illustrate our points.

WHY FOCUS ON BEHAVIORS?

When we begin to discuss the topic of "professionalism" during grand rounds, we often see that our audiences appear to be uninterested or even irritated. That reaction is understandable as our colleagues may think professionalism is some abstract concept, a theoretical aspirational goal, or a set of principles distant from clinical practice. They may believe they already have the right attitude toward patients and that this attitude will guide them to do the right thing when the circumstances require them to do so. They may be thinking, "What could this grand rounds speaker teach us that has any practical application to our daily lives?"

Thinking about professionalism as a set of behaviors that can be demonstrated in our everyday work has helped us to make "professionalism" much more practical and relevant. Behaviors, enabled by specific skills, are observable and can be learned (Lucey & Souba, 2010). The skills can be practiced and improved. When adult learners enter medical school with the desire to exhibit the values of professionalism (Leach, 2004), they have no experience in maintaining professional behavior under the challenging circumstances that confront practicing clinicians. Achieving professionalism in practice requires the capacity to navigate competing priorities and make sound judgments, often under pressure. Simply knowing right from wrong or having an internal compass does not suffice. Demonstrating professionalism is based on a set of practiced skills honed over time—skills we call on daily. The critical message of the framework is that professionalism is not a static or amorphous construct. Rather, it can be defined in concrete behaviors and should be understood as a lived approach to the practice of medicine that emanates, from physicians, to many varied interactions in the healthcare delivery system.

IDENTIFYING PROFESSIONALISM BEHAVIORS

In order to articulate a key set of behaviors, we revisit the Physician Charter on Medical Professionalism developed by the ABIM Foundation, American College of Physicians, and the European Federation of Internal Medicine. Since the creation of the Charter in 2002, it has become widely accepted around the world, and more than 300 medical organizations worldwide have endorsed it. The Charter offers a definition of professionalism based on three principles and a set of 10 commitments (Table 1-1) (ABIM Foundation, 2002).

Most physicians agree with the Charter's core commitments. For example, in a 2007 survey, 96% of physicians agreed with the principle of putting the patient's welfare above the physician's financial interest, and 98% agreed with the commitment to minimize healthcare disparities due to patient race or

Table 1-1   **THE PHYSICIAN CHARTER**
Three Fundamental Principles • Primacy of patient welfare • Patient autonomy • Social justice
Ten Commitments (commitments to…) • Competence • Honesty with patients • Patient confidentiality • Appropriate relations with patients • Improving quality of care • Improving access to care • Just distribution of finite resources • Scientific knowledge • Maintaining trust by managing conflicts of interest • Professional responsibilities

From ABIM Foundation. American Board of Internal Medicine; ACP-ASIM Foundation. American College of Physicians-American Society of Internal Medicine; European Federation of Internal Medicine. Medical professionalism in the new millennium: a physician charter. *Ann Intern Med*. 2002 Feb 5;136(3):243–246.

sex (Campbell et al, 2007). Because most physicians agree with the principles and commitments, this is a good starting point for articulating a set of behaviors that demonstrate professionalism in action. In order to operationalize the Charter into observable behaviors that can be demonstrated, we grouped the 10 commitments into four core values (Figure 1-1).

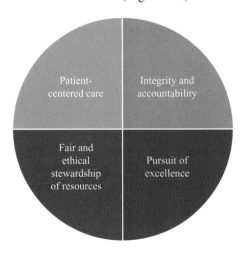

Figure 1-1 ▪ Four core values of medical professionalism.

	Core values			
Table 1-2 **RELATIONSHIP OF PROFESSIONALISM COMMITMENTS FROM CHARTER AND CORE VALUES**	Patient-centered care	Integrity and accountability	Pursuit of excellence	Fair and ethical stewardship of healthcare resources
Professional competence	*		*	
Honesty with patients	*	*		
Patient confidentiality		*		
Maintaining appropriate relations with patients		*		
Improving quality of care		*	*	
Improving access to care				*
Just distribution of finite resources				*
Scientific knowledge			*	
Maintaining trust by managing conflicts of interest		*		
Professional responsibility to maintain standards of care		*		

(Row label group: Commitments of the Physician Charter)

* Indicates the primary relationship between the values and the commitments of the Charter.

Table 1-2 displays the 10 commitments and how we grouped them into the four core values. Our goal is to make it clear that healthcare professionals can live the values of professionalism every day by exhibiting these behaviors.

THE SYSTEMS VIEW OF PROFESSIONALISM

During a teaching session on the topic of professionalism, anesthesia residents described a difficult situation that they did not know how to handle. The residents reported that during operations, one particular senior surgeon routinely berated surgical residents, criticizing them as incompetent and humiliating them in front of the operating room staff. The anesthesia residents were not personally attacked by this surgeon, but they were embarrassed for their surgical colleagues and were angry at the surgeon for this behavior. They felt uncomfortable speaking up about it, but they wanted the behavior to stop.

Many physicians think that upholding professionalism is their personal responsibility alone—a heavy burden to bear. These anesthesia residents each felt upset about being silent but also felt isolated individually with the problem. They did not talk to one another, except in quiet innuendos or jokes, and did not know how to share the problem with the surgeon himself, the team, or other leaders in the institution. The residents did not have the skills to analyze the problem or consider how best to demonstrate their professionalism by speaking up in some way. We understand their reticence and their uncertainty about what to do. However, they can learn the knowledge and skills needed to analyze and manage this difficult situation.

The anesthesia residents' case illustrates another important issue: that physicians typically think "being a professional" means they personally need to solve challenging dilemmas or use their time and energy to fix an entrenched and difficult problem in the working environment. The anesthesia residents may feel that they personally have to approach the surgeon and ask him to change his behavior—an approach that would be very intimidating for most residents and one that would likely not be successful. They may think a good physician should be able to "fix" these kinds of problems by some appropriate actions—as they would treat a patient with the right drug. Physicians may have the misconception that professionalism is being a hero who upholds professional values against all odds—a "professionalism superman".

The systems view of professionalism reframes a problem, like the one in the operating room, from a "hero" image to a team effort. The case may be analyzed in a different way using the systems view. In this case, the professionalism value at risk is respect for the surgery residents and for the members of the team witnessing the disrespectful behaviors of the surgeon. The anesthesia residents need to demonstrate their professionalism by speaking up in some way that has the potential to change the situation. They need the skills to reflect on the situation and decide who to talk with about the situation—their anesthesia residency program director, the surgery program director, the particular surgeon himself, or the chair of the department of surgery. The residents need effective communication skills to have these difficult and sensitive conversations.

However, the responsibility to uphold the value of respect in the operation room not only belongs to the anesthesia residents, but also to other players in the scene: the surgical residents who are experiencing the disrespectful treatment, the operating room nurses, and the staff anesthesiologist. The team itself can demonstrate professionalism by discussing the situation together and collectively determining a course of action. It is likely that all of the healthcare professionals in the operating room (nurses, residents, and staff physicians) are uncomfortable but afraid to speak up alone.

In addition, the hospital has a responsibility to create a working environment that supports collegiality and intervenes when there is a difficult problem, like this one. The hospital medical staff affairs office could intervene and meet with the surgeon to tell him directly that his behavior is disruptive and unacceptable. The hospital could provide support to the surgeon to remediate his performance (see Chapter 11, When Things Go Wrong: The Challenge of Self-Regulation). Professional organizations, in this case the American College of Surgeons and the American Board of Surgery, set standards for professional behaviors and provide tools to help assess appropriate behaviors in surgeons. These organizations actively engage in supporting the professionalism of surgeons.

The point of this is that all parties—individual physicians, team members, hospital administrators, and professional organizations—can demonstrate their commitment to professionalism and to the value of respect. Professionalism truly is a team effort.

In the tables below, we describe sample behaviors that can be demonstrated by individual physicians with patients and family members, and by colleagues and team members interacting together (Table 1-3). Table 1-4 describes behaviors that can be demonstrated by practice settings (i.e., hospitals, healthcare systems), professional organizations, and external stakeholders. The behaviors presented are intended to be illustrative but certainly not exhaustive. The tables are organized into the set of values described previously (patient-centered care; integrity and accountability; pursuit of excellence; and fair and ethical stewardship of healthcare resources).

For example, what behaviors (by individual clinicians, teams, healthcare systems, and professional organizations) demonstrate the value of patient-centered care? One core component of patient-centered care is listening to patients' concerns and feelings and, when appropriate, expressing empathy. The individual clinician (physician, nurse, physical therapist, and so on) needs to demonstrate empathy with patients and families, particularly during times of stress. Specific communication skills are required to do this effectively (see Chapter 4, Fostering Patient-Centered Care). At the healthcare team level, team members need to work collaboratively so they are able to focus on patient needs. This entails expressing support and empathy for one another as stressful situations occur in the workplace and in clinicians' personal lives. Supportive teams can help each team member by creating a culture of caring and respect for one another. Hospitals can also demonstrate the behaviors that support the value of patient-centered care by providing communication skills training for staff. Training programs can teach staff communication skills including expressing empathy, breaking bad news, or dealing with angry patients. Hospital administrators can model the same behaviors by demonstrating respect and support for clinicians in daily interactions. Lastly, professional organizations can also support the delivery of patient-centered care. For example, professional organizations, such as certifying boards, can set standards for communication skills as part of the competencies required of trainees and practicing clinicians. Certifying boards can require assessment of these skills for

Table 1-3	**FRAMEWORK FOR CONCEPTUALIZING PROFESSIONALISM—INDIVIDUAL CLINICIAN BEHAVIORS IN INTERACTIONS WITH PATIENTS AND FAMILY MEMBERS AND OTHER HEALTHCARE PROFESSIONALS**	
	Examples of individual physician behaviors	
Values	Interactions with patients and family members	Interactions with colleagues and other members of the healthcare team
Patient-centered care	Communicate effectively demonstrating empathy, compassion, and actively working to build rapport	Work collaboratively with other members of the care team to facilitate effective service to the patient
	Promote autonomy of the patient; eliciting and respecting patient preferences, and including patient in decision-making	Demonstrate respect for other team members in all interactions
	Be accessible to patients to ensure timely access to care and continuity of providers	
	Act to benefit the patient when a conflict of interest exists	
Integrity and accountability	Maintain patient confidentiality	Report impaired or incompetent colleagues
	Maintain appropriate relationships with patients	Participate in peer-review and 360 degree evaluations of team
	Promptly disclose medical errors; take responsibility for and steps to remedy mistakes	Specify standards and procedures for hand-offs across settings of care to ensure coordination and continuity of care
	Actively manage conflicts of interest and publicly disclose any relationships that may affect the physician's recommendations related to diagnosis and treatment (e.g., part ownership of surgery center)	

Table 1-3	FRAMEWORK FOR CONCEPTUALIZING PROFESSIONALISM—INDIVIDUAL CLINICIAN BEHAVIORS IN INTERACTIONS WITH PATIENTS AND FAMILY MEMBERS AND OTHER HEALTHCARE PROFESSIONALS (*Continued*)

	Examples of individual physician behaviors	
Values	Interactions with patients and family members	Interactions with colleagues and other members of the healthcare team
Pursuit of excellence	Adhere to nationally recognized evidence-based guidelines (e.g., guidelines issued by the Agency for Healthcare Research and Quality and/or U.S. Preventive Services Task Force), individualizing as needed for particular patients, but conforming with guidelines for the majority of patients Engage in lifelong learning and professional development Apply system-level continuous quality improvement to patient care	Participate in collaborative efforts to improve system-level factors contributing to quality of care Develop and participate in local educational conferences on quality improvement
Fair and ethical stewardship of healthcare resources	Do no harm; do not provide unnecessary/unwarranted care Commit to deliver emergent care equitably, respecting the different needs and preferences of subpopulations, but without regard to insurance status or ability to pay Deliver care in a culturally sensitive manner	Establish mechanisms for feedback from peers on resource use and appropriateness of care Work with clinical and nonclinical staff to continuously improve efficiency of care delivery process and ensure that all members of the care team are optimizing their contributions to care delivery and administration Actively work with colleagues to coordinate care, avoid redundant testing, and maximize prudent resource use across settings

From Lesser CS, Lucey CR, Egener B, Braddock CH 3rd, Linas SL, Levinson W. A behavioral and systems view of professionalism. *JAMA.* 2010 Dec 22;304(24):2732–2737.

certification in the discipline. In other words, all the players in the healthcare system can demonstrate their professionalism by fostering the delivery of patient-centered care.

Subsequent chapters in the book discuss each of these four values and the behaviors of professionalism related to each one of the values.

Table 1-4   FRAMEWORK FOR CONCEPTUALIZING PROFESSIONALISM—ORGANIZATIONAL BEHAVIORS IN PRACTICE SETTINGS AND PHYSICIAN ADVOCACY AND PROFESSIONAL ORGANIZATIONS

| | Examples of organizational behaviors | |
Values	Practice settings (e.g., hospitals, healthcare systems, clinics)	Physician advocacy and professional organizations
Patient-centered care	Support ongoing development of communication skills and cultural competency to foster effective interactions with patients, families, and care team members	Advocate payment policy that supports clinician time with patients to build rapport, engage in shared decision-making, and be accessible to patients to provide timely care
	Invest in shared decision-making supports and actively encourage patient engagement in care decisions	Actively promote ongoing development of competencies related to patient engagement and teamwork
	Establish mechanisms to engage representatives of patients and family caregivers in organizational management and governance	
	Adopt policies and practices that support timely access to patients' providers of choice	
	Foster creation of a physical environment that promotes healing	
Integrity and accountability	Provide peer and organizational support for disclosure of medical errors and reporting impaired or incompetent clinicians	Develop and encourage organizational strategies to foster a "culture of professionalism"
	Adopt clear and stringent policies regarding conflict of interest and maintaining patient confidentiality	Participate in development of professional standards and establish mechanisms for remediation and discipline of members who fail to meet those standards
	Provide performance feedback to care team and hold the team accountable for results for a defined population, e.g., via compensation and/or public reporting	Commit to disclosure of meaningful performance information
	Discourage provision of services without an evidence base to support value to the patient	Encourage development of systems to report and analyze medical mistakes to inform prevention and improvement strategies
		Develop conflict of interest policies
		Use benefit to patients as the metric to guide resolution of conflicts of interest

| Table 1-4 | **FRAMEWORK FOR CONCEPTUALIZING PROFESSIONALISM—ORGANIZATIONAL BEHAVIORS IN PRACTICE SETTINGS AND PHYSICIAN ADVOCACY AND PROFESSIONAL ORGANIZATIONS (Continued)** | |

	Examples of organizational behaviors	
Values	Practice settings (e.g., hospitals, healthcare systems, clinics)	Physician advocacy and professional organizations
Pursuit of excellence	Invest in system-level supports for organization-wide quality improvement, e.g., electronic health records, registries Establish clear targets for improvement and continuously monitor and raise the bar for performance	Develop and encourage use of meaningful measures of clinical quality of care and sound guidelines for clinical practice Establish ambitious targets and support actions to achieve significant and rapid system-wide improvements in quality of care Advance scientific knowledge
Fair and ethical stewardship of healthcare resources	Encourage judicious use of resources to care for a patient population, e.g., by providing information on system-level costs and outcomes Implement mechanisms for supporting cultural competency and continuous quality improvement focused on reducing disparities in care	Advocate for development and adoption of tools to support cost-effective care and judicious use of healthcare resources Promote public health and advocate on behalf of societal interests with respect to health and healthcare, without concern for the self-interest of the individual physician or the profession Advocate for payment policies that drive a focus on total cost of care rather than discrete encounters and individual clinician inputs Support development of tools to facilitate reflection on disparities in care and drive down unwarranted variation in quality and resource use

From Lesser CS, Lucey CR, Egener B, Braddock CH 3rd, Linas SL, Levinson W. A behavioral and systems view of professionalism. *JAMA*. 2010 Dec 22;304(24):2732–2737.

THE ROLE OF CONTEXT

Dr. Kramer is a primary care physician practicing in a small group. She has been in practice for 10 years and has loved her relationships with patients but recently has been thinking of quitting her work.

She feels that the practice has changed dramatically with intense pressures to see more patients in briefer visits, new financial incentives for "productivity," increasing documentation demands, and requirements to measure her performance in multiple different ways for different insurers. The clinic has recently bought a new electronic medical record, which she knows is going to be very helpful, but it is not the same one as the one that the local hospital uses and she is frustrated by the time she spends getting medical information she needs to care for patients.

The context in which physicians and other healthcare providers work strongly influences their ability to do their professional work. The individual interaction of a physician and a patient occurs in a context of the team and the team occurs in the context of the healthcare setting. In the case of Dr. Kramer, the clinic physicians are working under pressure to increase their productivity, but it is likely that many members of the team feel that this pressure is eroding some of their time to interact with patients. Yet, it is also likely that the team is not discussing the impact of these pressures on their work or considering how they might improve the environment. Furthermore, the managers of the clinic may not have fully considered the effect that the new incentive payments have on the wellbeing and retention of the staff. The point is that the environment shapes the norms and the culture of the work.

LEARNING EXERCISE 1-1

1. Select one of the four values that you consider personally important in your work.
2. Describe how this value is supported by each component of the system in which you work:
   - individual patient/physician interactions
   - team interactions
   - healthcare system (hospital, healthcare system, clinic)
   - your professional organizations
3. Do you have all of the data necessary to assess the behaviors in each of these components? If not, what data could you collect to assess this (consider patient surveys, team assessments, and so on)?
4. Is there one behavior that you are particularly proud of? How could you share this strength with others?
5. Is there one behavior that could be improved? What strategy might you undertake to improve it and measure the impact?

Professional behaviors are also profoundly influenced by the organizational and environmental context in which care is delivered and, likewise, the environmental context is shaped by the behaviors of healthcare professionals who work in it. The important implication is that healthcare professionals, particularly physicians, have the responsibility to improve both their individual competencies (their knowledge, communication skills, and so on), but also to improve the context in which they practice. If the external factors, such as the new incentives in the clinic, are inhibiting the professionalism of the staff, then physicians and others have the responsibility to discuss the problem and to try to improve it. It is not good enough to be silently unhappy. Solving this problem will require considering the competing forces of the need to increase the number of patients seen in the clinic and to ensure that each patient has enough time with the physicians and nurses. There are always competing demands in the real world. Even if these are challenging situations, physicians have a responsibility to press for changes across the spheres of influence that define the environment—from the immediate microsystem in which they practice (i.e., their own clinic) to the broader external environment that shapes how care is delivered (Figure 1-2).

Figure 1-2 illustrates the nested circles of influence on professionalism ranging from individual interactions with patients to the external environment, which includes the payment system, regulations influencing care

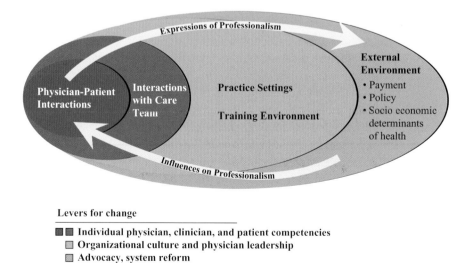

Figure 1-2 ▪ Systems views of professionalism.

From Lesser CS, Lucey CR, Egener B, Braddock CH 3rd, Linas SL, Levinson W. A behavioral and systems view of professionalism. *JAMA*. 2010 Dec 22;304(24):2732–2737.

delivery, and the social and economic conditions of the community. Furthermore, the arrows illustrate that the environment influences the interactions between patients and physicians and teams, and that physicians express their professionalism by pushing and forcing changes in the environment. Physicians have a responsibility to strive to create environments that foster professionalism in practice. Gruen and colleagues (2004) referred to this as "civic professionalism."

IS IT POSSIBLE FOR PHYSICIANS TO INFLUENCE THE SYSTEM?

You might be wondering how it is possible for individual physicians and nurses to change the system. How can busy physicians possibly be expected to do this? Is this view of professionalism asking too much? These are reasonable questions. However, three points are critically important.

1. Individual physicians need to recognize that the environment can be changed and need to raise the awareness of the need for change. No culture is static and fixed.
2. Small actions can have an impact.
3. These actions are often initiated and implemented by a group, rather than one person alone.

A medical school example follows (also see Chapter 12, Organizational Professionalism).

A 3rd-year medical student was on a rotation in a women's health clinic located in a community serving a low income population. She heard from several patients that they had not scheduled their screening mammograms, and she astutely learned that the cost of the mammogram in the local hospital was too expensive for these uninsured patients. In discussion with a group of her student colleagues, they decided to do a bit of investigating as part of their class on population-based health. The students called a variety of local mammogram centers in the community and pretended to be a patient without health insurance seeking a screening mammogram. Their investigation revealed that it was almost impossible to successfully schedule an appointment for a mammogram, even if the patient could afford it, within a 5-mile radius of the clinic—including at their own medical school facility. Armed with the data, the students approached the administration of the hospital and asked them to help create a

LEARNING EXERCISE 1-2

1. Consider one aspect of your practice environment (or one you have worked in) that is creating a barrier to optimizing care for patients.

2. Are there conflicting goals among different members of the healthcare team or healthcare system?

3. What data can be collected to assess the extent of the problem (consider survey data, administrative data already available, and so on)?

4. What possible approaches could you and your colleagues take to address the barrier and improve care? How could you measure the impact?

program to facilitate the appropriate care of these patients. The administrative staff, after being made aware of the data, was able to create a compelling rationale and a business case to provide the service to their patients.

We think that this true story of medical students recognizing a problem for their patients, collecting data to assess the extent of the issue, and presenting the case to the administrators, is an example of how physicians can influence and improve the professionalism value of fair and ethical use of resources. They did not do this alone but rather as a group, making the effort feasible and more likely to be successful than if one student alone had tried to undertake this project.

CONCLUSION

We have found this behavioral and systems approach to professionalism particularly helpful in our everyday work. Although prior codes of ethics have provided an important theoretical framework, it is often difficult to translate this into behaviors and actions on the front line. By framing professionalism in a behavioral and systems approach, it is easier to identify professionalism at its best and to recognize lapses when they inevitably occur. Furthermore, the systems approach helps individual physicians feel that upholding high standards of professionalism is truly a team responsibility in which we each have a part, but are not responsible for all by ourselves. This has given us the freedom to explore problems when they occur in a more positive and less judgmental fashion.

KEY LEARNING POINTS

1. Professionalism is demonstrated in everyday work through a set of behaviors that can be observed.
2. These behaviors can be demonstrated by multiple players in the system; the individual physicians interacting with patients, the healthcare team, the administrators in the practice setting, and the professional organizations and stakeholders in the external environment.
3. The ability of physicians to demonstrate professionalism is influenced by the setting in which they work and by the external environment that shapes care.
4. Physicians can and should identify barriers in the environment (microsystem or broader environment) that interfere with delivering the highest quality care to patients, and work with colleagues to improve the system.
5. Physicians and teams have a responsibility to strive to create environments that foster professionalism in practice.

REFERENCES

1. ABIM Foundation. American Board of Internal Medicine; ACP-ASIM Foundation. American College of Physicians-American Society of Internal Medicine; European Federation of Internal Medicine. Medical professionalism in the new millennium: a physician charter. *Ann Intern Med.* 2002 Feb 5;136(3):243–246.
2. Campbell EG, Regan S, Gruen RL, Ferris TG, Rao SR, Cleary PD, Blumenthal D. Professionalism in medicine: results of a national survey of physicians. *Ann Intern Med.* 2007 Dec 4;147(11):795–802.
3. Gruen RL, Pearson SD, Brennan TA. Physician-citizens—public roles and professional obligations. *JAMA.* 2004 Jan 7;291(1):94–98.
4. Leach DC. Professionalism: the formation of physicians. *Am J Bioeth.* 2004 spring;4(2):11–12.
5. Lesser CS, Lucey CR, Egener B, Braddock CH 3rd, Linas SL, Levinson W. A behavioral and systems view of professionalism. *JAMA.* 2010 Dec 22;304(24):2732–2737.
6. Lucey C, Souba W. Perspective: the problem with the problem of professionalism. *Acad Med.* 2010 Jun;85(6):1018–1024.

RESILIENCE IN FACING PROFESSIONALISM CHALLENGES

2

LEARNING OBJECTIVES

1. To convey the pitfalls of assuming professionalism is a character trait.
2. To articulate the advantages of viewing professionalism as a multifaceted competency.
3. To explain the connection between personal wellbeing and professional resiliency.
4. To describe skills set needed to maintain professionalism in stressful circumstances.

Joan kicked off her shoes and sank into her chair. It had been such a bad day. She has been on a clinical rotation for only a week and already she is thinking that she won't be able to be a good doctor. It's not taking the history or doing the physical examinations or even fielding the rapid-fire questions on rounds. It's the professionalism issues that worry her. Almost every day this week she has seen doctors and nurses lose their tempers with one another— responding sarcastically, leaving in anger, and yelling at the team for a bad outcome that wasn't their fault. Even worse, today, she found herself getting really angry at a patient who just refused to talk with her and then complained about her on rounds. She actually went back after rounds to tell him off, but fortunately his granddaughter was in the room, which made her think twice. She came into medical school to be a caring and compassionate physician and thought that the professionalism stuff would be easy—you know, just follow the golden rule and you will be fine. She realizes now that all of those professionalism lectures in the first 2 years were there for a reason—to drill into her head the need to work to ensure that she is the doctor her patients need her to be. But she had no idea it would be so hard— just reminding people to be professional doesn't seem to be enough. How do the best doctors do it?

Professionalism is at the heart of all that we as physicians aspire to be. When we enter medical school, we imagine ourselves calmly and compassionately ministering to the suffering by selflessly using our carefully honed skills and knowledge to determine and carry out the best treatment plan possible for the patient in front of us. In return, we would be appreciated and feel gratification.

In today's environment, professionalism appears to be under threat. On the national level, reports of unprofessional physician behavior—ranging from overt crimes, to abuse of power, to conflicts of interest—are easily disseminated using today's web-based communication tools. Each sensational story raises questions about why such a person was allowed into the medical profession and why the profession itself hasn't fulfilled its obligation to oversee its members and deal with the rogue physicians who are the subject of national headlines. At the state level, medical boards receiving complaints about physicians have few options other than to sanction with license suspension or revocation and publicize the names of the transgressors. At the institutional level, hospitals are struggling with physicians who exhibit disruptive behavior, like those witnessed by Joan. Repeated instances of ineffective interprofessional communication; disrespect for peers, patients, and trainees; and failure to adhere to evidence-based safety practices are tied to high staff turnover, low employee morale, and poor safety cultures (Hickson et al, 2007). At the individual level, medical students who experience a disconnect between classroom lessons on professionalism and the behaviors they witness in the clinical environment become cynical and lose empathy (Hafferty & Franks, 1994; Testerman et al, 1996) (see Chapter 8, The Hidden Curriculum and Professionalism). Residents and practicing physicians experience burnout as they find themselves ineffective in their daily work (Shanafelt et al, 2002; Billings et al, 2011; Zwack & Schweitzer, 2013).

IS PROFESSIONALISM A CHARACTER TRAIT?

The conventional approach to professionalism—an assumption that professionalism is a character trait of the good physician—reinforces the problem. With this approach, our role as educators and peers is to screen people entering the profession to make sure that they possess that trait, then to monitor them over time and remove them if they exhibit behaviors that suggest that the professionalism trait either never was or no longer is present. This disciplinary approach to professionalism often leads to inaction on the part of physicians who witness trainees or peers behaving in a manner incompatible with our professional values (Burack et al, 1999). Physicians may not know how to intervene to fix a problem that is linked to a trait rather than a competency. They may be fearful that the disciplinary sanction that may result if they intervene or report a colleague is too extreme for the behavior they witnessed. They may be also be fearful that their own behavior is at times not compatible with professionalism and worry that they too may someday be subject to a high stakes intervention. As a result, physicians are often silent when they witness colleagues who demonstrate unprofessional behaviors.

PROFESSIONALISM IS A COMPETENCY

A new set of assumptions is emerging as a useful paradigm to help all healthcare professionals deliver on the promise of professionalism for our patients (Lucey & Souba, 2010) (Table 2-1).

The practice of medicine is stressful and complex, and challenges to professionalism arise predictably on a daily basis. Physicians must be committed to living the values of professionalism. But rather than viewing

Table 2-1	NEW ASSUMPTIONS ABOUT PROFESSIONALISM TO GUIDE FUTURE PROBLEM SOLVING	
Aspects of professionalism	Old assumptions	New assumptions
Professionalism as a competency	Professionalism is an attitudinal competency based on character traits present at the start of medical school.	Professionalism is a multidimensional competency with elements of knowledge, attitudes, judgment, and skills.
Professionalism in an individual	Physicians who lapse are unprofessional. The competency of professionalism is dichotomous and fixed at the time of completion of formal education.	Lapses in professionalism can occur in physicians who are good professionals. The competency of professionalism follows a developmental curve from beginner to expert, and it is continuously shaped over the lifetime of a career.
Professionalism challenges	Challenges to professionalism are infrequent and unpredictable.	Challenges to professionalism are common and can be anticipated.

(Continued)

Table 2-1	NEW ASSUMPTIONS ABOUT PROFESSIONALISM TO GUIDE FUTURE PROBLEM SOLVING (*Continued*)	
Aspects of professionalism	Old assumptions	New assumptions
Response to a lapse in professionalism	The response to a lapse in professionalism is commonly punitive, relying on negative labels, sanctions, and the threat of removal from the profession.	The response to a lapse in professionalism should be pedagogical, using active, targeted coaching based on root-cause analysis of the lapse. Sanctions should be reserved for those who fail to respond to the pedagogical approach.
Role of the healthcare system	The healthcare system is simply the setting in which lapses in professionalism occur.	The organization and operations of a healthcare system can increase the likelihood that a lapse will occur. Changes in the healthcare system can support physicians as they strive to live out their professional values.
Responsibility for stewardship of professionalism	The educational system owns the primary responsibility for ensuring that physicians remain professional by selecting the right individuals and training them well.	The community of practicing physicians, inclusive of educational and healthcare system leaders must assume responsibility for supporting, reinforcing, and guiding physicians to remain professional throughout their careers.

From Lucey C, Souba W. Perspective: the problem with the problem of professionalism. *Acad Med.* 2010 Jun;85(6):1018–1024.

professionalism as an immutable trait, we view professionalism as a true competency; a set of knowledge, attitudes, and skills that can and should be the subject of professional development. Viewing professionalism as a competency means that we assume that transient episodes of unprofessional behavior are "performance lapses" rather than character flaws, and that we adopt an educational rather than a disciplinary approach to manage them. The role of educators and professionals within our environments should be to help build and sustain a commitment to professionalism by all within our community and to foster resilience in our students, our trainees, and our peers so that all may be "habitually faithful to professionalism values in highly complex situations" (Leach, 2004). This means not only ensuring that people intend to be professional (self-intent), but also that they have confidence that they can act in a professional manner (self-efficacy). The presence of positive role models who demonstrate professional behaviors reinforces and supports the ability of individual physicians to act in a professional manner. It is important to note that the likelihood of behaving in the desired manner decreases if people who the student admires conduct themselves in an unprofessional manner or if the

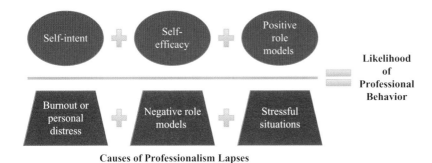

Causes of Professionalism Lapses

Figure 2-1 ▪ Many variables influence the likelihood of professional behavior.

context in which the behaviors are expected is too challenging for the individual's skills (Regehr, 2006; Hafferty & Franks, 1994). Figure 2-1 illustrates the relationship between these variables.

CAUSES OF PROFESSIONALISM LAPSES

> *Dr. Hernandez, the associate program director, sighed. He had just fielded a complaint from one of the ICU nurses who said that Dr. Miller, one of his residents, screamed at her in the middle of the night when she notified him that an error had occurred and a critically ill, 24-year-old patient with bacterial meningitis had missed a dose of antibiotics. Shaking his head, he wondered what to do. "If they don't know how to be nice to people by the time they are 26, how am I supposed to teach them? Who let this type of a person into medical school anyway?"*

Dr. Hernandez's view of a professionalism lapse is common, and his sense of futility is understandable. However, a closer analysis of this professionalism lapse might help turn this lapse into a learning opportunity for the resident in question by pinpointing the competencies that are needed to maintain professionalism in our complex, and at times stressful, healthcare environment.

In our view, few physicians are inherently unprofessional. Instead, professionalism challenges can lead to professionalism lapses if the individual in question lacks the knowledge, judgment or skills to be able to successfully navigate those challenges.

In this brief case, one can envision a resident on call covering for many patients. He is managing a patient who is doing poorly, and along with the nurses and other health professionals in the intensive care unit, he is trying desperately to save this young patient's life. It is likely that he is tired, possible

DEFINITIONS

Professionalism challenges: situations that may make it difficult for an individual physician or physician in training to remain true to professionalism values.

Professionalism lapse: an error in judgment, skill, or attitude that leads an otherwise competent physician or physician-in-training to behave in a manner contrary to established professionalism norms.

that he hasn't eaten, probable that there are other sick patients for whom he was responsible, and conceivable that an ill patient close to his own age is evoking some feelings of transference. He may be worried that he will be held responsible for the error, and the fact that it happened on his watch may reflect poorly on his reputation. He responded to the nurse in the heat of the moment in a manner that was both unprofessional and understandable.

The purpose of this analysis exercise is not to justify or excuse the behavior. If Dr. Hernandez simply attributes the resident's behavior to a stressful situation and chooses not to counsel or intervene with the resident, the resident will not get the opportunity to learn from the encounter. Bad behavior that is not corrected is likely to be repeated. Similarly, simply reminding the resident that he shouldn't yell at the nurses and not to do so in the future is unlikely to be successful in the long term. What is needed is a strategy that helps the resident to understand why he responded unprofessionally, how he can work to develop skills to ensure he can respond more professionally when he faces any another similarly challenging encounter in the future, and why remaining professional is so important to the healthcare environment and should be important to him.

> *Dr. Miller has felt terrible since he yelled at the ICU nurse. He knows he shouldn't have taken his frustrations out on her but he felt like he couldn't help it. Now Dr. Hernandez has called and said he wanted to talk with him about his interaction with the nurse. Dr. Miller worries that his poor handling of this situation will damage his reputation for good.*

Dr. Miller's feelings are also typical. Nobody feels good about acting inappropriately and yet, most of us have done this in one way or the other. Typically, we hope the episode will go unaddressed and be forgotten. We fear, as Dr. Miller does, discussing the behavior with our peers or supervisors. However, a training setting can develop a culture that fosters feedback and learning—even if at times these conversations can be difficult. If Dr. Hernandez provides feedback and support to Dr. Miller, this can be a critically important learning experience both in this situation and for his future ability to handle these types of situations.

DEFICIT NEEDS AND PROFESSIONALISM CHALLENGES

Behaving professionally may be sometimes counter to human nature. Abraham Maslow's hierarchy of needs theory states that humans will behave predictably to fulfill, in sequence, physiologic needs for food and shelter, safety needs for security and stability, belonging needs for friends and family, and self-esteem needs for achievement and recognition before they can behave in a self-actualized manner (Bryan, 2005) (Figure 2-2).

Despite this awareness of instinctive human behavior, we expect medical students, residents, practicing physicians, and other health professionals to behave in a self-actualized manner despite having unmet deficit needs. Dr. Miller is expected to respond calmly, respectfully, and in a problem-solving mode despite being tired and hungry (physiologic needs unmet), alone (belonging need unmet), and insecure (self-esteem need unmet). Work in cognitive psychology also reminds us that when human beings feel their ability to meet their essential needs is threatened, they respond predictably with fight or flight reactions. In the clinical environment, fight reactions are represented in yelling, intimidation, sarcasm, and physical violence. Flight reactions include ignoring questions, refusing to answer pages, and other forms of passive-aggressive behavior.

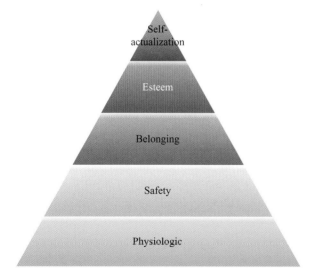

Figure 2-2 ■ Maslow's hierarchy of needs.

Maslow AH. A theory of human motivation. *Psychological Review* 1943;50(4):370–396. This material as a whole is now in the public domain. American Psychological Association.

It is inevitable that physicians in training and in practice will have times when they are not at their personal best when they are called upon to handle a professionalism challenge. Anticipating these situations and identifying coping strategies prior to their occurrence is a strategy that can help individuals remain professional in challenging circumstances.

VALUES, CONFLICTS, AND PROFESSIONALISM CHALLENGES

Third year medical student Yakira was in tears. She had prepared diligently all week to present the case at surgery grand rounds. She arrived at work early so that she could see her patients before the conference started. One of her patients, Mrs. Nida, looked terrible, so Yakira called the cross-covering resident to help. When Yakira tried to sign the patient over to her, the resident said, "You can't leave your patient when she is crashing—that's so unprofessional!" She stayed and helped transfer Mrs. Nida to the ICU but by the time she got to grand rounds, they had started without her. The attending physician took her aside and told her she was not demonstrating the professional values of excellence and accountability. What was she supposed to do?

LEARNING EXERCISE 2-1

Think of a recent circumstance when you feel you interacted with a patient, colleague, trainee, or staff member in a way that you thought afterward was not ideal.

1. What were the reactions of your colleague or staff member?
2. Did you debrief the interaction afterwards? If so, what did you learn? If not, why not?
3. What was your physical and emotional state going into the encounter? Might you have handled the situation better if your physical or emotional state at the start was better?
4. If so, what options existed for you to optimize your physical or emotional state before starting the encounter?
5. What can you do during your work day if you recognize that your physical or emotional state is such that it may negatively affect your ability to live the values of professionalism?
6. What might you do if a colleague appeared to be at risk of behaving unprofessionally because they were hungry, angry, lonely, or tired?

Ginsburg et al (2000) suggest that professionalism lapses may result when physicians in training or in practice experience a situation in which remaining true to one professionalism value means subjugating another professionalism value. To add to the complexity of the situation, empiric studies have also shown that different physicians disagree about what is the "correct" decision to make in a situation where professionalism values conflict, as illustrated in the preceding case (Ginsburg et al, 2004). For Yakira to behave professionally in this situation requires not only knowledge about relevant professionalism tenets but also judgment in deciding how to prioritize two competing demands and the skills to handle the challenge.

This type of dilemma of two competing demands often arises when the care of one patient requires delaying the needs of another patient. The case below illustrates this point and is a common professionalism challenge.

> *Dr. Chiang, a cardiology resident, felt like he was on a rollercoaster. He hadn't expected Mrs. Durrett's simple follow-up visit for hypertension to last so long. Asked if anything was worrying her, Mrs. Durrett burst into tears and talked about the stress she had been under as she cared for her dying mother. After 30 minutes of supportive listening and a bit of advice, Mrs. Durrett had calmed down, developed a plan to ask for help from her sister, and thanked Dr. Chiang profusely for listening and caring. Dr. Chiang hurried to the next exam room and found that his 2:15 patient was now irate about being kept waiting. She told Dr. Chiang that she felt disrespected and she wouldn't be returning to see such an unprofessional physician. Dr. Chiang felt badly about making the second patient wait but he felt good about helping Mrs. Durrett. Was there a way to be professional in everyone's eyes?*

Both Yakira and Dr. Chiang are in situations that happen frequently in our work lives. Educating for resilience means helping our students and residents anticipate, recognize, and prepare to handle common and predictable professionalism challenges. Effective management of professionalism challenges requires that physicians and physicians in training navigate a series of iterative steps (these are summarized in Figure 2-3).

Navigating these steps starts with knowledge and commitment but then requires insight (assessing the situation, and recognizing that values, patients, and self may be in conflict), judgment (identifying and analyzing options for action), and skill (carrying out that action). Yakira may have recognized the conflict between caring for the patient versus being on time for grand rounds but perhaps she did not fully take stock of the situation to realize the effect

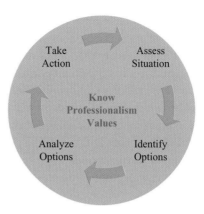

Figure 2-3 ▪ Managing a professionalism challenge requires knowledge, judgment, and skills.

LEARNING EXERCISE 2-2

Consider the situation that Dr. Chiang is experiencing. He knows he is running behind and keeping his next patient waiting, but he is uncomfortable interrupting Mrs. Durrett who is expressing her distress.

1. If you were his attending physician, how would you use this situation to teach him about competing professional demands?
2. What questions would you ask him to help him reflect on the situation and consider alternate strategies to handle the situation?

---

that this conflict had on her personally. Furthermore, she needed the judgment to consider options to handle the situation. She could have asked the resident to call the surgeon who was running grand rounds and advise him of the situation. She could have asked the resident to give the surgeon her written notes. Alternatively, she could have explained the dilemma to the resident and asked the resident to care for the patient for the first 10 minutes of grand rounds so she could present the case. It is likely that this type of reflection and analysis would have led to a better outcome for Dr. Yakira and her colleagues.

PROFESSIONALISM AS A COMPLEX COMPETENCY

As with other complex competencies, the ability to remain professional in difficult situations follows a developmental trajectory from novice to expert. Dreyfus, an aviation engineer, recognized a difference between novices and experts (Dreyfus & Dreyfus, 1980). *Novices*, those who had attended class but who had little practical experience, were good at and felt responsibility for following the rules, but had limited ability to deal with circumstances in which rules conflicted. With experience and feedback, the novice develops competency, learning how to apply the rules in the dynamic work environment. A *competent* professional takes responsibility for actively thinking through situations and making decisions about when and how to apply which rules. An *expert* professional intuitively recognizes a wide set of circumstances that call for sophisticated judgment and relies on the principles behind the rules. They feel responsible not only for their personal actions but also for the actions of others.

The application of this competency development theory to professionalism explains why beginning medical students who can voice an understanding of and commitment to professionalism in the abstract (novice level of competency), may not be able to operationalize professionalism values in the complex clinical environments (competent or proficient level of professionalism). The complexity of professionalism challenges increases when multiple people are involved in one situation, when there is a conflict or perceived conflict between patients or between professionalism values, and when the professional in question must navigate the challenge while not at their personal best. Indeed, many professionalism lapses occur when the developmental competency of a given student or trainee is insufficient to manage a uniquely complex or nuanced situation. Figure 2-4 summarizes a developmental curve for professionalism, moving from novice expectations to expertise.

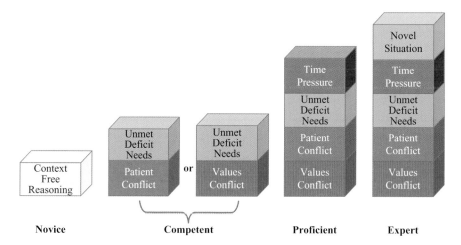

Figure 2-4 ▪ The ability to handle professionalism challenges follows a developmental curve, with higher level of competency required in situations with greater numbers of professionalism challenges.

RESILIENCE IN FACING PROFESSIONALISM CHALLENGES: INDIVIDUAL COMPETENCIES

As is the case with optimizing performance in any competency domain, remaining true to the values of professionalism requires that the student, resident, and practicing physician maintain personal wellbeing and what some authors have called "personal resilience." A number of authors have analyzed the habits and attitudes of physicians who demonstrate resilience despite the stress inherent in a career in medicine (Epstein & Krasner, 2013; Zwack & Schweitzer, 2013). Physicians who attend to personal wellbeing build a bank of emotional capacity that they can call upon when dealing with challenging situations (Figure 2-5). For example, activities that might enhance personal wellbeing (or personal resilience) include celebrating small and large successes or ensuring time for personal relationships outside of the work environment. Conversely, activities that may decrease personal reserves include being physically inactive or allowing work hours to expand without limits. In other words, we can engage in activities that either enhance or diminish our personal wellbeing and emotional reserves.

However, building resilience in the face of professionalism challenges requires one to develop additional competencies, beyond personal wellbeing, to effectively manage a spectrum of challenges. The theories of emotional intelligence arise from the field of cognitive psychology and have been adopted by experts working to improve the resilience of healthcare professionals (Epstein & Krasner, 2013). Strategies that can be taught and modeled are listed in Table 2-2.

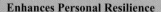

Enhances Personal Resilience
- Remaining interested in role
- Celebrating small and large successes
- Limiting working hours
- Accepting personal intellectual limitations
- Engaging in continuous development
- Participating in supportive relationships
- Ensuring regular contact with colleagues
- Control over work environment
- Engaging in personal reflection

Diminishes Personal Resilience
- Unrealistic expectations about the role
- Boredom with routine or simple cases
- No time limitations on availability
- Devalues time spent on leisure or alternate activities
- Prioritizes work over supporting personal or professional relationships
- Doesn't take time for professional development
- Physically inactive
- Doesn't take time to reflect on work

Figure 2-5 ▪ Attributes and activities associated with personal wellbeing and resilience.

Table 2-2 **SKILLS THAT CAN ENHANCE PROFESSIONALISM**		
Categories	Competencies	Activating competencies during professionalism challenges
Self-awareness	Recognize personal emotions, triggers, and transference that may interfere with optimal behavior. Understand personal limitations in skills and knowledge.	What are my emotions now? Does this other individual remind me of someone I have struggled with in the past? Do I have the knowledge and skills I need to manage this encounter?
Self-regulation	Manage strong emotions. Access assistance for complex tasks.	What can I do to ensure that I remain in control of my emotions? Do I need to take a time out? Who might be able to help me?
Social awareness	Analyze situations for professionalism challenges. Recognize the importance of considering the needs and state of all people in the encounter.	What values are at risk here? Where might different values conflict? Whose needs should I prioritize? Who besides the patient might be struggling and need help? What might others be thinking and feeling?
Social regulation	Habitually seek to identify more than one option for action. Use the strategy of assuming positive intent to understand others' behaviors. Develop crisis communication strategies to calm strong emotions. Use negotiation skills to create new options for moving forward. Be empowered to coach others to avoid or stop unprofessional behavior.	What options, other than my first instinct, may exist for managing this situation? Why might a reasonable person feel differently than I do about this encounter? Why might they be acting in a manner that is counter to professionalism? How can I de-escalate the emotions in this environment? How can I make sure that all feel respected and heard? How might I create a win-win situation? If they knew the way they were being perceived, would they be happy with it? How can I preserve my relationship with this individual but also help them improve?

Self-awareness requires an understanding of how personal biases and emotional triggers might hijack otherwise good intentions in high stress environments. It also requires that the physician-in-training or in-practice understand his or her limitations of expertise and knowledge when confronting a difficult situation. This means that physicians must recognize the warning signs of impending problems, such as irritability, annoyance, disengagement, or flashes of anger. Meditation, mindfulness, and Balint groups are formal ways for physicians to develop self-awareness (Epstein, 1999; Zwack & Schweitzer, 2013). Informal strategies for building and using self-awareness may take the form of simple habits of the mind, such as taking a deep breath or a quick walk to clear your mind before embarking on a tough encounter or stopping to think during a complicated surgical procedure (Moulton & Epstein, 2011; Borrell-Carrió & Epstein, 2004).

Self-awareness must be followed with **self-regulation**. Self-regulation is the ability to take control of counterproductive emotions or recognize when it is best to ask for help from someone else in the environment. Self-awareness and self-regulation in stressful professionalism situations might result in a physician asking a colleague with whom he is getting angry if they could continue the conversation at a later time. It is reflected in the intern who realizes that she gets irritable when she skips meals and plans ahead to always have food in her pockets. It is demonstrated by a physician who asks a colleague to cover for him so he can get a breath of fresh air when he is feeling out of control. Mentors can help junior colleagues reflect on and begin to regulate dysfunctional emotions through role modeling.

> *Matt, a 4th year medical student, felt like he had been let in on a secret. Today on rounds, his attending, Dr. Landerjol, called the team together to talk about Mr. Washington, a 50-year-old man who had just been given a diagnosis of stage IV lung cancer. Mr. Washington was terribly angry and either yelled, complained, or threatened Matt every time he went into the room. Matt was embarrassed to admit that he had been finding ways to avoid Mr. Washington altogether, because he frequently came close to responding inappropriately. Matt was sure that his attending, Dr. Landerjol, was going to lecture them either on chemotherapy or being nice. Instead, she started the conversation by saying, "Is anyone other than I finding it difficult to control their emotions when they visit Mr. Washington?", and then proceeded to talk about how she often finds it difficult to maintain empathy and professionalism when dealing with a patient who was manifesting his suffering by lashing out. The team was so relieved. Once the topic was out in the open, many ideas for helping Mr. Washington and each other became apparent. Matt decided then and there that if he felt like he was going to get angry with a patient, he would reach out and ask others for help, like Dr. Landerjol did.*

Professionalism lapses almost always involve more than one person. A truly resilient professional is one who accepts responsibility for understanding and managing the social dynamics of professionalism challenges. *Social awareness* in professionalism challenges describes the ability to recognize that a professionalism challenge is present and analyze why that might be so. Rather than simply responding instinctively, the resilient professional takes time to identify alternate strategies for action that preserve professionalism while managing the emotions and needs of other healthcare professionals in the encounter. The resilient professional also takes a moment to understand why others in the environment (physicians, nurses, students, family members) might be acting in way that is causing a problem. *Social regulation* is the action component of social awareness. Highly resilient physicians don't have to remove themselves from difficult situations. They use crisis communication techniques, including empathic listening, negotiation, conflict resolution, and de-escalation of emotional peers and patients. They are successful in engaging others in mutual problem solving. They look for ways to devise strategies for minimizing stress on others and supporting others as they navigate challenges. Physicians with strong social regulation skills also are able to effectively coach peers to improved professionalism in a manner that maintains their relationship with others while reinforcing the aspirational goals of professionalism.

Unlike yesterday, Dr. Weinstein, a junior resident, felt good at the end of her day about something she had observed. She had been on call with Dr. Hunt, a senior resident who had just taken over the service. Dr. Weinstein watched Dr. Hunt do amazing things all night. But one thing really stuck in her mind. Dr. Hunt had been very busy with a sick patient and she was paged numerous times by a nurse on another floor about Mrs. Waldren, who needed her pain medications adjusted. Dr. Weinstein had answered some of the pages to tell the nurse that Dr. Hunt was busy and would be up soon, but the nurse was getting more and more frustrated because the patient kept calling her. Even Dr. Weinstein felt anxious when Dr. Hunt's pager went off the fifth time. Dr. Hunt answered the call and calmly said, "I can hear how worried you are about Mrs. Waldren and I appreciate that you are keeping me posted. I am going to walk upstairs so we can talk together about how to help her with her pain. Can you give me 15 minutes to finish up what is happening here?" Dr. Hunt turned to Dr. Weinstein and said, "if people in the clinical environment call you with increasing frequency, it means that something is going to happen unless you intervene—just like unstable angina! I find it best

LEARNING EXERCISE 2-3

1. Think of a time when one of your learners (or colleagues) seemed like they were burning out.
2. Did you talk to him or her about your concerns? If so, what did you say? If not, what might you say now if you had the chance?
3. What do you think is contributing to his or her diminished resilience?
4. When thinking about how to help enhance his or her resilience, which factors do you think would resonate or work best for this person at this time?
5. How might you help your student or colleague develop a strategy to optimize their resilience?
6. Does your institution have resources available to help you approach this situation? If not, what sorts of resources do you think would be helpful?

to acknowledge and thank them for their concerns and then plan to work together to solve the problem. They feel heard, respected, and responsible for helping rather than just passing off the problem. Think about it."

RESILIENCE IN FACING PROFESSIONALISM CHALLENGES: TEAM–BASED COMPETENCIES

The culture of our institutions, reflected in units or patient care teams, can either undermine or augment professional resilience in their members. Leape and colleagues (2012) have described categories of disrespect that undermine professionalism and jeopardize patient care and patient caring (Table 2-3). Teams that undermine the resilience of professionals may do so by creating a culture in which negative emotions like anger, fear, and intolerance result in overtly unprofessional behaviors like yelling, abuse of power, or other forms of mistreatment directed at patients, students, and other healthcare professionals. Team-based undermining of resilience may take more surreptitious forms as well. Covertly, disruptive teams may behave professionally in the presence of a patient but then make disparaging comments out of earshot of those who are the subjects of the barbs. Whether overt or covert, unprofessional behavior in the clinical environment that is counter to the professionalism values taught in the classroom is known as the hidden curriculum. Students exposed to the hidden curriculum develop cynicism about whether professionalism values

Table 2-3 **CATEGORIES OF UNPROFESSIONAL BEHAVIOR**	
Unprofessional behaviors	Examples
Disruptive* behavior	Yelling, abusive or foul language, violent actions, or threatened violence.
Humiliating or demeaning treatment of others	Mocking, derisive comments, intimidation, belittlement, exploitation, articulating, and perpetuating stereotypes about other specialties, professions, or people; dismissing other's concerns as insignificant or ignorant.
Passive-aggressive behavior	Refusing to participate in problem solving and then criticizing the identified solutions, making others look bad, demand for unreasonably perfect proof before making changes in practice.
Passive disrespect	Chronic lateness, missed pages, failure to meet deadlines for documentation, failure to complete assigned committee work, or turning in work that is substandard but on time.
Dismissive treatment of patients	Ignoring patient requests, talking down to patients, disbelief of patient stories, and disregard for patient concerns.

*Disruptive: the characteristic of any behavior that interferes with the smooth functioning of the health-care team or institution.

From Leape LL, Shore MF, Dienstag JL, Mayer RJ, Edgman-Levitan S, Meyer GS, Healy GB. Perspective: a culture of respect, part 1: the nature and causes of disrespectful behavior by physicians. *Acad Med.* 2012 Jul;87(7):845–852.

can be truly lived in real world clinical environments and subsequently may manifest the unprofessional behaviors that were role modeled by their supervisors. The hidden curriculum can be particularly powerful if attending physicians fail to intervene to stop unprofessional behavior (see Chapter 8, The Hidden Curriculum and Professionalism).

Conversely, team behaviors can augment resilience. Acknowledging challenging situations, providing support to colleagues struggling under heavy workloads, and attending to the need for team members to be well rested and well fed, are all behaviors that can help individuals maintain their resilience. Teams that support professionalism can commit to intervening when they feel that a team member is at risk for a professionalism lapse. Sometimes an offer to hold someone's pager while they take a walk outside may help someone maintain their commitment to professionalism values. Strong teams also courageously address episodes of unprofessional behavior in their members rather than simply ignoring them. Professionally resilient members will accept a gentle correction from a colleague. Enacting this kind of professional behavior can be difficult and can require individual courage if the team is not used to doing this regularly.

> *Dr. Sharma swallowed hard. He had just come from a talk about the hidden curriculum. It made him think about how often he, as a new attending physician, just ignored unpleasant or frankly disrespectful comments on rounds. At the end of the talk, he vowed that he would try the intervention strategy that the expert recommended the next time he heard something that seemed to be contrary to the team's professionalism values. And here it was, the chief resident was making a joke about a patient's obesity on rounds. Dr. Sharma said, "I know that it is challenging to take care of this patient because of her size, but let's not forget that she is suffering and needs her doctors to be on her side, treating her like we would want to be treated. Now, let's figure out what to do about her elevated glucose." The chief resident looked up, shocked, and said, "You're right. I shouldn't have said that. Thanks for reminding me."*

It can be productive to reflect on the culture in our own team settings. Is our environment one that supports and fosters discussion of the types of professionalism challenges discussed in this chapter? Productive teams build interpersonal communication to facilitate exploration of these issues. Similar to the patient safety literature that encourages fostering a "just culture" where open discussion of errors is feasible and welcomed, developing a culture to foster professionalism is a team effort.

CONCLUSION

Professionalism is more than the golden rule, more than civility, and more than good citizenship. It means building and bringing your best self to incredibly complex environments where suffering, strong emotions, and controversies are the norm, rather than the exception. The development of resilience involves knowledge, attitudes, and skills that can be taught, practiced, modeled, and refreshed over a lifetime in medicine. Individuals can enhance their resilience by surrounding themselves with team members who are also committed to professionalism and by constructing systems that support adherence to professionalism values.

ADDITIONAL EXERCISES

1. What are the top three professionalism lapses you have witnessed? If you were asked to develop a curriculum to help students and residents prepare to deal with these challenges, what would you recommend?

2. Think of a time when you saw someone lose his or her temper with a patient, a family, or a colleague. What emotional or physical challenges might they have been dealing with BEFORE they entered into the challenging situation? In retrospect, what might they have done to prevent losing their temper with the patient? How might others have helped? How do you think they felt after they lost their temper?

3. Remember a time when you felt conflicted about fulfilling your obligations to a patient and fulfilling your obligations to a loved one. How did you navigate the challenge? What alternatives did you consider that might allow you to meet everyone's expectations of you?

4. Have you ever had to counsel someone about a professionalism lapse? What did you know about the challenges that individual was facing? What advice did you give the individual to help them to avoid repeating the same mistake?

5. What three things could you start to do tomorrow to help others avoid making professionalism mistakes?

KEY LEARNING POINTS

1. Demonstrating professionalism depends on multiple competencies including knowledge, attitudes, and skills necessary to navigate complex situations.

2. The ability to reflect, analyze options, and act professionally in challenging situations can be developed throughout a career: from medical student, to resident, to practicing physician.

3. Professionalism lapses are common in daily practice and can be viewed as opportunities for learning, rather than requiring punishment.

4. Professional resilience, the ability to handle these complex situations, can be enhanced by addressing issues in both the work and personal environments.

5. Teams can develop a culture to support and foster the ability of the team members to manage professionalism challenges.

REFERENCES

1. Billings ME, Lazarus ME, Wenrich M, Curtis JR, Engelberg RA. The effect of the hidden curriculum on resident burnout and cynicism. *J Grad Med Educ*. 2011 Dec;3(4):503–510.
2. Borrell-Carrió F, Epstein RM. Preventing errors in clinical practice: a call for self-awareness. *Ann Fam Med*. 2004 Jul-Aug;2(4):310–316.
3. Bryan CS. Medical professionalism and Maslow's needs hierarchy. *Pharos Alpha Omega Alpha Honor Med Soc*. 2005 spring;68(2):4–10.
4. Burack JH, Irby DM, Carline JD, Root RK, Larson EB. Teaching compassion and respect. Attending physicians' responses to problematic behaviors. *J Gen Intern Med*. 1999 Jan;14(1):49–55.
5. Dreyfus SE, Dreyfus HL. *A five-stage model of the mental activities involved in directed skill acquisition*. February, 1980. Available at: http://www.stormingmedia.us/15/1554/A155480.html
6. Epstein RM. Mindful practice. *JAMA*. 1999 Sep 1;282(9):833–839.
7. Epstein RM, Krasner MS. Physician resilience: what it means, why it matters, and how to promote it. *Acad Med*. 2013 Mar;88(3):301–303.
8. Ginsburg S, Regehr G, Hatala R, McNaughton N, Frohna A, Hodges B, Lingard L, Stern D. Context, conflict, and resolution: a new conceptual framework for evaluating professionalism. *Acad Med*. 2000 Oct;75(10 Suppl):S6–S11.
9. Ginsburg S, Regehr G, Lingard L. Basing the evaluation of professionalism on observable behaviors: a cautionary tale. *Acad Med*. 2004 Oct;79(10 Suppl):S1–S4.
10. Hafferty FW, Franks R. The hidden curriculum, ethics teaching, and the structure of medical education. *Acad Med*. 1994 Nov;69(11):861–871.
11. Hickson GB, Pichert JW, Webb LE, Gabbe SG. A complementary approach to promoting professionalism: identifying, measuring, and addressing unprofessional behaviors. *Acad Med*. 2007 Nov;82(11):1040–1048.
12. Leach DC. Professionalism: the formation of physicians. *Am J Bioeth*. 2004 spring;4(2):11–12.
13. Leape LL, Shore MF, Dienstag JL, Mayer RJ, Edgman-Levitan S, Meyer GS, Healy GB. Perspective: a culture of respect, part 1: the nature and causes of disrespectful behavior by physicians. *Acad Med*. 2012 Jul;87(7):845–852.
14. Lucey C, Souba W. Perspective: the problem with the problem of professionalism. *Acad Med*. 2010 Jun;85(6):1018–1024.
15. Moulton CA, Epstein RM. Self-monitoring in surgical practice: slowing down when you should. In: Fry H, Kneebone R, eds. *Surgical Education: Theorising an Emerging Domain*. Dordrecht, The Netherlands: Springer; 2011:169–182.
16. Regehr G. The persistent myth of stability. On the chronic underestimation of the role of context in behavior. *J Gen Intern Med*. 2006 May;21(5):544–545.
17. Shanafelt TD, Bradley KA, Wipf JE, Back AL. Burnout and self-reported patient care in an internal medicine residency program. *Ann Intern Med*. 2002 Mar 5;136(5):358–367.
18. Testerman JK, Morton KR, Loo LK, Worthley JS, Lamberton HH. The natural history of cynicism in physicians. *Acad Med*. 1996 Oct;71(10 Suppl):S43–S45.
19. Zwack J, Schweitzer J. If every fifth physician is affected by burnout, what about the other four? Resilience strategies of experienced physicians. *Acad Med*. 2013 Mar;88(3):382–389.

A BRIEF HISTORY OF MEDICINE'S MODERN-DAY PROFESSIONALISM MOVEMENT

3

LEARNING OBJECTIVES

1. To understand the history and evolution of medical professionalism.
2. To review key efforts to institutionalize professionalism within the arenas of medical education and clinical practice.
3. To frame some of the modern issues of conflict-of-interest, duty hours, and social media in the light of professionalism.
4. To link the concepts of professionalism with that of the hidden curriculum.

This chapter examines the history and evolution of medicine's modern-day professionalism movement. The brief discussion in this chapter is partial and not comprehensive, and is intended to provide readers with some historical context. In particular, we think it is useful to realize that medical professionalism, while it has roots back into the 1600s, has only recently received a good deal of attention in medical literature and medical education. Furthermore, understanding this history may allow readers to reflect on the present day challenges facing medicine and consider how professionalism will continue to evolve.

ROOTS

For the last several hundred years, medicine has been considered, and considered itself to be, a profession. Historical documents reflect this view. During the Great Plague of London in 1666, an apothecary William Boghurst argued:

> Every man that undertakes to be of a profession, or takes upon himself an office must take all parts of it, the good and the evil, the pleasure and the pain, the profit and the inconveniences all together and not pick and choose; for Ministers must preach, Captains must fight and Physicians attend upon the sick (Huber & Wynia, 2004).

In 1803, Thomas Percival published his pivotal book entitled *Medical Ethics* (Percival, 1803). Percival labeled medicine as a "profession," and he characterized the practice of medicine as a "public trust." Percival recast medical ethics as a collective rather than an individual physician responsibility "essentially creating the notion of medical professionalism" (Wynia & Kurlander, 2007). Although the term "profession" would not be a common descriptor for most of the second millennium, the historical connections of medicine to the guild structure of medieval Europe and to the notions of skilled labor and apprenticeship training, is well documented (Sox, 2007).

Occupational claims of expertise were not always supported by the public. By the 1700s and 1800s, there were widespread signs that the public held a deep distrust of trade and professional groups over the tendency of such groups toward self-interest. Writers as disparate as Adam Smith and George Bernard Shaw framed professions as "conspiracies against the public" (Smith, 1991) or against the "laity" (Shaw, 1946), with Shaw adding an occupationally specific dagger in characterizing medicine as "a conspiracy to hide its own shortcomings." Over time, and as documented in Paul Starr's book *The Social Transformation of American Medicine* (Starr, 1984), organized medicine became strategic and proactive in its attempts to reclaim its image and to solidify its claims to professional powers and privileges—a process Starr characterized in the subtitle of his book as "the rise of a sovereign profession." By the 1950s, medicine's efforts were so successful that the terms "medicine" and "profession" had become linked. Physicians were viewed as professionals by virtue of their training and degree. The state and the status had become one.

Today, we live in more critical times. Questions about the legitimacy of medicine's status as a profession have become more challenging. In this chapter, we briefly trace the history of medicine's modern-day professionalism movement, beginning with its conceptual origins in the field of sociology and moving through more contemporary concerns with issues such as conflict-of-interest, duty hours, and social media. The professionalism movement itself is in its early adolescence, and the kinds of discord we see taking place across the current professionalism landscape speaks to the movement's nascent status. At the same time, it is equally true that medicine's future as a profession is not guaranteed. If present challenges are not properly addressed, organized medicine may well experience significant curtailments of its professional powers and privileges.

THE PROFESSION OF MEDICINE AND PROFESSIONALISM

Whether we are discussing historical origins or modern expressions, it is critical to differentiate between *profession* and *professionalism*. Profession is a sociological construct and a way of organizing work. Each profession is controlled by skilled workers and has its own knowledge base, organizational forms, career paths, education, and ideology, and thus its own logic for how work is carried out and valued (Freidson, 2001). Understanding how work is organized and executed, however, is different from examining the underlying ethos driving that work—and thus how *professionalism* functions as an occupationally specific moral imperative. Professionalism describes the core values (e.g., altruism, conscientiousness, and so on) that are shared by physicians.

Historically, attention to issues of professions predates those of professionalism. During the early 1900s, social scientists began to examine a number of occupational groups for their (potentially) professional characteristics, including accountancy, life insurance, and "handing men" (a.k.a. hiring managers) (Bloomfield, 1915). Medicine was just one of many occupations subject to such sociological scrutiny. In 1915, Abraham Flexner, whose earlier and scathing study of North American medical schools (the Flexner Report) would revolutionize medical training, published a piercing dissection of claims to professional status (Flexner, 1915). In his article, Flexner applied six criteria to analyze the professional status of a range of occupational groups, including banking, engineering, medicine, nursing, pharmacy, plumbing, and social work. He concluded that medicine had yet to realize its professional potentials because its altruistic aspirations were being undercut by its commercialist tendencies—a conclusion no doubt influenced by Flexner's earlier encounters with the shameful state of proprietary, for-profit medical schools.

> All activities may be prosecuted in the genuine professional spirit. Insofar as accepted professions are prosecuted at a mercenary or selfish level, law and medicine are ethically no better than trades.
>
> Abraham Flexner 1915 (page 165)

In the next decade, authors continued to raise concerns about the "inherent conflict" in medicine between the need to maintain standards to protect the public and actions taken to promote the interests of the profession and individual professionals (Parsons, 1939). In 1970, Eliot Freidson began to examine how medicine as a profession operated in a protectionist and self-interested manner.

> ". . . the critical flaw in professional autonomy . . . [is that] . . . it develops and maintains in the profession a self-deceiving view of the objectivity and reliability of knowledge and the virtues of its members. Furthermore, it encourages the profession to see itself as the sole possessor of knowledge and virtue, to be somewhat suspicious of the technical and moral capacity of other occupations, and to be at best patronizing and at worst contemptuous of its clientele . . . . Its very autonomy has led to insularity and a mistaken arrogance about its mission in the world. . . [and] . . . [to] . . . sanctimonious myths of the inherently superior qualities of themselves as professionals – of their knowledge and their work."
>
> Eliot Freidson 1970 (pages 369–370)

Freidson's analyses helped to launch an extensive debate within sociology about the nature of profession and, in particular, whether medicine was losing or maintaining its professional powers and prerogatives (Hafferty, 1988). Like Freidson, Starr adopted a critical view of medicine by documenting medicine's potential for both self-interest and self-deception—something perfectly captured in the evocative opening sentence of *The Social Transformation of American Medicine*—"The dream of reason did not take power into account" (Starr, 1984). Starr also saw medicine as initially successful in efforts to resist corporate control, but that success waned over time in the face of an omnivorous march by corporate forces.

> Unless there is a radical turnabout in economic conditions and American politics, the last decades of the twentieth century are likely to be a time of diminished resources and autonomy for many physicians, voluntary hospitals, and medical schools . . . [with the] . . . rise of corporate enterprise in health services, which is already having a profound impact on the ethics and politics of medical care as well as its institutions.
>
> Paul Starr 1984 (pages 420–421)

Sociologists, particularly Freidson and Starr, gained the attention of medical readers and highlighted the challenge to medicine as a profession about whose interests came first—the public or the physicians. The public might well have started to question whether the profession could be trusted.

Attention to issues of *professionalism* (as opposed to profession) has a similar, but more contemporary history. One early article entitled, "Culture and professionalism in education," was authored by the famous educationalist and philosopher John Dewey (1923). However, articles on professionalism were few and far between during most of the 1900s, and very few focused on medicine. Aside from one article each in the nursing, hospital administration, and pharmacy literatures, it would not be until the early 1990s before a reasonable substantive (more than 20 citations) professionalism literature began to take shape within medicine. The first three of these articles were, "Yellow professionalism. Advertising by physicians in the yellow pages," published in the *The New England Journal of Medicine* (Reade, 1987) and, "Countdown to millennium: balancing the professionalism and business of medicine: medicine's rocking horse," published in *The Journal of the American Medical Association (JAMA)* (Lundberg, 1990), and, "Conflicts of interest: physician ownership of medical facilities," also published in *JAMA* (Clarke et al, 1992).

These three exemplars notwithstanding, professionalism articles within medicine would remain scanty for much of the 1990s. Figure 3-1, compiled from Web of Science data, traces the publication of articles on professionalism since the early 1970s and illustrates that a substantive literature using the word "professionalism" did not emerge until the late 1990 to early 2000s.

This historical window into the rise of a professionalism literature within medicine highlights several important points. First, this publication-centric view helps us to date the rise of a *professionalism* movement within medicine to the turn of the twenty-first century. In other words, the movement, at best, is no more than 25 years old. In fact there were other terms being used to describe problems including communication difficulties, student attitudes of cynicism, and ethical problems, but they were not gathered under the umbrella of "professionalism."

Second, there have been shifts over time in the kinds of topics or issues addressed under the banner of professionalism. The three articles mentioned

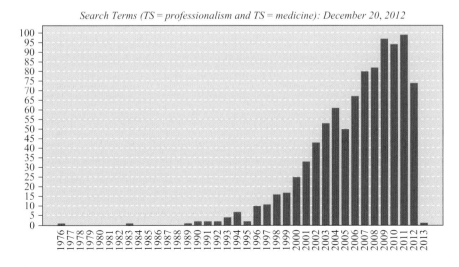

Search Terms (TS = professionalism and TS = medicine): December 20, 2012

Figure 3-1 ▪ Articles on medicine and professionalism by Year: Thomson Reuters's Web of Science.

focus on advertising, the relationship of commercialism and medicine, and conflicts-of-interest, respectively. Other "professionalism issues," such as duty hours and social media, did not appear until 2000.

Third, issues of professionalism reflect political and economic environments (Hafferty & McKinlay, 1993). It is not surprising to see the theme of commercialism and conflict of interest in medicine as a key issue in these U.S. publications, since the "business" side of medicine was emerging as a strong influence. The idea of dual agency, that is, working for the public interests versus the interest of the profession, did not have the same resonance within a U.K., Canadian, or German healthcare environment, where the "business" side of medicine was less evident.

THE MOVEMENT: OPENING SALVOS

Medicine's modern day professionalism movement was well underway by the late 1990s. Editorials began to address the threats of commercialism to values of professionalism. Articles emerged about the medical-industrial complex (Relman, 1980) and the rise of for-profit medicine; "big business" could be antithetical to *professional* ideals. What followed was a flurry of calls, first to define professionalism, given the widely circulating observation that the medical community lacked a definitional consensus (Swick, 2000); then to teach professionalism principles to trainees, given the emerging conclusion that the best route to salvation would come via the newest generation of providers (Swick et al, 1999); and finally to measure and assess professionalism, given the widely circulating belief that any efforts to pass on these "new" ideals to trainees would be futile unless assessment was part of the package (Lynch, Surdyk, & Eiser, 2004). In turn, there was a variety of efforts to institutionalize professionalism within medical settings with the creation of professionalism codes, charters, curriculum, and competencies (Hafferty & Levinson, 2008).

The development of the professionalism movement was not linear. Although it is true that calls for definitions preceded calls for curricula or assessment, it also is true that assessment efforts have come to function as implicit definitions of professionalism and that the establishment of codes, charters, and competencies have spilled "backward" into the creation of new definitions. For these reasons, it is more accurate to think of professionalism pulses or waves—each having its moment, only to be recycled and renewed in some other form within a dynamic of interdependent and continuously evolving profiles. Table 3-1 lists examples of both early and more contemporary pulses.

As medical schools and other organizations began to operationalize and deploy their own definitions, assessment tools, and institutionalization efforts, these initiatives began to trigger a range of "flash points" where conflicts emerged (e.g., collegiality and responsiveness to the work demands of

Table 3-1   **PROFESSIONALISM PULSES**
• Calls to define professionalism • Calls to measure and assess professionalism • Calls to teach professionalism (particularly within undergraduate medical education) • Institutionalization efforts (the development of professionalism codes, competencies and charters, curriculum) • A shift from individuals and their motives to occupational settings, structures, and processes • An emerging consideration of professionalism as a complex adaptive system with social actors, social structures, and environmental forces as interactive, interdependent, and adaptive

From Hafferty FW, Levinson D. Moving beyond nostalgia and motives: towards a complexity science view of medical professionalism. *Perspect Biol Med.* 2008 Autumn;51(4):599–615.

colleagues versus patient care responsibilities), clashes between professionalism and organizational prerogatives (e.g., the need to standardize physician work practices versus the need for physician autonomy in decision-making), or clashes between professionalism and broader environmental factors (e.g., how medicine is practiced versus how it is paid for).

Basically, flash points reflect the tensions that arose in these settings as the "new professionalism ideals" represented in these definitions, assessment tools, and institutionalization efforts came into conflict with the more entrenched organizational and normative practices of clinical and educational work. Therefore, students began to hear one set of professionalism messages in the classroom while seeing another being role modeled on the wards or in clinic situations. Similarly, although students might be formally introduced to their medical school's conflict-of-interest policies within these new professionalism curricula, they also were seeing faculty engaged in what clearly appeared to students as "conflicted" behaviors. Even attempts to assess professionalism appeared to students to reflect more the politics-of-power than the operationalization of core professionalism principles. Faculty often resisted efforts to have their professionalism evaluated, while at the same time insisting that student assessment was critical to the educational mission of the school. New rules about what students could and could not post on social media sites such as Facebook also drew students' ire. Students began to complain about all the new professionalism teachings, the professionalism rules, and requirement to "jump through hoops" to demonstrate professionalism. Cynicism about professionalism began to emerge and students began to push back against what faculty thought were rather straightforward and noncontroversial issues.

In short, one unintended consequence of medicine's modern-day professionalism movement was the creation of a rift between the "ideal" and the "real"—a rift that was not there prior to the ideal becoming more formalized. Moreover, these rifts were being labeled as "professionalism issues." For example, the evolution of the Accreditation Council for Graduate Medical Education (ACGME) duty hour regulations governing the number of hours residents can work has been framed within the medical literature, not only as a "not-enough-time-to-properly-educate-residents" issue, but also as a "professionalism" issue with explicit references to the work ethic of new residents, and to the quality and safety issues embedded in patient care handoffs (Coverdill et al, 2010). Similarly, concerns about the types of materials being posted by trainees and physicians on Facebook and other social media sites have been framed as "important professionalism issues" (MacDonald, Sohn, & Ellis, 2010). Results from a survey of physicians about attitudes and actual behaviors toward professional and ethical standards articulated in The Physician Charter, such as honesty with patients, physician impairment, and self-referral, found that attitudes and behaviors very often failed to align. For example, 93% said all medical errors should be reported, but 46% of physicians who knew about a medical error did not report it on at least one occasion (Campbell et al, 2007). In short, the arrival of medicine's modern-day professionalism movement helped both to uncover, but also to create and label, the very tensions between professionalism-as-an-ideal and professionalism-in-practice. In turn, the perceived need among medical leaders to address the professionalism issues being identified in these flash points further raised the visibility of professionalism within the academic and clinical communities, thereby accelerating efforts to create ever better definitions, more valid and reliable assessment tools, more effective curricula, and ever more robust institutionalization efforts within educational and clinical settings. In these interesting and intersecting ways, flash points fueled new interactions of professionalism pulses, which, in turn, helped to ignite new flash points. Examples of key flash points are listed in Table 3-2.

Table 3-2   **PROFESSIONALISM FLASH POINTS**
• Conflicts of interest
• Duty hours
• Student push back
• Social media
• Teamwork and interprofessional education
• Physician performance measurement
• Self-regulation

As this groundswell of interactive forces gathered steam, notions of professionalism began to shift as well. What had been an almost exclusive focus on professionalism as a characteristic of individuals, and thus something tied to the motives and motivations of individual practitioners and trainees, slowly began to be reframed as an organizational issue, thus drawing attention to how various forms of organizational structure might either facilitate or hinder the expression of professionalism among trainees and practicing clinicians. In this way, terms like "organizational professionalism" began to creep into the literature (Evetts, 2010; Egener et al, 2012).

> Organizational professionalism is the ability of an organization to develop and sustain a culture and related institutional structures that align personal and organizational conduct around competency standards and ethical principles and thereby assure the public it is trustworthy in the execution of its work.

Taken as a whole, this swirl of definitional, assessment, institutionalization initiatives, and flashpoints continue to fuel and form the evolution of medicine's modern-day professionalism movement. What follows are some observations on professionalism issues that have surfaced within the intersections of these pulses and flashpoints.

THE "PROBLEM OF DEFINITION"

One of the more interesting aspects of medicine's modern-day professionalism movement is the concern expressed by many physicians that medicine continues to suffer from the lack of a *singular* definition of professionalism—and thus a core and/or consensual sense of what it means to be a professional. Although it may be true that medicine lacks a literally *singular* definition, it is not true that medicine is besieged by definitional chaos. Therefore, although multiple definitions exist, there also is considerable homogeneity across those definitions (Cruess & Cruess, 2008; Van De Camp et al, 2004).

However, in the last decade, a definition has emerged that is widely accepted and has become the most commonly used one. "Medical Professionalism in the New Millennium: A Physician Charter," is the definition we have used in this book (see Chapter 1, A Practical Approach to "Professionalism"). The Charter quickly became the de facto definition for many medical organizations—particularly in medical training and with specialty boards and medical societies.

MAJOR INSTITUTIONALIZATION INITIATIVES: TWO EXAMPLES

Its short history notwithstanding, medicine's modern-day professionalism movement is marked by a cadre of notable efforts to embed professionalism into the routines of medical education and clinical practice. Definitions have been created; assessment tools developed; articles and books written; symposia organized; foundation initiatives launched; and codes, charters, competencies, and curricula formulated. Although we lack the space to critically examine even one of these pulses, it is important to at least mention two examples of specific initiatives to give context to this narrative:

1. The Association of American Medical College's (AAMC) *Medial School Objectives Project* (MSOP); and
2. The Accreditation Council of Graduate Medical Education's (ACGME) *Six Core Competencies.*

The AAMC's MSOP

In 1998, the AAMC released the first of several reports on medical education. The inaugural report showcased what the AAMC considered to be the four key learning objectives that should underscore undergraduate medical education. Although each of the objectives came with a bevy of clarifying subtext, the AAMC's basic message was that: "physicians must be . . . altruistic, knowledgeable, skillful, and dutiful" and that medical schools must ensure that students internalize and master these objectives "to the satisfaction of the faculty" (Association of American Medical Colleges, 1998). The objectives are listed in Table 3-3.

Over time, the first (altruism) and fourth (dutifulness) objectives came to be identified as the MSOP's professionalism objectives. However, and once again reflecting the fact that this report was released early in medicine's modern-day movement, there was only one direct reference to professionalism in this report—a bullet-point within the altruism section calling for

Table 3-3 **THE MSOP OBJECTIVES**
Physicians must be . . .
• Altruistic
• Knowledgeable
• Skillful
• Dutiful

Data from the Association of American Medical Colleges. Retrieved from https://www.aamc.org/initiatives/msop/.

students to "understand the threats to medical professionalism posed by conflicts of interest inherent in various financial and organizational arrangements
for the practice of medicine." Once again, we see, conflict of interest (COI)
issues (as a flash point) assuming a prominent position in this early framing
of professionalism.

The ACGME's six core competencies

In 1999, the ACGME released its six core competencies and ushered in a new
era in residency education (in Canada, the CanMEDS framework described
similar competencies). In adopting a competency framework, the ACGME
shifted the focus of residency education from its previous preoccupation with
structure and process (what was taught, how, and when) to a focus emphasizing performance and outcomes (what residents actually can do). One of the
six competencies is "professionalism" (the ACGME framework is discussed
further in the Chapter 11, Evaluating Professionalism). In specifying these
competencies, the ACGME also provided residency programs with guidance
as to how these competencies might be defined and assessed. In the case of
professionalism, the ACGME created a definition (Table 3-4).

Looking across these documents, the first (MSOP) targets undergraduate
medical education, the second (ACGME competencies) graduate medical
education, whereas the Physician Charter described earlier targets clinical
practice. As is characteristic of U.S. medical education, and in contrast to
medical education in other countries such as the United Kingdom, each of
these reports and the educational domains they represent, operates independently of the others. Therefore, although it is true that some medical schools
have adopted a competency-based curricular framework (thus borrowing a
standard from the ACGME), or a definition of professionalism borrowed

---

Table 3-4 ACGME LONG-FORM DEFINITION OF PROFESSIONALISM

Residents must demonstrate a commitment to carrying out professional responsibilities
and an adherence to ethical principles. Residents are expected to demonstrate:

- Compassion, integrity, and respect for others;
- Responsiveness to patient needs that supersedes self-interest;
- Respect for patient privacy and autonomy;
- Accountability to patients, society, and the profession; and
- Sensitivity and responsiveness to a diverse patient population, including but not
  limited to diversity in gender, age, culture, race, religion, disabilities, and sexual
  orientation.

From Accreditation Council for Graduate Medical Education (ACGME). Program Director Guide to the
   Common Program Requirements, September 2012.

from the Charter, medical school accreditation requirements do not mandate that individual schools adopt the framings or tools from these other realms of medical education. Instead, the accreditation of medical schools, residency programs, and clinical practitioners (via licensure, specialty certification, and maintenance of certification) operate largely independent of each other.

MEDICAL STUDENT PUSH BACK

One particular sign that all was not well within medicine's modern-day professionalism movement was a growing disquietude and resistance among medical students to the various institutionalization practices being implemented within their medical schools (Skiles, 2005). The reasons for these tensions and pushbacks are varied:

1. A growing awareness by students that the professionalism being taught in the classroom was not the same professionalism being role modeled in the clinic or on the wards—and thus the appearance of "double standards" or organizational hypocrisy, (see Chapter 8, The Hidden Curriculum and Professionalism) (Brainard & Brislen, 2007);
2. The initial tendency by faculty to endorse "professionalism rules" for students, while rejecting similar rules/guidelines for themselves—with students sensing, once again, the power of hierarchy and privilege dominating the ethic of professionalism;
3. The tendency for professionalism to embrace a "nostalgic" version of professionalism; and
4. The continuing cloud of faculty relations with industry and institutional conflicts-of-interest.

As noted earlier, one of the most volatile professionalism issues within medicine's modern-day professionalism movement is medical school and faculty relations with industry and the potential for conflicts-of-interest within those relationships. The issue is both contentious and nuanced, with some critics calling for a "ban," and others arguing that conflicts-of-interest (COIs) are best "managed." The Physician Charter contains the term "manage" COI. A second key point is that many COI reforms have been driven by student initiatives—not by faculty. A prime example is the American Medical Student Association's (AMSA) PharmFree Campaign (http://www.pharmfree.org), and in particular, their PharmFree Scorecard (http://www.amsascorecard.org). What began as an in-house and relatively crude ranking of U.S. medical schools and the COI policies, has developed, in partnership with the Pew Foundation and its Prescription Project, into a continuously updateable, interactive/searchable, web-based reporting system that tracks medical school COI policies along a number of dimensions. Over its lifetime, the Pharm-Free project has had a noticeable impact on medical schools—despite school denials that this initiative has influenced their policies. When the ranking first came out, a majority of medical schools received grades of "D" or "F." Today, a majority of medical schools are rated B or higher with many more schools either implementing policies for the first time or substantially updating policies already in place (Krupa, 2011).

Policy improvements notwithstanding, tensions between students and their schools continue to bubble as students resist "being lectured to" about professionalism or finding themselves the object of new professionalism initiatives that appear to target students, but not faculty. In some cases, figurative blood has been spilled. A recent case at Harvard Medical School illustrates how contentious "professionalism issues" can become (Cooney, 2009a, 2009b). Faced with concerns about faculty financial ties to industry, students aired their concerns in the media—drawing administrative ire. In response, administration created a formal policy requiring students to clear contact with media through the school. Harvard subsequently rescinded its policy after the entire episode went public, but the relational damage between students and administration was not as easily repaired.

THE RISE OF A HIDDEN CURRICULUM OF PROFESSIONALISM (ALSO SEE CHAPTER 8, THE HIDDEN CURRICULUM AND PROFESSIONALISM)

For what is yet another set of complicated reasons, it turned out to be much easier to write definitions, create assessment tools, and develop curriculum codes and charters than to change physician practice behaviors. For this reason—and with a certain degree of irony—one early consequence of medicine's modern-day professionalism movement was the emergence of a hidden curriculum of professionalism, including a literature specifically linking the hidden curriculum of medical education with a literature on medical professionalism. Until the professionalism movement, there had been few disjunctures between what students were being formally taught in the classroom (at least about professionalism) and what they were seeing on the wards and in the clinic. Until the rise of medicine's modern-day professionalism movement, what it meant to be a profession, or to act professionally, was more an implicit than explicit part of the medical school curriculum. However, now students find themselves having to grapple with formally taught and institutionally sanctioned professionalism definitions and/or being tested on the content of formal codes and charters. Residents, driven by the new ACGME competencies, were expected to demonstrate competence in professionalism and to be assessed on their performance. Nonetheless, and in many respects, all of these competencies, content, and assessment exist somewhat peripherally to what trainees see in the "real world" of clinical practice—a world in which something other than the ideal is being role modeled. Trainees found themselves trapped between formal/explicit rules and the "rules of the road." Cynicism about professionalism percolated, and they began to rebel (Finn, Garner, & Sawdon, 2010).

> I know he stands at the absolute top of surgery here at "X." I mean everybody knows his name, and not just here but nationally. Even still, what he preaches about professionalism and caring for the patient just isn't done any more. He may still come in on weekends, but you won't find any of the other surgeons coming by on their days off to check on their patients.
>
> A First Year Surgical Intern

Fissures emerged along a number of fronts as well. In 2005, the University of Washington School of Medicine essentially banned the term professionalism—substituting the phrase "professional values" because of student complaints that they were tired of "lectured at" on this topic (Goldstein et al, 2006). Similarly, and at other schools, policies about social media have drawn student wrath along with student and faculty debates about issues of lifestyle, balance, and the difference between work and personal time (Chretien et al, 2010). Sometimes there is little joy in Mudville (Thayer, 1888).

| CONCLUSION

None of the data about fissures and points of conflict should be taken as evidence that medicine's modern-day professionalism movement is in trouble or is otherwise fatally flawed. Instead the interjection of definitions, assessment tools, and curricula into an educational and practice environment that was less-than-fully professional has led to inevitable confusion, consternation, and conflict. That medicine continues to wrestle with these conundrums is a mark of professionalism's success as a movement—not failure. This is not to imply that all flashpoints are ultimately resolvable. As we have seen earlier in this chapter, COI was one of the earliest flashpoints, remains an area of concern today, and is likely to continue in the future. In short, this particular flashpoint may never be fully resolved.

At the same time, the emerging examination and understanding of how different organizational forms may either hinder or facilitate professionalism directly challenges organizations to be more professionalism-friendly and supportive. Furthermore, we may also begin to see how organizations themselves may be thought of as being more—or less—professional. This, in turn, could call for new definitions, charters, and professionalism assessment tools, this time for organizations rather than individuals. All this should add new fuel and robustness to the movement.

Finally, we wish to note that the movement is not only dynamic and adaptive, but also not all that predictable. Not that long ago, social media was not on the professionalism radar—in large part because Facebook and other social media platforms did not exist. In 2003, therefore, medical educators had no idea that healthcare professional postings on such sites would be a huge professionalism issue. In this same way, other issues will emerge and other discussions, debates, and definitions, and so on, will continue to fuel the movement. This is what makes professionalism a dynamic and relational enterprise.

KEY LEARNING POINTS

1. Professionalism needs to be recognized as a dynamic and evolving concept with a past, present, and future.
2. Efforts by organized medicine to shape definitions, assessment tools, and related institutionalization efforts (via the creation of professionalism curricula, codes, charters, competencies, and so on) have played a pivotal role in this evolution.
3. Within this evolution, particular issues (e.g., "flash points") such as duty hours and conflicts-of-interest have generated intense discussions within medicine about the meaning and operationalization of professionalism.
4. Despite the rise of formal professionalism curricula, along with related codes, charters, and competencies, much of the learning that trainees undergo regarding what it means to be a good professional is embedded in the hidden curriculum.

REFERENCES

1. Association of American Medical Colleges. *Report 1. Learning Objectives for Medical Student Education: Guidelines for Medical Schools. Medical School Objectives Project.* Washington, DC: Association of American Medical Colleges; 1998.
2. Bloomfield M. The new profession of handling men. *Annals of the American Academy of Political and Social Science.* 1915 Sep;61:121–126.

3. Brainard AH, Brislen HC. Viewpoint: learning professionalism: a view from the trenches. *Acad Med*. 2007 Nov;82(11):1010–1014.

4. Campbell EG, Regan S, Gruen RL, Ferris TG, Rao SR, Cleary PD, Blumenthal D. Professionalism in medicine: results of a national survey of physicians. *Ann Intern Med*. 2007 Dec 4;147(11):795–802.

5. Chretien KC, Goldman EF, Beckman L, Kind T. It's your own risk: medical students' perspectives on online professionalism. *Acad Med*. 2010 Oct;85(10 Suppl):S68–S71.

6. Clarke OW, Glasson J, August AM, Barrasso JA, Epps CH, McQuillan R, Plows CW, Puzak, MA, Wilkins GT, Orentlicher D, Halkola KA, Johnson KB, Conley RB. Conflicts of interest. Physician ownership of medical facilities. Council on Ethical and Judicial Affairs, American Medical Association. *JAMA*. 1992 May 6;267(17): 2366–2369.

7. Cooney E. *Harvard Medical students, administrators revising media policy.* 2009a Sep. Available at: http://www.boston.com/news/health/blog/2009/09/harvard_medical_3.html

8. Cooney E. *Harvard rethinks media policy: Medical students had bristled at rule.* 2009b Sep. Available at: http://www.boston.com/news/education/k_12/articles/2009/09/03/harvard_rethinks_media_policy/

9. Coverdill JE, Carbonell AM, Fryer J, Fuhrman GM, Harold KL, Hiatt JR, Jarman BT, Moore RA, Nakayama DK, Nelson MT, Schlatter M, Sidwell RA, Tarpley JL, Termuhlen PM, Wohltmann C, Mellinger JD. A new professionalism? Surgical residents, duty hours restrictions, and shift transitions. *Acad Med*. 2010 Oct;85(10 Suppl): S72–S75.

10. Cruess SR, Cruess RL. The cognitive base of professionalism. In Cruess RL, Cruess SR, Steinert Y (Eds.), *Teaching Medical Professionalism*. New York, NY: Cambridge University Press; 2008, 7–31.

11. Dewey J. Culture and professionalism in education. *Bulletin of the American Association of University Professors*. 1923 Dec:9(8);51–53.

12. Egener B, McDonald W, Rosof B, Gullen D. Perspective: organizational professionalism: relevant competencies and behaviors. *Acad Med*. 2012 May;87(5):668–674.

13. Evetts J. *Organizational Professionalism: Changes, challenges and opportunities.* Proceedings from DPU Conference. Copenhagen, Denmark; 2010.

14. Finn G, Garner J, Sawdon M. "You're judged all the time!" Students' views on professionalism: a multicentre study. *Med Educ*. 2010 Aug;44(8):814–825.

15. Flexner A. Is social work a profession? *Research on Social Work Practice.* 1915:11(2);152–165.

16. Freidson E. *Profession of Medicine: A Study of the Sociology of Applied Knowledge.* New York, NY: Harper & Row; 1970.

17. Freidson E. *Professionalism: The Third Logic.* Chicago, IL: University of Chicago Press; 2001.

18. Goldstein EA, Maestas RR, Fryer-Edwards K, Wenrich MD, Oelschlager AM, Baernstein A, Kimball HR. Professionalism in medical education: an institutional challenge. *Acad Med*. 2006 Oct;81(10):871–876.

19. Hafferty FW. Theories at the crossroads: a discussion of evolving views on medicine as a profession. *Milbank Q*. 1988;66 (Suppl 2):202–225.

20. Hafferty FW, Levinson D. Moving beyond nostalgia and motives: towards a complexity science view of medical professionalism. *Perspect Biol Med.* 2008 Autumn;51(4):599–615.

21. Hafferty FW, McKinlay JB. *The Changing Medical Profession: An International Perspective.* New York, NY: Oxford University Press; 1993.

22. Huber SJ, Wynia MK. When pestilence prevails...physician responsibilities in epidemics. *Am J Bioeth.* 2004 Winter;4(1):W5–W11.

23. Krupa C. *Medical schools get high marks on conflict-of-interest policies: More than half earn an A or B for their rules governing drug industry interaction with students and faculty.* January, 2011. Available at http://www.ama-assn.org/amednews/2011/01/03/prsc0104.htm

24. Lundberg GD. Countdown to millennium—balancing the professionalism and business of medicine. Medicine's Rocking Horse. *JAMA.* 1990 Jan 5;263(1):86–87.

25. Lynch DC, Surdyk PM, Eiser AR. Assessing professionalism: a review of the literature. *Med Teach.* 2004 Jun;26(4):366–373.

26. MacDonald J, Sohn S, Ellis P. Privacy, professionalism and Facebook: a dilemma for young doctors. *Med Educ.* 2010 Aug;44(8):805–813.

27. Parsons T. The professions and social structure. *Social Forces.* 1939 May 17;(4): 457–467.

28. Percival T. *Medical Ethics: Or, a Code of Institutes and Precepts, Adapted to the Professional Conduct of Physicians and Surgeons.* Oxford, UK: I. Shrimpton; 1803.

29. Reade JM, Ratzan RM. Yellow professionalism. Advertising by physicians in the Yellow Pages. *N Engl J Med.* 1987 May 21;316(21):1315–1319.

30. Relman AS. The new medical-industrial complex. *N Engl J Med.* 1980 Oct 23;303(17):963–970.

31. Shaw GB. *The Doctor's Dilemma.* New York, NY: Penguin; 1946.

32. Skiles J. Teaching professionalism: a medical student's opinion. *The Clinical Teacher.* 2005 Dec:2(2);66–71.

33. Smith A. *The Wealth of Nations.* Amherst, MA: Prometheus Books; 1991.

34. Sox HC. Medical professionalism and the parable of the craft guilds. *Ann Intern Med.* 2007 Dec 4;147(11):809–810.

35. Starr PE. *The Social Transformation of American Medicine: The Rise of a Sovereign Profession and the Making of a Vast Industry.* New York, NY: Basic Books; 1984.

36. Swick HM. Toward a normative definition of medical professionalism. *Acad Med.* 2000 Jun;75(6):612–616.

37. Swick HM, Szenas P, Danoff D, Whitcomb ME. Teaching professionalism in undergraduate medical education. *JAMA.* 1999 Sep 1;282(9):830–832.

38. Thayer E. Casey At Bat. *San Francisco Examiner;* 1888.

39. Van De Camp K, Vernooij-Dassen MJ, Grol RP, Bottema BJ. How to conceptualize professionalism: a qualitative study. *Med Teach.* 2004 Dec;26(8):696–702.

40. Wilson D. Harvard backs off media policy. *New York Times,* 2009, p. B4.

41. Wynia MK, Kurlander JE. Physician ethics and participation in quality improvement: renewing a professional obligation. In Jennings B, Baily MA, Bottrell M, Lynn J (Eds.), *Quality Improvement: Ethical and Regulatory Issues.* Garrison, NY: The Hastings Center; 2007.

FOSTERING PATIENT-CENTERED CARE

4

LEARNING OBJECTIVES

1. To define patient-centered care.
2. To explain the importance of patient-centered care as a primary component of medical professionalism.
3. To outline the behaviors and skills needed to demonstrate caring and to build trust.
4. To describe the behaviors and skills needed to conduct informed decision-making conversations.
5. To explain the role individual physicians, healthcare teams, the healthcare setting, and the external environment play in fostering the delivery of patient-centered care.

John and Helen are 65 years old and have been married for 30 years. Recently they were recounting to a friend their vivid memories of the day Dr. Owen, an oncologist, told Helen that she had breast cancer. Although this event took place 20 years ago when Helen was 45 years old, both of them remember in great detail the visit with Dr. Owen when he broke the news. What Helen remembers most is how he told her he had bad news but he was going to be with her every moment of the journey ahead—that she was going to be okay. She remembers him holding her hand when she cried. She remembers the silence in the room that hung there for what seemed like a long time while she sobbed and couldn't speak. She remembers the warmth in his voice when he said, "I am so sorry you have to deal with this."

John remembers similar moments, and he also recalls how Dr. Owen checked to see how he was feeling. He remembers how Dr. Owen answered his questions about the next steps in the work-up and the possible treatment options (Helen doesn't remember that part of the conversation at all). John remembers that he called Dr. Owen later the same day to clarify a question and that Dr. Owen called back at 8 pm and addressed his concerns. John and Helen told their friend how much Dr. Owen meant to them over the next years of treatment and that even though Helen does not need him anymore they will always remember how much he cared.

Medical care ideally is delivered by caring professionals who are seeking to meet patients' physical, psychological, and social needs. Patients and families all want a physician like Dr. Owen who demonstrates compassion in times of stress and who helps them to understand the complex and confusing world of healthcare. Although we feel comfortable in medical settings, the medical environment can be a scary, overwhelming, and sometimes intimidating place for patients. Despite our best intentions, we sometimes forget what it feels like to be a patient. Many patients do not feel that they have encountered a physician like Dr. Owen.

Excellent medical care combines sophistication in scientific knowledge with equally sophisticated communication skills to understand the needs of patients, to address their emotions, and to educate patients about their choices in care. These communication skills underpin our ability to deliver "patient-centered care"—the term used by the Institute of Medicine to describe the model of care widely accepted as the goal of excellent care (Institute of Medicine, 2001). Many authors have written about this model using slightly different terms, but most agree about the functions of communication (Figure 4-1).

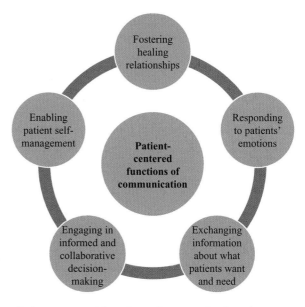

Figure 4-1 ▪ Patient-centered functions of communication.

Patient-centered communication is characterized by continuous healing relationships, shared understanding, emotional support, trust, patient enablement and activation, and informed choices. Physicians need specific communication skills to realize each of the components of patient-centered care. Learning and improving these skills is a critical component of professionalism.

Consistent with our systems view of professionalism, delivering patient-centered care depends not only on individuals but also on the healthcare team, the setting in which they work, and the broader external environment. All of these players either foster or inhibit the delivery of patient-centered care. In this chapter, we describe examples of how each player can demonstrate their professionalism in this domain.

WHY DOES COMMUNICATION MATTER?

The delivery of patient-centered care depends on the communication skills of all members of the healthcare team. There is a vast body of literature on the relationship between effective communication and outcomes of care (Epstein & Street, 2007; Stacey et al, 2011). Figure 4-2 is a representation of the relationship between patient-centered care, communication, and health outcomes. It illustrates our point that patient-centered care requires all the players—patients who participate actively in their care; skilled clinicians; and a well-organized care delivery system—to communicate effectively, and in turn, to optimize patient outcomes. A systematic review published in 2012 reviewed 40 studies assessing the relationship between patient-centered care and a variety of different clinical outcomes. Most of the studies demonstrated a positive relationship, particularly with patient satisfaction and wellbeing (Rathert & Wyrich, 2012; Epstein & Street, 2007; Mead & Bower, 2002). In addition, longitudinal studies were reviewed that found positive relationships between patient-centered care and clinical outcomes in diseases like diabetes and myocardial infarction (Meterko et al, 2010; Rocco et al, 2011).

Conversely, breakdowns in communication often lead to patient dissatisfaction with their care and sometimes to patients seeking legal recourse, and possible to malpractice litigation (Levinson et al, 1997). Patients complain that physicians are too rushed, do not listen to their concerns, and do not provide adequate information about their problem or options. The literature also abounds with stories of patient disappointment in care (Levinson & Shojania, 2011). When we tell people that we are interested in improving communication between physicians and patients, they all have a story to tell—and usually they are not complimentary to our profession.

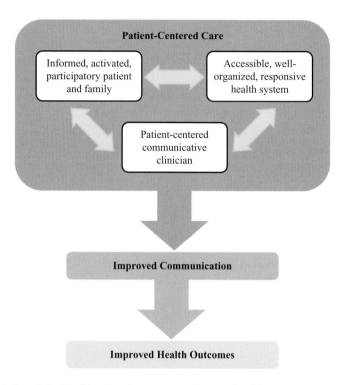

Figure 4-2 ■ Relationship of patient-centered care to health outcomes.

From Epstein RM, Street RL. Patient-centered communication in cancer care: promoting healing and reducing suffering. Bethesda, MD: National Cancer Institute; 2007, page 2. Available at: http://outcomes.cancer.gov/areas/pcc/communication/monograph.html

MISCONCEPTIONS ABOUT COMMUNICATION SKILLS

Adam Santos, a 1st-year medical student at a prestigious medical school, went to a lecture designed to set the stage for a course on clinical skills. At the end of the lecture he wrote on the evaluation form, "Why do I need to learn this stuff? If I didn't have good communication skills I would never have been admitted to this medical school. What a waste of my time."

Gut check—are you feeling the same way while reading a chapter on communication in a book on professionalism? This is not surprising. Medical education and our medical culture have suffered from several misconceptions.

Misconception #1: communication is simple—there is nothing to learn or to teach.

Misconception #2: communication is less important than the real stuff of medical care—knowing scientific facts. We hear the phrase,

"Ignore his bedside manner. *He is a really good surgeon and he knows how to cut.*"

Misconception #3: communication cannot be taught—you either have it or you don't.

Evidence does not support any of these statements but the culture of medical education and practice has fostered these beliefs.

BEHAVIORS AND SKILLS OF INDIVIDUAL PHYSICIANS

Delivering high quality patient-centered care requires many sophisticated communication skills. Extensive literature describes these skills. In this chapter we describe skills in two components of communication: demonstrating caring and building trust, and conducting informed decision-making conversations. Although delivering compassionate care requires a broader array of communication skills, these two components are critically important and commonly used in daily practice.

Demonstrating Caring and Building Trust

Trusting relationships between physicians and patients depends on both parties engaging in effective communication (Table 4-1). Patients need to share the details of their problems and their concerns and, in turn, physicians need to listen carefully without interrupting. An often quoted study of primary care physicians found that physicians interrupted patients an average of 18 seconds from when they began to speak (Beckman & Frankel, 1984). Patients often express their worries and distress subtly, and clinicians need to be attentive to hear and respond to these clues. Physicians often do not notice or even ignore these "clues," and they miss the opportunity to really connect with patients (Levinson, Gorawara-Bhat, & Lamb, 2000).

A 3rd-year medical student wrote about her experience on the medicine wards. "I remember as our team was rounding one day, we came across a patient who was upset and confused concerning her care. She felt unsure of what was being done to help her illness and why. The attending sat down on her bed and began explaining to her all that had been going on concerning her treatment. He told her what our team was doing, and he explained what all the consulting teams were recommending. After spending 10 to 15 minutes with the patient, I could tell how much better she felt about the situation and that she felt cared for. I was impressed by just how a few minutes can make a world of difference for a scared and confused patient, or any patient."

Table 4-1	EXAMPLES OF BEHAVIORS THAT CLINICIANS AND PATIENTS/FAMILY MUST ENGAGE IN FOR EFFECTIVE COMMUNICATION	
Clinicians	**Patients / Family**
Listen	Disclose needs
Avoid interruptions	Share information about symptoms and concerns
Organize the visit	Share information about family, culture, and context
Solicit patient's beliefs and preferences	Discuss expectations
Elicit and validate patient's emotions	Voice concerns
Provide clear and jargon-free explanations	Discuss options

From Epstein RM, Street RL. *Patient-centered communication in cancer care: promoting healing and reducing suffering.* Bethesda, MD: National Cancer Institute; 2007, page 100. Available at: http://outcomes.cancer.gov/areas/pcc/communication/monograph.html

This student astutely observed an attending physician demonstrate compassionate care by noticing the concerns of the patient, indicating he had the time to sit down with the patient, and spending the necessary time to explain the medical situation. The patient was noticeably reassured. Furthermore, the student observed that it did not take long to provide this care for the patient. Physicians often think it will take too long and that they are too busy to sit down and discuss the problem. This attending physician served as a role model for the student by demonstrating professionalism in this domain.

The skills demonstrated by the attending require training and practice. Empathy is a key skill and requires that a physician truly understands how the patient feels and that he or she expresses this understanding verbally and/or nonverbally. Patients do not know that the physician feels concern and care unless it is expressed in some tangible way; when patients are distressed they may miss subtle indications of caring. Genuine expressions of empathy are powerful in building trust and communicating caring. As in the case of Dr. Owen and the patient with breast cancer, patients feel deeply cared for by physicians who express empathy, and they remember these experiences as the most powerful ones on their medical journey. However, it is particularly challenging to express empathy when the patient is frustrated, or even angry. Responding to these negative emotions requires physicians to maintain their composure, "listen actively" even when feeling attacked, and respond with caring—this is sometimes really tough to do. Maintaining a sense of composure in difficult interactions is even more challenging when physicians or nurses are tired, stressed, or frustrated with the situation themselves.

> *A new gynecology intern was attending to one of her patients late at night. She overheard an interaction between one of the night nurses and the patient in the next bed. The nurse was yelling at the patient to get up and go to the bathroom. Finally sounding at her wits end with frustration, the nurse threatened to give the patient an enema if she didn't get up right then and go to the bathroom.*

Let's face it, we all get frustrated and say things we shouldn't. This nurse was likely feeling hurried and probably under pressure to get her work done—including getting this patient to the bathroom. The professional challenge is to have the ability to take a breath in these stressful situations, get help if needed, and respond to patients—even ones who are frustrating us—with care. It is not always easy. Expressing empathy for patients' distress requires sincere concern in addition to use of the right words. It requires understanding of our own emotional reactions, particularly when we are stressed. What if the nurse had confessed that she was frustrated and asked the patient to help resolve the problem in this fashion: "Mrs. Regan, I am sorry for being irritable and persistent. I have an order to get you to the bathroom but you don't want to get up. Please explain to me your concerns and maybe we can figure this out together." This type of emotional work is part of our role and responsibility as a professional.

LEARNING EXERCISE 4-1

Think of a recent encounter with a patient during which you felt a negative emotion.

1. What were your feelings specifically?
2. What was happening in the encounter that led to your feeling this way? What do you think the patient was feeling?
3. Where there any other influences on you (hungry, tired, and so on) that influenced your feelings?
4. What did you say to the patient and what was the impact of your response? What were your other options?
5. Is your response in this situation one that you experience more generally? Could there be something in the situation that triggers this type of response in you?

HELPING PATIENTS MAKE DECISIONS—INFORMED DECISION-MAKING

A 55-year-old nonsmoking patient is found to have a small (0.5 cm) nodule on a routine chest X-ray. The finding was confirmed on chest computerized tomography (CT). The radiologist recommends following up with repeat imaging in 1 year based on the benign appearance of the nodule and in concordance with current guidelines. However, the patient insists that Dr. Smith order a repeat scan earlier.

In this example, Dr. Smith needs to understand why the patient wants a CT scan sooner. Was there a family member who had lung cancer? Is his insurance expiring and he is hoping to get the test covered? What is the underlying reason for the request? Furthermore, Dr. Smith will need to have a conversation, incorporating the patient's concerns, about the potential risks and benefits of CT scans in this situation. The patient is unlikely to know about the radiation risk associated with frequent CT scans or the potential risk of false positives and subsequent invasive investigations. This conversation requires skills in informed decision-making (IDM). Informed decision-making skills are particularly important in the procedural specialties in which physicians need to help patients make complicated decisions about whether to undergo a major procedure, such as hip replacement or cardiac surgery.

Patients want information that will help them make informed decisions that are tailored to their own personal values. This requires that physicians understand what a particular patient believes is most important in his or her life and to be able to describe treatment options in sufficient detail to help patients make wise choices. For example, some patients want to avoid side effects of treatment at all costs, whereas others will tolerate uncomfortable symptoms if they believe it may increase the chance of a cure of their disease. To assess patients' wants and needs, the physician must ask questions about patients' concerns, priorities, and values using follow-up questions if the answers need clarification and deeper understanding. For example, a patient might say that he wants to have "everything possible" done to treat a life-threatening condition. The astute physician would realize the "everything possible" could have a number of different meanings and that correct understanding of what this patient wants will require exploration of the patient's fears about illness and opinions about possible treatment options. In addition, further questioning may be needed to explore what the patient hopes to achieve, to correct unrealistic expectations, and to explore the possibility that treatment might result in increased suffering. Only after the patient's values and preferences have been clarified will the physician and patient be able to make a truly collaborative decision that is in the patient's best interest. Fully informed decisions are associated with both patient satisfaction and outcomes of care (Stacey et al, 2011; Barry & Edgman-Levitan, 2012). For example, after such discussions, patients with terminal illnesses receive fewer intensive interventions in the last week of life, generate lower healthcare spending, and report better quality of life in their final days (Lautrette et al, 2007; Wright et al, 2008; Zhang et al, 2009).

The skills required to conduct effective informed decision-making conversations are shown in Table 4-2. Extensive literature describes elements of informed decision-making conversations including the following: describing the clinical issues related to the decision; discussing the alternative risks of

Table 4-2 **ELEMENTS OF INFORMED DECISION-MAKING**		
Elements of informed decision-making	**Rationale**	**Examples**
1. Discussion of the patient's role in decision making	Many patients are not aware that they can and should participate in decision-making.	"I'd like us to make this decision together." "It helps me to know how you feel about this."
2. Discussion of the clinical issue of nature of the decision	A clear statement of what is at issue helps clarify what is being decided on and allows the physician to share some of his/her thinking about it.	"This is medication that would help with…" "The blood test will tell us…"
3. Discussion of alternatives	A decision is always a choice among certain options, including doing nothing at all. This is not always clear to the patient without an explicit discussion.	"You could try the new medication or continue the one you are on now."
4. Discussion of the pros (potential benefits) and cons (risks) of the alternatives	We frequently discuss the pros of one option and the cons of another without fully exploring the pros and cons of each. A more balanced presentation allows the patient's decision to be more informed.	"The new medication is more expensive, but you only need to take it once a day." "Screening for colon cancer using the stool cards is easier for you but the flexible sigmoidoscopy is more precise."
5. Discussion of uncertainties associated with the decision	While often difficult, a discussion of uncertainties is crucial for a patient's comprehensive understanding of the options. Thoughtful discussion can promote trust and encourage adherence.	"The chance that this will help is excellent." "Most patients with this condition respond well to this medication, but not all."

(Continued)

Table 4-2	ELEMENTS OF INFORMED DECISION-MAKING (*Continued*)	
Elements of informed decision-making	Rationale	Examples
6. Assessment of the patient's understanding	Once the core disclosures are made, the physician must check in with the patient to know if what he/she has said so far makes sense. Fostering understanding is really the central goal of informed decision-making.	"Does that make sense to you?" "Are you with me so far?"
7. Exploration of patient preference	Physicians may assume that patients will speak up if they disagree with a decision, but patients often need to be asked for their opinion. If should be clear to the patient that it is appropriate to disagree or ask for more time.	"Does that sound reasonable?" "What do you think?"

From Braddock CH 3rd, Edwards KA, Hasenberg NM, Laidley TL, Levinson W. Informed decision making in outpatient practice: time to get back to basics. *JAMA*. 1999 Dec 22–29;282(24):2313–2320, page 2314.

each; explaining the uncertainties; and assessing patients' understanding of the choices and their preferences. Although Table 4-2 presents an overview and examples, multiple skills are required to accomplish these communication tasks successfully. Studies often demonstrate that even experienced clinicians fall short in demonstrating these skills. For example, Braddock has audiotaped surgeons having IDM conversations with patients who are considering major surgical procedures such as hip replacements. In these conversations, surgeons frequently describe the nature of the decision (92% of the time), sometimes discuss the risks (62%), and rarely assess whether the patient understands (12%). Furthermore, although clinicians worry that these conversations will take too much time, the researchers found that the adequacy of IDM was only modestly related to the duration of the visit (Braddock et al, 1999). Conducting a high-quality IDM conversation depends less on time than on sophisticated clinician communication skills.

The bottom line is that clinicians need sophisticated communication skills to deliver patient-centered care. Clinicians can learn and improve these skills throughout their career. A systematic review, published in 2007, examined 36 randomized trials designed to improve verbal communication skills and demonstrated that training could improve skills, including expressing empathy and explaining patients' illnesses and treatments (Rao et al, 2007; Levinson, Lesser, & Epstein, 2010).

However, the link between teaching communication skills and improved outcomes for patients is not a direct one. The new skills need to be incorporated into a physician's routine behavior, in turn affecting intermediate

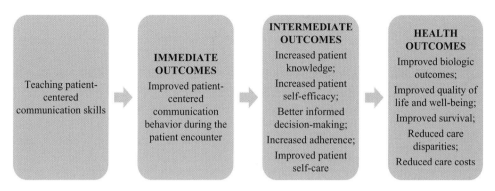

Figure 4-3 ▪ Link between teaching patient-centered communication skills and outcomes.

From Levinson W, Lesser CS, Epstein RM. Developing physician communication skills for patient-centered care. *Health Aff (Millwood).* 2010 Jul;29(7):1310–1318.

outcomes (such as increased patient knowledge or increased engagement in healthy lifestyle) and ultimately improving biologic outcomes (such as diabetes control) (Figure 4-3).

THE ROLE OF THE TEAM

> *Shortly after her rotation started, Samantha, a 3rd-year medical student, overheard her resident talking poorly about their attending physician to the nephrology fellow. The resident was sitting at the computer next to Samantha and was speaking loudly so it was not difficult for Samantha to hear her. The resident was questioning the attending's intelligence and mocking some of the treatment suggestions he had made. Samantha thought it was extremely disrespectful of her to talk about him behind his back in such a belittling way, especially in a public setting, and knowing that a medical student, who is supposed to look to her for leadership and guidance, was close. If she had problems with the attending, she should have talked directly to him privately.*

This medical student is put in an uncomfortable position by overhearing this and must wonder what the resident will say about *her* in the future. She is very unlikely to say anything about what she heard to the resident directly and even less likely to tell the attending physician. Sadly, these types of disparaging comments about another team member are not uncommon.

This example illustrates a key team behavior—demonstrating respect in team interactions. If team members don't treat each other with respect, they create a negative work environment and risk that these same negative behaviors will occur with patients, for example, using disparaging language about patients. Patient-centered care, which depends on respect, can only thrive if the team members practice the same respect with one another.

Healthcare teams need communication skills to respectfully talk to one another, including about difficult issues. Particularly when team members disagree with each other or when team members are stressed by long work hours, they need skills to demonstrate compassion for one another. For example, when errors occur and patients are harmed inadvertently in the course of care, team members tend to blame one another and fail to recognize or acknowledge the distress that errors cause for the individual physicians and nurses. Stressed by a medical error, they lack the necessary skills to discuss the error as a team in a nonjudgmental and supportive fashion. Team communication that is respectful and provides support for one another creates the environment for delivering the same kind of respectful and supportive care of patients.

Well-functioning multidisciplinary teams are essential to the provision of high quality care. The attention to the importance of teamwork has increased with the quality and safety movement over the last decade. Evidence shows that teams with effective communication between team members lead to better outcomes and fewer errors. The same principles of effective communication in the patient safety movement apply to delivering high quality patient-centered care (Wynia, Von Kohorn, & Mitchell, 2012; Mitchell et al, 2012). Effective teams encourage each member of the team to share their perspective freely without a hierarchy that inhibits the flow of information. For example, a nurse may think that a patient is worried about a planned surgical procedure and may know that the patient and family are considering not proceeding with the surgery. Can that nurse tell the surgeon without feeling intimidated or concerned that she is overstepping her authority? In fact, understanding how best to meet a patient's needs requires involvement of the full team to discuss the details of management—often patients tell one member of the team, and not another, about their worries and fears. The values and principles that characterize well-functioning teams are summarized in Figure 4-4.

LEARNING EXERCISE 4-2

1. Think of a recent challenge your team experienced in caring for patients.
2. How would you describe the team's communication among members, the team's problem solving, and the creativity of the solutions?
3. How did you personally feel in the process?
4. Are there aspects of the team's communication that could be improved?
5. Are there opportunities to discuss these ideas with the team?

Shared values among team members	Principles to guide team-based care
Honesty Put a high value on open communication within the team, including transparency about aims, decisions, uncertainty, and mistakes.	*Clear roles* Have clear expectations for each member's functions, responsibilities, and accountabilities.
Discipline Carry out roles and responsibilities even when inconvenient, and seek out and share information to improve even when it is uncomfortable.	*Mutual trust* Earn each other's trust, creating strong norms of reciprocity and greater opportunities for shared achievement.
Creativity Be excited by the possibility of tackling new or emerging problems, seeing errors and unanticipated bad outcomes as potential opportunities to learn and improve.	*Effective communication* Prioritize and continuously refine communication skills using consistent channels for candid and complete communication.
Humility Recognize differences in training but do not believe that one type of training or perspective is uniformly superior; recognize that team members are human and will make mistakes.	*Shared goals* Work to establish shared goals that reflect patient and family priorities and that can be clearly articulated, understood, and supported by all members.
Curiosity Delight in seeking out and reflecting on lessons learned and using those insights for continuous improvement.	*Measurable processes and outcomes* Agree on and implement reliable and timely feedback on successes and failures in both the overall functioning of the team and achievement of specific goals.

Figure 4-4 ▪ Values and principles of high-functioning health care teams.

From Wynia MK, Von Kohorn I, Mitchell PH. Challenges at the intersection of team-based and patient-centered health care: insights from an IOM working group. *JAMA.* 2012 Oct 3;308(13):1327–1328.

THE ROLE OF THE HEALTHCARE SETTING

The hospitals and offices in which we work are not just passive places but rather settings that substantially influence our ability to deliver patient-centered care. Hospitals and healthcare systems are especially influential by indicating that patient-centered care is truly valued by providing training, measuring how well it is delivered, and providing incentives to increase the performance.

Dr. Smith is a surgeon and the medical director of a large multidisciplinary group practice. She has been monitoring the patient satisfaction ratings of the group compared to available regional data and also routinely investigates all patient complaints. She recently noticed that the percentage of patients who would recommend their clinic to friends had fallen during the last 2 years. Analysis of the data indicated that the majority of complaints were about communication with clinicians. In discussion with the medical staff, the leadership group has decided to start giving physicians and teams feedback on their patient satisfaction ratings compared to others and to reward the highest performing teams with a financial bonus. Dr. Smith realizes that the clinic must support this program with training and is seeking resources to do this effectively. She is not certain how best to implement this program or how to measure its success.

The context in which we work strongly influences whether we can collectively deliver patient-centered care. Dr. Smith recognizes this based on the group's patient experience data. She is implementing improvement strategies through patient feedback, clinician education, and payment incentives. These are all potentially useful approaches. In some settings, introducing these kinds of changes represents a culture change and requires multiple strategies implemented over time. Leaders of these efforts must be patient and persistent.

There are many approaches that clinics and hospitals can use to enhance and support the delivery of patient-centered care. Table 4-3 provides an overview of some potential strategies, the goals of each strategy, the national resources available to support the efforts, and what these resources provide. It is designed to be a useful resource for healthcare organizations that are considering approaches to enhance the patient-centered care they provide through communication training, cultural competence programs, use of tools to enhance patient decision-making, and even architectural approaches to building spaces designed to support patient-centered care.

During the last decade, with the increased attention on patient-centered care, training programs have been designed and implemented to teach patient-centered communication skills to clinicians. These programs are provided by a variety of groups including medical societies with a particular interest in communication training (e.g., the Society of General Internal Medicine, the American Academy of Orthopedic Surgeons), national training organizations (the American Academy on Communication in Healthcare), or by some large medical groups that have created their own programs tailored to their setting (Kaiser Permanente in Northern California or Park Nicollet in Minneapolis). These programs have led to improvements in physicians' self-confidence and self-assessed communication skills as well as improvements in patient

Table 4-3	**HEALTHCARE STRATEGIES TO IMPROVE PATIENT-CENTERED CARE**		
Strategy	Goals	Resources	What they provide
1. Communication Skills Training	• Increase staff competence • Increase patient satisfaction • Improve team communication	1. American Academy on Communication in Healthcare (AACH) (http://www.aachonline.org) 2. American Medical Association Ethical Force Program (http://www.ama-assn.org/ama/pub/physician-resources/medical-ethics/the-ethical-force-program/patient-centered-communication.page?) 3. DocCom website (http://www.aachonline.org/?page=doccom) 4. Institute for Patient- and Family-Centered Care (http://www.ipfcc.org/) 5. Medical specialty societies. e.g., American Academy of Orthopedic Surgeons (http://www6.aaos.org/member/pemr/COAP/pcc.cfm)	1. Publications and training modules 2. Communication Climate Assessment Toolkit (C-CAT) 3. Multimedia communication skills learning modules 4. Self-assessment tools and guidance documents 5. Presentations and publications
2. Cultural Competence	• Increased ability to address needs of variety of patient populations	1. AMA (http://www.a,a-assn.org) 2. Joint Commission cultural competence resources (http://www.jointcommission.org/Advancing_Effective_Communication/) 3. National Center for Cultural Competence (http://nccc.georgetown.edu/resources/publicationstype.html) 4. U.S. Department of Health and Human Services Office of Minority Health (https://www.thinkculturalhealth.hhs.gov/)	1. Communication Climate Assessment Toolkit (C-CAT); Health Disparities Toolkit 2. Organizational tools and best practices 3. Organizational assessments, planning tools, training modules, best practices 4. Cultural competency training modules for physicians and other providers

(Continued)

Table 4-3   HEALTHCARE STRATEGIES TO IMPROVE PATIENT-CENTERED CARE (*Continued*)

Strategy	Goals	Resources	What they provide
3. Shared Decision-Making Support	• Enhanced IDM for complex decisions (cancer treatment, surgical procedures)	1. Dartmouth-Hitchcock Center for Shared Decision Making (http://med.dartmouth-hitchcock.org/csdm_toolkits.html) 2. Informed Medical Decisions Foundation (http://informedmedicaldecisions.org/) 3. Ottawa Hospital Research Institute Patient Decision Aids (http://decisionaid.ohri.ca/index.html)	1. Decision support toolkits and training modules 2. Decision aids for common conditions 3. Inventory of patient decision aids with International Patient Decision Aid Standards (IPDAS) ratings, development, and implementation toolkits
4. Physical Environment to Support Patient-Centered Care	• Improved patient outcomes through healthcare facility design	1. Center for Health Design (http://ripple.healthdesign.org/) 2. Institute for Patient-Centered Design (http://patientcentereddesign.org/index.html) 3. Planetree (http://planetree.org)	1. Evidence-based design database, technical assistance 2. Educational materials for healthcare professionals, patients, and designers 3. Patient-centered design case studies, consultation services
5. Measurement of Patient Feedback	• Understand and improve patient experiences	1. Consumer Assessment of Healthcare Providers and Systems (CAHPS) (http://cahps.ahrq.gov/surveysguidance.htm) 2. HCAHPS (http://www.hcahpsonline.org/home.aspx) 3. NRC Picker (http://www.nrcpicker.com/home/)	1. Patient surveys for recent office visits, information on measures and reporting 2. Patient surveys for hospital care experience, information on measures and reporting 3. Patient survey administration, feedback

satisfaction (Brown et al, 1999; Rao et al, 2007; Stein & Kwan, 1999; Stein, Frankel, & Krupat, 2005). The programs are usually conducted over a short period of time—typically half a day to three days. They typically include an opportunity for a physician to practice communication skills while being observed by colleagues. Role playing exercises, in which learners "act" the physician role and receive feedback on their performance, are commonly used, since they are low cost and effective for learning these skills. When practicing physicians play the roles of patients, they often increase their understanding of patients' feelings and experiences and can then try new approaches in the role of a physician. For example, a role playing exercise might script the "patient" to insist that the physician order a magnetic resonance imaging (MRI) study to evaluate his headache when the physician explains that it is not necessary in his case. In this scenario, the challenge for the physician would be to understand the reason for the patient's demand and to negotiate a mutually acceptable plan of diagnosis and treatment.

The use of standardized patients, actors trained to play the role of patients, is also common in these programs in order to allow physicians to practice difficult communication skills such as breaking bad news, disclosing medical errors, and discussing end of life issues. Experienced standardized patients become "connoisseurs of care" who can provide credible feedback about how a particular question or a statement made them feel. Workshops allow the opportunity for physicians to role play a scenario, receive feedback from the standardized patient, and try the scenario again using a different approach.

Training programs require expert teachers and are most effective if the training period is longer, includes practice and feedback, and is reinforced over time with the opportunity to try new skills in practice. Most physicians are not accustomed to receiving feedback on their communication skills—in fact, most have never received any feedback about their communication since they were in medical school. Some physicians resist participating in these types of programs, as they question the value compared to learning biomedical information, feel uncomfortable demonstrating their skills publicly, or think they already have obtained mastery of communication. Healthcare leaders need to recognize this as a potential barrier and create a safe environment to support this kind of learning. Launching communication skills training requires a significant commitment on the part of a healthcare organization. National resources are available, including groups that provide tailored on-site educational programs (Table 4-3).

Beyond communication training, patient-centered care can be supported by many other strategies. Training specifically in cultural competence is particularly important in settings with a multicultural patient population. This would include translation services so that language barriers are decreased. In addition, patient decision-making support tools have grown over the years.

These tools are designed to help patients understand the pros and cons of different treatment choices, typically from the perspective of other patients who have previously made these choices themselves. The Informed Medical Decisions Foundation has developed a variety of tools that are focused on helping patients make complex decisions, like what type of treatment to choose for prostate cancer or certain types of cardiac disease. A recent Cochrane review of 86 randomized trials of shared decision-making tools demonstrated that these tools increase patient knowledge, and increase comfort with decisions that align with patient values, with fewer patients remaining undecided (Stacey et al, 2011). The Institute for Patient- and Family-Centered Care offers a variety of services, including consultation, courses, and networking for institutions invested in creating a patient-centered care model.

One essential element of any effort to improve patient-centered care is ongoing measurement and feedback to providers. The most commonly used instrument is the CAHPS (Consumer Assessment of Healthcare Providers and Systems) survey, which captures many of the dimensions of patient-centered care, is well validated, and easy to administer. Because many institutions use the survey, it is relatively easy to compare results in specific settings. Table 4-4 provides a variety of instruments designed to measure patient-centered communication, sample questions, and patient outcomes associated with the measure.

ROLE OF THE EXTERNAL ENVIRONMENT

Healthcare settings, such as hospitals and clinics, work in the environment created by the external world of regulators, accreditors, and payers. These forces strongly influence organizations in their ability to deliver patient-centered care.

Dr. Brossard is a practicing internist and endocrinologist. He practices in an academic medical center that recently made the decision to require all new faculty members to enroll in the Maintenance of Certification (MOC) program of the American Board of Medical Specialties (ABMS). Although he is not new to the medical center, he realizes that he should set a model and do the MOC program himself. Taking the secure examination was anxiety provoking, since he hadn't written an examination in many years. Fortunately he passed. The more challenging part of the MOC process for Dr. Brossard is the component where he is required to assess and improve his practice. As part of that practice improvement work he had to give surveys to his patients and they sent their responses to the Board. He just received his survey results from the Board and was surprised to learn that he did not

Table 4-4 VALIDATED PATIENT SURVEY MEASURES TO ASSESS PATIENT-CENTERED COMMUNICATION (PCC)

Name of measure (Reference)	Summary	What is being measured	Sample items	Outcomes associated with the measures
Clinician and Group Consumer Assessment of Healthcare Providers and Systems (CG-CAHPS) (Agency for Healthcare Research and Quality, 2012)	Developed by the Agency for Healthcare Research and Quality (AHRQ) to provide standardized measures of patient experience to allow comparisons (1) between providers and (2) within providers over time All CAHPS surveys are in the public domain; other outpatient surveys include the Home Health Care Survey, Health Plan, and In-Center Hemodialysis Surveys	How well providers communicated with patients during a recent office visit	Provider explained things in a way that was easy to understand Provider listened carefully to patient Provider gave easy to understand information about health questions or concerns Provider knew important information about patient's medical history Provider showed respect for what patient had to say Provider spent enough time with patient Response options • Never • Sometimes • Usually • Always	Patient satisfaction Less symptom burden; fewer referrals
Hospital Consumer Assessment of Healthcare Providers and Systems (HCAHPS, 2012)	Developed by AHRQ and the Centers for Medicare & Medicaid Services (CMS) National, standardized, publicly reported survey of patient experiences with hospital care HCAHPS surveys are in the public domain; survey results are reported four times per year on the *Hospital Compare* Web site (www.hospitalcompare.hhs.gov)	How well providers communicated with patients during a recent hospital stay	During this hospital stay, how often did nurses/doctors treat you with courtesy and respect? During this hospital stay, how often did nurses/doctors listen carefully to you? During this hospital stay, how often did nurses/doctors explain things in a way you could understand? During this hospital stay, did doctors, nurses or other hospital staff talk with you about whether you would have the help you needed when you left the hospital? Response options • Never • Sometimes • Usually • Always	Patient satisfaction Understanding of illness and treatment plan Adherence

(Continued)

Table 4-4 VALIDATED PATIENT SURVEY MEASURES TO ASSESS PATIENT-CENTERED COMMUNICATION (PCC) (*Continued*)

Name of measure (Reference)	Summary	What is being measured	Sample items	Outcomes associated with the measures
NRC Picker survey (NRC Picker, 2013)	Patient experience surveys originally developed by the Picker Institute and Harvard researchers; acquired by the National Research Corporation (NRC) in 2001 Commercially available, but not in the public domain	Measures eight dimensions of patient-centered care, including: Respect for patients' values, preferences and expressed needs Information and education Emotional support and alleviation of fear and anxiety Continuity and transition	Questions are proprietary	Patient satisfaction Understanding of illness and treatment plan Adherence

From Agency for Healthcare Research and Quality. Patient Experience Measures From the CAHPS® Clinician & Group Surveys. May 1, 2012. Available at: http://cahps.ahrq.gov/clinician_group/cgsurvey/patientexperiencemeasurescgsurveys.pdf *compare favorably to his peers on elements of the patient satisfaction questionnaire. For example, only 25% of his patients with diabetes said that they got the information they needed on diet and exercise. Dr. Brossard brought the results to a meeting of his team with the nurse, patient educator, trainees, and hospital administrators to discuss how they could improve.*

Accrediting bodies, like the ABMS, influence patient-centered care by requiring measurement of patient feedback. This is part of a broader recognition in the external environment that medical education and medical care should increase their knowledge and skills on dimensions important to the public. In the recent decades, medical education has focused on developing knowledge and skills related to scientific information, and less attention has been given to other competencies including patient-centered communication, population-based health, awareness of cost and value, and patient safety and quality. The Accreditation Council for Graduate Medical Education (ACGME) has recently dramatically changed its accreditation approach to ensure that trainees develop competencies in these areas. New ACGME standards are influencing training programs to enhance training in patient-centered communication and to require assessment of this competency (Nasca et al, 2012).

In the United States, the ABMS, which includes member boards in each of 24 specialties, sets the standards for certification of all specialty physicians and surgeons. Although the program is voluntary, more than 90% of graduates from accredited residency training programs in the United States choose to participate and become diplomates. The ABMS provides a voluntary program called Maintenance of Certification (MOC) to ensure that diplomates keep their knowledge and skills current throughout their practice. There are four components of the MOC program, including one component dedicated to professionalism (see also Chapter 6, Commitment to Excellence).

A patient survey, which includes patient reports of communication with physicians, is a required element of the MOC program. For example, the American Board of Internal Medicine includes patient feedback surveys in many of the MOC practice improvement activities. As part of MOC, physicians could choose a practice improvement exercise designed to improve the care of their patients with diabetes. As part of that exercise they receive feedback from patients on elements of their care and their communication, and their scores will be compared to those of other physicians. Figure 4-5 provides sample items from the patient survey. The key point is that a physician like Dr. Brossard will get performance feedback as seen through the eyes of patients. The external environment, through certification by the ABMS, is influencing practicing physicians to enhance their patient-centered care.

Primary Care Patient Survey

In the last 12 months…

1. How often did this doctor explain things in a way that was easy-to-understand?
2. How often did this doctor check to be sure you understood everything?
3. Sometimes doctors give instructions that are hard to follow. How often did this doctor ask you whether you would have any problems doing what you need to do to take care of this illness or health condition?
4. How often did this doctor encourage you to talk about all your health problems or concerns?
5. How often did this doctor listen carefully to you?
6. How often did this doctor interrupt you when you were talking?
7. How often did this doctor give you easy-to-understand instructions about taking care of these health problems or concerns?
8. Did you and this doctor talk about specific things you could do to prevent illness?
9. How often did this doctor seem to know the important information about your medical history?
10. How often did this doctor show respect for what you had to say?
11. How often did this doctor spend enough time with you?
12. How often did you feel this doctor really cared about you as a person?
13. Choices for treatment or healthcare can include choices about medicine, surgery, or other treatment. Did this doctor tell you there was more than one choice for your treatment or healthcare?
14. Did this doctor talk with you about the pros and cons of each choice for your treatment or healthcare?
15. When there was more than one choice for your treatment or healthcare, did this doctor ask which choice you thought was best for you?

Figure 4-5 ▪ Sample patient survey questions.

Credit: ABIM Primary Care Patient Survey. Available at: http://www.abim.org/sep2/60A1201p/html/survey.pdf. Copyright 2013 American Board of Internal Medicine. Used with permission.

Another external force that has influenced the delivery of patient-centered care is malpractice insurance companies.

George Tomasson is the CEO of a large medical malpractice insurance company. He has been working with the company for years and knows that most of their malpractice claims result from patients who are unhappy with the relationship with their physicians. He has reviewed the literature on the topic, and this corroborates his experience— patients seek advice about suing when they feel that the physician did not listen or provide them adequate information. He thinks many of the claims the companies sees could be avoided if physicians improved their communication, and so he is exploring the possibility of physician training. The company is willing to offer a 5% discount on physicians' malpractice insurance premium if they participate in the program.

The medical literature supports George Tomasson's view that physicians' communication is related to malpractice claims. For example, in research with two malpractice insurance companies in Colorado and Oregon, Levinson audio-taped actual encounters between physicians (primary care physicians and surgeons) and their patients during routine office visits (Levinson et al, 1997). She conducted an analysis of the communication patterns of physicians who had prior malpractice claims against them compared to those who had never had a claim, and she was able to differentiate between the two groups based on the content and the tone of voice of the physicians. For example, "no claims" primary care physicians compared to those who had prior claims, were more likely to educate patients about what to expect in their care, encourage patients to talk, solicit patients' opinions, and checked to see if they understood their problems or treatments. "No-claims" primary care physicians spent longer in routine office visits than claims primary care physicians (mean, 18.3 vs 15.0 minutes). As a result of this type of data, some malpractice insurance companies have offered both communication training programs and financial incentives in the form of premium reductions to their physicians. The actual impact of these programs on the delivery of care is not known, but malpractice companies signal the importance of patient-centered communication by offering these types of training programs.

In addition, payment systems can be used to reward or provide incentives to enhance patient-centered care. These types of "pay for performance" incentives are typically based on patient survey scores. For example, Rodriguez and colleagues reported on the use of financial incentives based on the CAHPS survey results in 25 California medical groups and more than 1400 primary care physicians (Rodriguez et al, 2009). They found that physician scores on the CAHPS improved over time while these incentives were in place, and that physicians with lower baseline scores demonstrated the greatest improvement. Also of note, they found that financial incentives tied to productivity and efficiency were associated with decreases in scores on the CAHPS survey. Reimbursement can also be designed to support communication through specific additional payment for complex conversations like advanced planning directive, breaking bad news, or patient counseling for smoking cessation. The point is that the reimbursement system in healthcare can and does influence the delivery of patient-centered care through a variety of mechanisms.

CONCLUSION

A core value of the profession is the delivery of compassionate patient-centered care. Patients highly value clinicians who listen to their concerns, express empathy, and help them make informed choices about their care. All the players on the healthcare team—the individual clinicians, the team, the healthcare setting, and the broader environment—have critical roles to play to demonstrate patient-centered care. We observe that this area of medical care often falls short of patients expectations and that there is room for considerable improvement.

CHALLENGE CASE

Dr. Rodriguez is having a difficult time. She is in the middle of her night float shift as a second year resident in internal medicine. Last evening, she admitted an elderly man with weight loss, confusion, and fever. A chest X-ray showed a massive lung tumor and his calcium level was 15.0. She started the patient on antibiotics and fluids, but despite this he has become hypotensive and short of breath. When she tried to move the patient to the intensive care unit (ICU), the ICU resident told her that a bed wouldn't be available for three hours and she would need to manage the patient on the floor.

While she is working on stabilizing her patient with sepsis, she is paged several times to another patient care unit. When she has a minute to answer, she is confronted by Walter Burns, a nurse on another floor who angrily demands to know why Dr. Rodriguez hasn't been up to evaluate a patient with chronic pain who has called repeatedly to ask for more pain medications. Walter demands to have a verbal order for an escalating dose of narcotics. While reviewing the sign out list, Dr. Rodriguez sees that this patient's primary team has recommended against giving the patient any more pain medications without a thorough evaluation. When she demurs and says she will be up soon, Walter responds by threatening to report her to her program director.

What professionalism challenges exist in this encounter?
This resident is facing several professionalism challenges. There is conflict between providing excellent patient care for one patient and compassionate patient care for another. She is torn between respecting the judgment and request of the nurse for more pain medications and respecting the judgment of the primary team that is caring for the patient. She has many personal challenges: she is undoubtedly tired, probably hungry, worried about her patient, and a nurse who is unaware of what else is transpiring is yelling at her.

What role does the system have in this situation?
There are many ways in which the system may be making it more difficult for Dr. Rodriguez to behave in a manner compatible with her professional values. The lack of an available ICU bed is placing a tremendous burden on the resident, who must singlehandedly provide care that is usually provided a team of dedicated caregivers in a specialized unit. The lack of geographically organized wards makes it more difficult for the resident to

simply walk next door and see the second patient, and makes it likely that she has no relationship with the nurse in question. There may be too few physicians and too few nurses available in the middle of the night, leading to a lack of staff to back up either the resident or the nurse.

What might the resident do?
It is common for clinicians to feel overworked, and unfortunately it is also common for some healthcare professionals (from all disciplines) to respond to stress and conflict with anger and threats. Common responses include fight—returning the anger by yelling at the nurse, or flight—slamming down the phone and ignoring subsequent pages.

What should this resident do?
Situational analysis: Dr. Rodriguez is an overworked, stressed resident who is being called upon to act in a mature manner when she is the recipient of anger and threats from a fellow healthcare professional.

A helpful template for working through dilemmas is found in Chapter 2, Resilience in Facing Professionalism Challenges, Table 2-2. Following the template, this situation calls for:

Self-awareness (recognizing personal emotions or triggers; understanding personal limitations in skills and knowledge)
- Dr. Rodriguez should realize that she is stressed and vulnerable to a possible professionalism lapse. In the moment, she might wonder if she has the expertise to respond professionally to Walter.

Self-regulation (managing strong emotions; accessing assistance for complex tasks)
- Dr. Rodriguez should do what she can to get a moment to think before responding. This will give her time to move beyond automatic flight or fight reactions and toward more thoughtful professionalism actions.

Social awareness (recognizing the importance of considering the needs and state of all participants)
- If she has time to think, she will realize that the nurse on the phone is probably either concerned about or frustrated by the patient in question and possibly worried that failing to escalate the patient's request will result in disciplinary action toward the nurse.

Social regulation (seek to identify more than one option for action, assume positive intent to understand others' behaviors, develop crisis communication strategies and negotiation skills, be empowered to coach others)
- Dr. Rodriguez needs to realize that to satisfy everyone in this environment, she needs to acknowledge their concerns, respect their priorities,

and ask for help in managing the situation. Ultimately she needs to try to deescalate the emotions involved in this situation. Assuming that everyone involved wants what's best for the patient(s) helps her understand their behaviors and helps reduce the tension.

Actions:

Dr. Rodriguez recalls advice given during their team leadership seminars. They were advised that situations like this can be deescalated if they acknowledge the emotion in the room and attempt to move the other person from blaming communication to problem-solving communication. Furthermore, she recalls that the teachers also said that it is good to take a few calming breaths before responding.

> *"I am so sorry that you have had to wait for me to return your page. I can hear how worried you are about this patient and he deserves to be evaluated. I am in working on a patient who needs to go to the ICU but I will find another doctor to come and evaluate Mr. Johnson. Can we brainstorm a minute about what we might do to help him before the other doctor gets there other than giving him more narcotics?"*

The two clinicians brainstorming together identify others who can help in this situation. Dr. Rodriguez realizes that this is a situation with which the Rapid Response Team can help. Mr. Burns offers also to call the night supervisor to see if someone can help him manage his other patients.

Dealing with systems issues:

Dr. Rodriguez learned a lot by reflecting about this case. One suggestion she makes in morning report is that they all agree in advance to respond promptly when any one in their residency program calls and says "I need help." She also joins a team to work on moving patients into geographic units, even if it means that sometimes their services are bigger.

KEY LEARNING POINTS

1. A component of professionalism is the ability to deliver compassionate, respectful patient-centered care. "Patient-centered care" style is defined by the Institute of Medicine as "Providing care that is respectful of and responsive to individual patient preferences, needs, and values, and ensuring that patient values guide all clinical decisions."

2. Delivering patient-centered care depends on a set of specific communication skills that can be learned. Patient-centered communication is associated with positive patient outcomes, particularly in patients with chronic diseases.

3. Individual clinicians require sophisticated communication skills including demonstrating empathy and building trust, and conducting informed decision-making conversations.

4. Healthcare teams must build a culture that demonstrates respect for team members and fosters open communication between team members, particularly when difficult situations arise, such as medical errors. Good communication between team members supports high quality patient-centered care.

5. The healthcare setting influences the delivery of patient-centered care and can enhance care by providing communication training, cultural competence programs, and informed decision-making tools.

6. The external environment also fosters the delivery of patient-centered care by setting standards through accreditation and rewarding effective communication based on patient surveys.

REFERENCES

1. ABIM Primary Care Patient Survey. Available at: http://www.abim.org/sep2/60A1201p/html/survey.pdf

2. Agency for Healthcare Research and Quality. Patient Experience Measures From the CAHPS® Clinician & Group Surveys. May 1, 2012. Available at: http://cahps.ahrq.gov/clinician_group/cgsurvey/patientexperiencemeasurescgsurveys.pdf

3. Barry MJ, Edgman-Levitan S. Shared decision making—pinnacle of patient-centered care. *N Engl J Med.* 2012 Mar 1;366(9):780-781.

4. Beckman HB, Frankel RM. The effect of physician behavior on the collection of data. *Ann Intern Med.* 1984 Nov;101(5):692–696.

5. Braddock CH 3rd, Edwards KA, Hasenberg NM, Laidley TL, Levinson W. Informed decision making in outpatient practice: time to get back to basics. *JAMA.* 1999 Dec 22–29;282(24):2313–2320.

6. Brown JB, Boles M, Mullooly JP, Levinson W. Effect of clinician communication skills training on patient satisfaction: a randomized, controlled trial. *Ann Intern Med.* 1999 Dec 7;131(11):822–829.

7. Epstein RM, Street RL. *Patient-centered communication in cancer care: promoting healing and reducing suffering.* Bethesda, MD: National Cancer Institute; 2007.

8. Institute of Medicine. *Crossing the Quality Chasm: A New Health System for the 21st Century*. Washington, DC: National Academies Press; 2001.

9. Lautrette A, Darmon M, Megarbane B, Joly LM, Chevret S, Adrie C, Barnoud D, Bleichner G, Bruel C, Choukroun G, Curtis JR, Fieux F, Galliot R, Garrouste-Orgeas M, Georges H, Goldgran-Toledano D, Jourdain M, Loubert G, Reignier J, Saidi F, Souweine B, Vincent F, Barnes NK, Pochard F, Schlemmer B, Azoulay E. A communication strategy and brochure for relatives of patients dying in the ICU. *N Engl J Med*. 2007 Feb 1;356(5):469–478.

10. Levinson W, Gorawara-Bhat R, Lamb J. A study of patient clues and physician responses in primary care and surgical settings. *JAMA*. 2000 Aug 23–30;284(8): 1021–1027.

11. Levinson W, Lesser CS, Epstein RM. Developing physician communication skills for patient-centered care. *Health Aff (Millwood)*. 2010 Jul;29(7):1310–1318.

12. Levinson W, Roter DL, Mullooly JP, Dull VT, Frankel RM. Physician-patient communication. The relationship with malpractice claims among primary care physicians and surgeons. *JAMA*. 1997 Feb 19;277(7):553–559.

13. Levinson W, Shojania KG. Bad experiences in the hospital: the stories keep coming. *BMJ Qual Saf*. 2011 Nov;20(11):911–913.

14. Mead N, Bower P. Patient-centred consultations and outcomes in primary care: a review of the literature. *Patient Educ Couns*. 2002 Sep;48(1):51–61.

15. Meterko M, Wright S, Lin H, Lowy E, Cleary PD. Mortality among patients with acute myocardial infarction: the influences of patient-centered care and evidence-based medicine. *Health Serv Res*. 2010 Oct;45(5 Pt 1):1188–1204.

16. Mitchell P, Wynia M, Golden R, McNellis B, Okun S, Webb CE, Rohrbach V, Von Kohorn I. *Core Principles and Values of Effective Team-Based Health Care: 2012*. Discussion paper. Institute of Medicine. Available at: http://www.iom.edu/tbc

17. Nasca TJ, Philibert I, Brigham T, Flynn TC. The next GME accreditation system-rationale and benefits. *N Engl J Med*. 2012 Mar 15;366(11):1051–1056.

18. Rao JK, Anderson LA, Inui TS, Frankel RM. Communication interventions make a difference in conversations between physicians and patients: a systematic review of the evidence. *Med Care*. 2007 Apr;45(4):340–349.

19. Rathert C, Wyrwich MD, Boren SA. Patient-centered care and outcomes: a systematic review of the literature. *Med Care Res Rev*. 2012 Nov 20. [Epub ahead of print]

20. Rocco N, Scher K, Basberg B, Yalamanchi S, Baker-Genaw K. Patient-centered plan-of-care tool for improving clinical outcomes. *Qual Manag Health Care*. 2011 Apr–Jun;20(2):89–97.

21. Rodriguez HP, von Glahn T, Elliott MN, Rogers WH, Safran DG. The effect of performance-based financial incentives on improving patient care experiences: a statewide evaluation. *J Gen Intern Med*. 2009 Dec;24(12):1281–1288.

22. Stacey D, Bennett CL, Barry MJ, Col NF, Eden KB, Holmes-Rovner M, Llewellyn-Thomas H, Lyddiatt A, Légaré F, Thomson R. Decision aids for people facing health treatment or screening decisions. *Cochrane Database Syst Rev*. 2011 Oct 5;(10).

23. Stein T, Frankel RM, Krupat E. Enhancing clinician communication skills in a large healthcare organization: a longitudinal case study. *Patient Educ Couns*. 2005 Jul;58(1):4–12.

24. Stein TS, Kwan J. Thriving in a busy practice: physician-patient communication training. *Eff Clin Pract*. 1999 Mar–Apr;2(2):63–70.

25. Wright AA, Zhang B, Ray A, Mack JW, Trice E, Balboni T, Mitchell SL, Jackson VA, Block SD, Maciejewski PK, Prigerson HG. Associations between end-of-life discussions, patient mental health, medical care near death, and caregiver bereavement adjustment. *JAMA*. 2008 Oct 8;300(14):1665–1673.

26. Wynia MK, Von Kohorn I, Mitchell PH. Challenges at the intersection of team-based and patient-centered health care: insights from an IOM working group. *JAMA*. 2012 Oct 3;308(13):1327–1328.

27. Zhang B, Wright AA, Huskamp HA, Nilsson ME, Maciejewski ML, Earle CC, Block SD, Maciejewski PK, Prigerson HG. Health care costs in the last week of life: associations with end-of-life conversations. *Arch Intern Med*. 2009 Mar 9;169(5):480–488.

INTEGRITY AND ACCOUNTABILITY | 5

LEARNING OBJECTIVES

1. To define integrity and accountability as they relate to the practice of medicine.
2. To describe the importance of integrity and accountability as core elements of the social contract between the profession and society.
3. To outline behaviors that demonstrate integrity and accountability.
4. To describe the contribution of the team and the system to integrity and accountability.

Dr. Porter was suddenly struck by an awful thought—he realized he had made a mistake on a prescription he wrote for a patient in the emergency department. It was toward the end of a very busy shift and one of the last patients he saw had a clear-cut case of cellulitis. As he has done dozens of times before, he wrote a prescription for cloxacillin, handed it to the patient, and carried on. While reviewing charts at the end of his shift he suddenly noticed that the patient had a documented penicillin allergy. In a panic, he asked the nurses whether the patient had left. One nurse thought she saw the patient heading toward the pharmacy, so Dr. Porter went to look. He saw the patient speaking with the pharmacist—they had caught the error and were just about to call Dr. Porter. He was so relieved! He thanked the pharmacist and apologized to the patient for the mistake. Together, they reviewed the patients' allergy history and selected a different antibiotic that was safe. The patient, although at first quite upset, was really pleased with the way the pharmacist and the doctor handled the issue, and appreciated Dr. Porter's apology.

WHAT ARE INTEGRITY AND ACCOUNTABILITY?

Integrity can be defined as, "A virtue consisting of soundness of and adherence to moral principles and character and standing up in their defense when they are threatened or under attack. This involves consistent, habitual honesty and a coherent integration of reasonably stable, justifiable moral values, with consistent judgment and action over time" (Miller-Keane & O'Toole, 2003). In healthcare settings we can define integrity as encompassing honesty, keeping one's word, and consistently adhering to principles of professionalism, even when it is not easy to do so. **Accountability** usually refers to reliability and answering to those who trust us, including our patients, colleagues, and society in general. Dr. Porter demonstrated these attributes when he took responsibility for the error, corrected it, and apologized to the patient.

WHY DO INTEGRITY AND ACCOUNTABILITY MATTER?

Integrity and accountability are fundamental to ensuring trust between the public and healthcare professionals. Physicians' integrity forms a foundation for patients' trust and fosters healthy therapeutic relationships that promote healing. Integrity and accountability form the basis of the "social contract" between physicians and society, which grants professionals the privilege of self-regulation. Indeed, as history has shown, this social contract is fragile—if we do not maintain this trust the contract can be rescinded. Perhaps the best-known example of the fragility of the social contract in medicine occurred in Bristol, UK, in the late 1980s, and led to great limitations in the ability of the medical profession to be self-regulating. A summary of the case can be found in Figure 5-1.

"In the late 1980s some clinical staff at the Bristol Royal Infirmary, particularly a recently appointed consultant anaesthetist named Stephen Bolsin, began to raise concerns about the quality of paediatric cardiac surgery undertaken at the hospital by two surgeons who were responsible for both adult and paediatric cardiac surgery. In essence, it was suggested that the results of paediatric cardiac surgery were less good than at other comparable specialist units in the UK and, in particular, that mortality was substantially higher, especially for some types of operation. Between 1989 and 1994 there was a continuing conflict at the hospital about the issue between surgeons, anaesthetists, cardiologists, and managers. The Royal College of Surgeons and the Department of Health both became involved in the increasingly acrimonious dispute, and the media became aware of the concerns. Agreement was eventually reached that a specialist paediatric cardiac surgeon should be appointed and that, in the meantime, a moratorium on certain procedures should be observed. In January 1995, before the new surgeon had taken up his post, a child called Joshua Loveday was scheduled for surgery against the advice of anaesthetists, some surgeons, and the Department of Health. He died and this led to further surgery being halted, an external inquiry being commissioned from experts from the Great Ormond Street Hospital for Children in London, and to extensive local and national media attention.

Parents of some of the children complained to the General Medical Council (GMC) which, in 1997, opened an investigation into events in Bristol and specifically examined the cases of 53 children, 29 of whom had died and four of whom suffered severe brain damage. The GMC inquiry, which concluded in 1998, found three doctors guilty of serious professional misconduct—James Wisheart and Janardan Dhasmana, the two cardiac surgeons involved in the operations, and John Roylance, a radiologist who was the chief executive of the hospital at the time. Mr. Wisheart and Dr. Roylance were struck off the medical register.

The Secretary of State for Health immediately established a full public inquiry, chaired by Professor Ian Kennedy, professor of health law, ethics and policy at University College London. The Inquiry, which cost about £14 million, began hearing evidence in October 1998 and finally published its report with almost 200 recommendations for the NHS in July 2001".

Figure 5-1 ▪ Brief outline of the events in pediatric cardiac surgery in Bristol.
Walshe K, Offen N. A very public failure: lessons for quality improvement in healthcare organisations from the Bristol Royal Infirmary. *Qual Health Care.* 2001 December;10(4):250–256.

There is much to be learned from what is known as the Bristol Affair, and many questions remain unanswered. In retrospect, it is hard to imagine why it took so long before action was taken. One can wonder why no one spoke up when children were dying, or why pediatricians still referred patients to a unit with such bad outcomes. Many health systems' problems contributed in addition to problems with individual doctors (the inquiry resulted in 109 recommendations for change). Further, data collection and reporting were not as widespread or robust as is the situation today. A full exploration of what happened in Bristol is beyond the scope of this chapter, but the important lesson is that the medical profession was seen by the Inquiry to have failed in its duty to self-regulate. The Bristol affair contributed significantly to major changes in the profession in the United Kingdom. The key change was that the General Medical Council (GMC), which had long been the principal regulatory body for the medical profession, is now itself overseen by the Council for the Regulation of Health Professions, which has the power to intervene if it feels the public interest is not being served, or if it feels that physician-imposed sanctions are too lenient. Therefore, the profession now has a regulatory body overseeing its work; the profession does have input into that process, but the Council (the GMC's governing body) now has half of its members from the lay community.

Many healthcare practitioners were involved in the poor outcomes in Bristol, but most of the public outrage focused on the surgeons, rather than the other members of the team such as the nurses or hospital. This may be reflective of the way in which physicians and surgeons have traditionally been viewed—as the tops of the hierarchy, or leaders of their teams. In the past, most patients considered their care to be the responsibility of a specific individual physician, who took "ownership" of the accountability to patients. However, increasingly, patient care is considered a team responsibility, with a physician perhaps in a "most responsible" position but with an integrated, multidisciplinary team that takes "ownership" collectively (Park et al, 2007). Individuals may rely more on teams to provide expertise and continuity, yet each person must maintain responsibility for their own behaviors and actions within these teams and systems. That is, the team or system does not dilute the responsibility each professional owes to the patient.

This chapter includes a discussion of the behaviors of individual physicians, healthcare teams, healthcare settings, and professional organizations that can promote the values of integrity and accountability. In the individual physician section, we have used examples in several areas to illustrate how individual physician behaviors can support the values of integrity and accountability. The illustrative topics include confidentiality, use of the Internet, inappropriate relationships with patients, medical error, and managing conflicts of interest.

BEHAVIORS AND SKILLS OF INDIVIDUAL CLINICIANS

Confidentiality

Confidentiality is of the utmost importance in patient care. Patients must feel free to discuss openly and without hesitation any aspect of their lives, including sensitive information, trusting completely that this information will be guarded safely by the physician or healthcare professional. We owe it to our patients to protect the information they share with us and, in fact, this is codified in legislation (such as the Health Insurance Portability and Accountability Act in the United States and the Personal Information Protection and Electronic Documents Act in Canada). But as easy as it is to outline the importance of maintaining patient confidentiality, it is just as easy to see how breaches can occur. Consider the following scenario:

> *A surgical team is on the elevator talking about their patient list for the day. At first they are the only ones present, but at one floor three people get on. The senior resident is in mid-sentence, and continues, "We'll just go in and hack out the bowel. That's how Dr. Roberts likes to do it—just hack it out. He'll need a colostomy after but it's no big deal." Two of the other residents chuckle, and the three onlookers stand in silence.*

Is there an issue of privacy or confidentiality in this scenario? At first you might not think so, as no patient's name is disclosed and there is no mention of any particular disease. But what if one of the people on the elevator was there to visit a friend or relative about to have bowel surgery? Or if another recognizes Dr. Robert's name, or is on her way to an appointment with him? The onlookers might reasonably wonder if it's their loved one being discussed, and may not know (or care to know) about details such as a colostomy. But even if they don't know anyone having surgery, how might they feel about the cavalier way they see doctors discussing—and laughing about—patients? They might now wonder if all doctors talk about patients this way, or worry that their own doctors might. This behavior is unprofessional not just because of a potential breach in private information, but because it undermines the confidence patients have in their healthcare providers. And it certainly does not speak well for the education system or the institution.

Inadvertent breaches in patient confidentiality may occur in many other ways. For example, we have seen patient sign-out lists left on cafeteria tables, or sticking out of pockets so that patients' names can be seen. We have all seen and heard patient-related discussions in the coffee line-ups, or hallway consults being conducted in crowded emergency departments. Although this section is about individual behavior, it is important to note that the team has a role to play here as well (e.g., to redirect or halt conversation, ensure sound privacy when presenting and discussing patients, and being careful to keep track of sign-out lists). The institution can also create and support policies that make these breaches less likely to occur, such as ensuring that all patients are seen and examined in private settings, and by not allowing patient lists to be emailed or printed from non-secure computers. In short, this too is a shared responsibility.

Use of the Internet

Karen is a 3rd-year medical student who just started on her first real clinical rotation. She used to have an active social life, but it has become increasingly apparent that being on call and working long hours will make it difficult for her to keep up with her friends. She maintains an active Facebook page and often shares her thoughts and feelings with her friends and followers. After a particularly rough shift in the emergency department she went home and posted about it, stating that, "The ER tonight was a complete zoo! People were coming in from all directions, with all sorts of issues that were not even real emergencies. They spend years smoking and drinking and not taking care of themselves and then expect us to pick up the pieces. They're burdening the system and it's really frustrating."

Has Karen done anything that might be considered unprofessional? In terms of confidentiality, she hasn't named anyone or given particularly specific information that could lead to the identification of a particular patient or healthcare provider. But it would not be difficult to figure out to which hospital and/or medical center she is referring. This is an issue of integrity. In a bygone era—before

LEARNING EXERCISE 5-1

1. Think of a recent time where you witnessed (or were party to) a breach in confidentiality.

2. Describe what happened. Who was involved? What was the nature of the information that was breached?

3. Was anything done or said at the time to interrupt or stop the breach from occurring? In retrospect can you think of anything that could have been done?

4. Was anything done or said after the fact, either to the individual(s) who lapsed or to others?

5. What strategies could your institution put in place to reduce the occurrence of these sorts of lapses?

the Internet—she might have said these same words to a friend or family member on the phone. Anyone from those previous generations may wince at remembering how we vented after difficult shifts ourselves. However, two key differences exist. The first is the public nature of the Internet. Although it is possible to restrict one's presence so that only "friends" can see postings, a recent study showed that only two thirds of medical students activated these settings (MacDonald, Sohn, & Ellis, 2010). Furthermore, because the concept of "friends" is so loose, family members and acquaintances not in the profession may see what's posted and can then choose to re-post or share with their "friends." So the information posted can never be thought of as being truly private. The other main issue is that of permanence because what is posted online can potentially be there forever. Tweets, for example, are all archived at the Library of Congress, even if they are later deleted from a user's account or timeline. Venting to a friend on the phone may have compromised some rules of professionalism (such as use of derogatory language about patients), but it did not have the staying power (or damaging potential) of a similar rant online.

Studies of medical students report that most students and residents have an online presence, and find it essential for keeping up with their social lives while on busy clinical rotations. Some try to resolve this by creating two online personae—one personal and one professional—but this can become burdensome and confusing, and it's easy to slip between them (just as it is unfortunately easy to hit "reply to all" when sending a private email). Students often report feeling constricted in developing identities as professionals, while struggling to maintain a sense of their old selves, and this tension can lead to lapses in professionalism. In one study, students felt that guidelines would be helpful to teach them about boundaries, confidentiality concerns, and other issues related to online professionalism—but they rejected the idea of "rules," as they did not think it

1. Establish and sustain an online professional presence that befits your responsibilities while representing your interests

2. Use privacy controls to manage more personal aspects of your profile and to not make anything public that you would not be comfortable defending as "professionally appropriate" in a court of law

3. Think carefully and critically about how what you say or do will be perceived by others and act with appropriate restraint while online

4. Think carefully and critically about how what you say or do reflects on others (individuals and organizations) and act accordingly

5. Think carefully and critically about how what you say or do will be perceived in years to come; consider every action online as permanent

6. Be aware of the potential for attack or impersonation, and know how to protect your online reputation and what resources are available to you in that event

7. An online community is still a community and you are still a professional within it

Figure 5-2 ▪ Principles for online professionalism in medicine.
Ellaway R. Digital Professionalism. *Med Teach* 2010;32(8):705–7.

was fair to attempt to regulate their social lives (Chretien et al, 2010). In their view, if we trust students to look after patients, we should trust them to know right from wrong when it comes to social networking. It is with this spirit in mind that many guidelines for "digital professionalism" have been created. Rather than attempting to restrict or regulate what healthcare professionals can and cannot do online, they provide information and guidelines for use (Figure 5-2). The idea is that these guidelines should be educational for all involved.

The preceding example focused on a medical student who used derogatory language about patients online, but similar issues arise when students post personal content about themselves. Studies have found that healthcare students and professionals often post personal information and photographs of themselves, including those from vacations, parties, and social occasions. Students have appeared intoxicated or partially undressed. Apart from the obvious concerns discussed previously about who might view these postings and the potential for permanence, this highlights another issue, that of the tension between the "person" and the "professional." Students often struggle when developing their new identities as healthcare professionals and sometimes chafe against new rules and constraints on their behaviors. But it is important to note that medical authorities and licensing bodies do not make this distinction, and precedents exist for physicians to be publicly sanctioned and reprimanded for behaviors that occur well outside the healthcare setting (e.g., incidents of "road rage" and personal income tax evasion).

Thus it is our duty as educators to teach and guide students and residents, and to ensure that they are fully aware of what is expected of them as they develop into professionals. A recently published policy statement from the American College of Physicians and the Federation of State Medical Boards included this helpful table to help guide physicians and trainees (Table 5-1) (Farnan et al, 2013).

Relationships with Patients

Clinicians have ample opportunity to demonstrate integrity and accountability when it comes to their relationships with patients. Maintaining appropriate

TABLE 5-1   ONLINE PHYSICIAN ACTIVITIES: BENEFITS, PITFALLS, AND RECOMMENDED SAFEGUARDS

Activity	Potential benefits	Potential pitfalls	Recommended safeguards
• Communications with patients using email, text, and instant messaging	• Greater accessibility • Immediate answers to nonurgent issue	• Confidentiality concerns • Replacement of face-to-face or telephone interaction • Ambiguity or misinterpretation of digital interactions	• Establish guidelines for types of issues appropriate for digital communication • Reserve digital communication only for patients who maintain face-to-face follow-up
• Use of social media sites to gather information about patients	• Observe and counsel patients on risk-taking or health-averse behaviors • Intervene in an emergency	• Sensitivity to source of information • Threaten trust in patient–physician relationship	• Consider intent of search and application of findings • Consider implications for ongoing care
• Use of online educational resources and related information with patients	• Encourage patient empowerment through self-education • Supplement resource-poor environments	• Non–peer-reviewed materials may provide inaccurate information • Scam "patient" sites that misrepresent therapies and outcomes	• Vet information to ensure accuracy of content • Refer patients only to reputable sites and sources
• Physician-produced blogs, microblogs, and physician posting of comments by others	• Advocacy and public health enhancement • Introduction of physician "voice" into such conversations	• Negative online content, such as "venting" or ranting, that disparages patients and colleagues	• "Pause before posting" • Consider the content and the message it sends about a physician as an individual and the profession

| | | | Recommended |
| TABLE 5-1 **ONLINE PHYSICIAN ACTIVITIES: BENEFITS, PITFALLS, AND RECOMMENDED SAFEGUARDS (Continued)** | | | |
Activity	Potential benefits	Potential pitfalls	safeguards
• Physician posting of physician personal information on public social media sites	• Networking and communications	• Blurring of professional and personal boundaries • Impact on representation of the individual and the profession	• Maintain separate personas, personal and professional, for online social behavior • Scrutinize material available for public consumption
• Physician use of digital venues (e.g. text and Web) for communicating with colleagues about patient care	• Ease of communication with colleagues	• Confidentiality concerns • Unsecured networks and accessibility of protected health information	• Implement health information technology solutions for secure messaging and information sharing • Follow institutional practice and policy for remote and mobile access of protected health information

Source: Farnan JM, Snyder Sulmasy L, Worster BK, Chaudhry HJ, Rhyne JA, Arora VM; American College of Physicians Ethics, Professionalism and Human Rights Committee; American College of Physicians Council of Associates; Federation of State Medical Boards Special Committee on Ethics and Professionalism*. Online medical professionalism: patient and public relationships: policy statement from the American College of Physicians and the Federation of State Medical Boards. *Ann Intern Med.* 2013 Apr 16;158(8):620–622.

boundaries is a fundamental skill that all healthcare professionals must learn, and it is an area in which lapses, when they occur, can be particularly serious and damaging. Everyone has heard or read of cases in which physicians have become sexually involved with their patients. Thankfully, these occurrences are relatively rare overall, but they are still one common reason for physicians to lose their license to practice medicine (Alam et al, 2011). All healthcare professionals will recognize that behaviors such as assaulting one's patients are clearly wrong, but some controversy exists around other types of boundary issues.

For example, although it is usually considered undesirable for a physician to enter into a friendship or social relationship with a patient, it is important to remember that context matters. If you are the only physician in a small or remote town it is inevitable that you will form friendships with your patients, otherwise you would be completely isolated. However, rules and policies exist for guidance and it is paramount that patients' needs remain the priority (American Medical Association, 2013a). Of interest, physicians' support for such relationships has been found to differ based on certain contextual factors. In one survey study of more than 1600 physicians, social and business relationships with patients were thought to be potentially acceptable by 91% and 65% of respondents, respectively, but it was much less supported by women, nonwhites, and international graduates (Regan, Ferris, & Campbell, 2010).

Some authors have drawn distinctions between boundary *violations* and boundary *crossings*, which are thought to be milder and more innocent, but which might, over time, develop into violations. One commonly cited example of a boundary crossing is an elderly patient who gives homemade cookies to her family doctor. Refusing such a gift may do more harm than good, by embarrassing the patient and making her feel self-conscious or uncomfortable. Instead, one might thank the patient, being sure to inform her that gifts are not necessary, and share the cookies with the entire office, making the gift seem less personal. On the other hand, if a patient brings gifts to every encounter, or the gifts are expensive or personal in nature, it is a different story. The physician should be aware that accepting such gifts is considered to be undesirable, because it runs the risk of altering the physician–patient relationship and contributes to a loss of objectivity. This can affect patient care by consciously (or unconsciously) treating that patient's symptoms as more or less serious, or being persuaded to order unnecessary tests or treatments.

Receiving gifts from patients is an example of the daily challenges to boundaries that occur in all practices. Although avoiding these challenges is desirable, it is not always possible, so the goal here is to learn how to respond to them in a professional manner. Figure 5-3 presents a sample self-assessment tool that can assist physicians handle such challenges.

Managing Conflicts of Interest

The Institute of Medicine has defined a conflict of interest (COI) as, "A set of circumstances that creates a risk that professional judgment or actions regarding a primary interest will be unduly influenced by a secondary interest" (Lo & Field, 2009). The primary interests usually refer to patients, but also can refer to protecting the integrity of research or the quality of medical education. Secondary interests usually mean financial gains but also can mean professional advancement, recognition for personal achievement, and favors to friends and family, among others. Consider the following example that takes place on a 3rd-year medical student's psychiatry rotation:

A prominent visiting professor is at the university and is giving an afterhours talk at a nice restaurant nearby. The clerkship supervisor invites the student group along. The other students decline, as

This self-assessment tool consists of 27 questions. The goals of using this tool are to help raise awareness and encourage self-reflection, as well as to promote open discussion among physicians about boundary issues.

When answering a question, try to think about how often some of the things mentioned below occur, i.e., seldom, routinely, occasionally or often. After you have finished, review the discussion points provided on the website of the College of Physicians of Ontario (reference below table). The discussion points will illuminate the reasoning behind the questions and how they relate to boundary issues.

1. How do I feel if certain patients leave my practice, and why do I feel that way?
2. Do I feel that I would like to discontinue treatment with patients that seem ungrateful?
3. Do I avoid terminating the physician–patient relationship with patients who are emotionally dependent on me?
4. Do I favour patients who comply with my recommendations?
5. How do I feel and act towards patients who get an expected treatment outcome but still complain?
6. How do I deal with cultural taboos that conflict with my opinion of effective treatment?
7. Do I spend a disproportionate amount of time thinking about particular patients?
8. Do I inadvertently or advertently, in words, tone, or attitude, prevent patients from participating in the decision-making process in relation to their healthcare?
9. Do I accept inappropriate gifts from patients?
10. Do I seek advice for personal benefit from a patient during a clinical encounter?
11. Do I pay more attention to my personal appearance if I know that I will be seeing a certain patient?
12. Do I seek more personal details than I clinically need to, in order to find out about a patient's personal life?
13. Do I routinely do favours or make special arrangements for certain patients (i.e., schedule off-hours or off-site appointments, extend usual appointment length, etc.) and why?
14. Do I treat patients differently if I find them physically attractive or important?
15. Do I share my personal problems with patients?
16. Do I have thoughts or fantasize about becoming personally involved with a certain patient?
17. Do I seek social contact with certain patients outside of clinically scheduled visits? If so, why?
18. Do I tell patients personal things about myself in order to impress them and if so, why?
19. Do I feel a sense of excitement or longing when I think of a patient or anticipate her/his visit?
20. When a patient has been seductive with me, do I experience this as a gratifying sign of my own sex appeal?
21. Do I find myself prescribing medication or making diagnoses for my social acquaintances?
22. Do I ask patients to do personal favours for me?
23. Do I undertake business deals with patients?
24. Do I explain what I am about to do before I examine patients or perform an intimate examination?
25. Do I ensure the patient's comfort and privacy by appropriate draping or by leaving the room when the patient undresses?
26. Do I ensure that the patient is comfortable during intimate procedures and exams?
27. Under appropriate situations, do I ask patients if they would like a third party present at an examination?

Figure 5-3 ■ Self-assessment tool.

From College of Physicians and Surgeons of Ontario. Members Dialogue: Maintaining Boundaries with Patients. September/October 2004. Available at: http://www.cpso.on.ca/uploadedFiles/downloads /cpsodocuments/members/Maintaining%20Boundaries.pdf *they are not particularly interested in the topic, and because they are concerned that a "drug talk" may violate their school's guidelines about medical student-industry interactions. But Lisa is interested in psychiatry as a career, and thinks this might be a good opportunity to learn more and to have an opportunity to interact with (and show her interest to) the residency director and other important faculty members. Furthermore, she worries that if she is the only one to decline she might draw negative attention to herself.*

Does this represent a conflict of interest, and for whom? If we focus on Lisa, we can appreciate her competing desires for not violating a school policy and not being exposed to potentially biased information, while also appreciating a unique opportunity to get to know influential people. Not to mention her concern about potentially making herself look bad if she declines the invitation. It is important to note that, at least so far, Lisa has done nothing wrong. It is not possible to avoid all conflicts of interest—this set of circumstances arose independently of the student—but she is now put in a difficult position. The professional responsibility we have is to negotiate conflicts such as this one in a way that protects the primary interests and is not unduly influenced by the secondary ones. The primary interest here might be the quality of medical education, in that Lisa may be exposed to biased clinical content from influential leaders. But she is also at risk of being unduly influenced by a desire for professional advancement or recognition. The other students may be correct about violating school policy, but it is not clear what role industry is actually playing in the dinner. Lisa should probably try to determine this first before making her decision. And she could also ask if there are other opportunities to meet this professor or other faculty members that do not involve industry at all.

From a systems perspective it is important to consider the roles that others have played in allowing this situation to occur, such as the department that invited the speaker and arranged the dinner, and the faculty member that invited the student's group along.

There is good evidence that accepting gifts such as meals and funding for continuing education activities has an effect on physicians, for example, by being linked to increased prescription costs and non–evidence-based prescribing (Wazana, 2000). Even small gifts can have an effect, although unfortunately the average gift is not exactly small—a recent study reported an average payment per physician of close to $5000 (Kesselheim et al, 2013). Because of these issues most universities and academic health centers have developed guidelines for students and faculty when it comes to interactions with industry, and the good news is that these policies can be effective (Ehringhaus et al, 2008). Some recent research has reported more restrictive policies on drug company involvement (such as restricting gifts) at some schools translates to better prescribing practices in its graduates (King et al, 2013). The American Medical Student Association (2012) publishes a scorecard that grades each medical school's policies on COI. In 2012, 18% of schools received an "A" and 49% received a "B," indicating at least the presence of a policy aligned with best practices. Very few schools failed by having either no policy or one that violates the guidelines. The Institute on Medicine as a Profession (IMAP) has sample medical school COI policies and curricular material on their Web site (http://www.imapny.org/).

> *Dr. Daniels is an internist working in a large multidisciplinary clinic, and she often refers her patients to one of the six cardiologists who work there. She has noticed that when her patients are seen by Dr. Wells, they almost always end up with stenting procedures, whereas with the other cardiologists a larger variety of treatment approaches are utilized. At first she thought it was a coincidence, or that maybe she was somehow sending the sicker patients to Dr. Wells. But then a colleague made an off-hand comment that, "Everybody knows that about Dr. Wells." It turns out that he alone performs and interprets the angiogram, decides whether or not the patient needs stents (and how many), and does the procedure himself. No one else even views the images. Dr. Daniels is further dismayed to learn that cardiologists are paid by the stent. She is now concerned that her patients may have been overtreated and subject to needless risk, and that Dr. Wells may not be acting in the best interests of his patients.*

It seems likely that there is a financial COI here for Dr. Wells. He may indeed be influenced by the secondary interest of financial gain and not acting in the best interests of his patients. Now that Dr. Daniels suspects this conflict what should she do? Unfortunately, although "everybody knows," no one has approached Dr. Wells or the clinic's medical director with their concerns. Dr. Daniels decides, as a first step, that she will not send any more patients to Dr. Wells. But she struggles over what to do next. She knows she should talk to someone about her concerns, but the clinic is otherwise a tight-knit group and she is worried about rocking the boat. If she's wrong she could damage relationships and reputations. But if she is right she knows that patients—and the system—will be better off. She also knows that if this came to light, and the public knew that doctors were aware and did not act, it would greatly undermine their trust in the healthcare system. She recognizes that this is an important concern related to integrity and accountability. As daunting as it seemed, she decided to discuss the issue with some of her close colleagues, and was surprised to hear their relief that someone was finally talking about this concern. They gathered some information and data from their own patients and

LEARNING EXERCISE 5-2

1. Potential conflicts of interest are ubiquitous. Think of a time where you experienced a potential conflict of interest, either as a student, resident or practicing physician.
2. Can you identify the primary interest? All secondary interests?
3. How did you resolve the conflict at the time?
4. What, if anything, would you do differently now? Why?

as a group went to the clinic's medical director. Although this was difficult for them to do, it did alert the director that there was a potential issue. In response the director decided to begin collecting relevant data from all invasive cardiologists in the group, in order to begin more rigorous documentation and evidence that would help him approach Dr. Wells.

In summary, COIs are probably unavoidable, but can be identified and managed. An excellent resource for physicians is the IMAP Web site, which contains a collection of resources, including tool-kits and an online curriculum, to help physicians learn about and manage COIs (Institute on Medicine as a Profession, 2012).

THE ROLE OF THE TEAM IN INTEGRITY AND ACCOUNTABILITY

What role do team members play when it comes to integrity and accountability? We have noted earlier that even when it comes to individuals' behaviors, other people in the team have roles to play, but specifically in this section we focus on four main areas of professional challenge that center on teams: reporting impaired or incompetent colleagues, participating in peer review and multisource feedback, disclosing and investigating medical errors, and the issues surrounding handoffs and sign-over.

Reporting an Impaired or Incompetent Colleague

A group of three medical students came to talk to the rotation coordinator on internal medicine during their 3rd-year clerkship. They were concerned about Mark, a fellow student who seemed to be struggling. In particular they felt that Mark was very anxious and not coping well, and they were worried not only about his safety but also his efficacy as a medical provider. They asked the rotation coordinator what they should do. The coordinator thanked them for bringing the issue forward, recognizing that it was not easy for them to do, and gathered more specific information. She then met with Mark and told him that others were a bit concerned that he wasn't doing well. At first, Mark was embarrassed, but after a few minutes he expressed relief that others had actually noticed and wanted to help. He disclosed that he had been having major personal stresses and had struggled on previous rotations, and suggested that a leave of absence might be appropriate. The rotation coordinator liaised with the student affairs and student wellness offices and Mark was able to receive appropriate care before returning.

This situation is notable for the insight and courage of the students who came forward. All too often a colleague in distress is ignored or avoided, as we have recently found in a study of practicing internists. In that study, when responding to hypothetical scenarios, internists were often reluctant to approach a colleague in apparent difficulty, expressing concern about crossing boundaries, being uncertain or incorrect regarding their suspicions, and believing that other people (or "the system") would take care of it (DesRoches et al, 2010; Ginsburg et al, 2012). Furthermore, their responses were different—and more avoidant—if there was concern that there might be a mental illness or addiction as compared to physical ailments like cancer. In these situations, coming forward is difficult but necessary in order to protect the student or colleague from potential harm to themselves—and to their patients.

The American Medical Association provides guidance for physicians regarding the duty to report impaired or incompetent colleagues (American Medical Association, 2013b). This is considered an ethical obligation in order to protect the public. Impairment is loosely defined as a condition that "interferes with a physician's ability to engage safely in professional activities." Legal requirements may vary by jurisdiction, but the basic premise is that physicians are in a position to intervene when unsafe care may result from impairment or incompetence, and thus they can help the physician in question obtain help or remediation where appropriate. This may take the form of addiction or mental health diagnosis and treatment, remediation of particular skill sets, or even removal from practice if no improvement is possible.

Peer Review and Multisource Feedback

All too often, evaluation is unidirectional, and nearly always from the top down. Medical students are usually evaluated by their residents and staff, nursing students by their supervisors, and residents by their attending staff and program directors. But significant evidence suggests that peers and members of other healthcare professions can provide valuable feedback on performance. In studies of medical students, researchers have found that students are willing to participate in peer assessment, provided that their needs and concerns are met. In one study, students were more likely to participate in peer assessment if they could remain anonymous, if immediate feedback and action would be taken, and if it focused on positive as well as negative behaviors. Students preferred giving formative feedback and stressed that a supportive climate was essential (Arnold et al, 2007). In other studies, peer assessments were found to correlate with other related measures, such as faculty evaluations (Kovach, 2009), or a measure of students' conscientiousness (Finn, 2009).

As with peers, other healthcare professionals can provide invaluable feedback on performance, especially regarding behaviors that may not be visible or apparent to faculty, and this may be especially true for feedback about humanistic care (Woolliscroft et al, 1994). Gathering assessments from different people who observe a variety of behaviors in diverse settings, adds to the richness of formative feedback. However, despite the apparent value of such feedback, healthcare professionals have also been shown to be reluctant to provide feedback on their peers, even at the faculty level.

> *The surgical nurses and residents have noticed that a senior and well-respected surgeon, Dr. Rasul, continues to use a particular surgical instrument that all of the other surgeons stopped using because of evidence suggesting that it was associated with more complications of a particular procedure. It is not clear to the team, who have discussed this in hallway conversation, whether Dr. Rasul knows that she is the only one still using this instrument, and it is not clear whether someone should mention it, or who should do so. The hospital has created standard surgical sets for a variety of different procedures, but not for this one.*

The team members may feel uncomfortable and therefore avoid the topic completely. However, this could be detrimental to the patients, subjecting them to unnecessary risk, and to the surgeon herself. If Dr. Rasul is unaware that she is using the equipment differently than others are, depriving her of such feedback does not allow her to change her practice in a positive way. She also would not have the opportunity to explain to the team potential reasons for her practice. If this team had a system of multisource feedback in place, it would provide a safe opportunity for concerns to be raised and for appropriate feedback to be given and received. In most cases, because power differentials and hierarchies exist, it might be best to have an anonymous system so that team members would feel protected in giving their feedback.

Receiving and acting on feedback is a skill highly relevant to professionalism. Research has suggested that resistance to feedback may be a particularly important red flag that is linked to unprofessional behavior in practice (Teherani et al, 2005). Being able to give and receive feedback in a professional manner is key to learning and growth, yet understandably it can be distressing to receive negative feedback. In one study, students recalled specifics of both positive and negative feedback they had received in the past, and often reported strong emotional reactions (Nofziger et al, 2010). Yet students also reported transformations to their behavior based on feedback received from peers, and nearly all of them found it a valuable process. As echoed in many other studies, feedback was seen to be most helpful when it was specific, when it came from a credible source, when it was consistent across multiple raters (lending it further credibility and validity), and when there was an opportunity to discuss it with a trusted advisor.

As professionals, if we explicitly open ourselves up to feedback, and act on what we hear, we demonstrate our commitment to excellence and show our accountability to the public and to our patients. One well-established example of this is the Physician Achievement Review (PAR) program through the College of Physicians and Surgeons of Alberta, Canada. Every 5 years physicians must gather ratings on their performance from patients and colleagues from a range of healthcare professions (Physician Achievement Review, 2011). Similarly some of the certifying boards, for example, the American Board of Orthopaedic Surgery, have begun to mandate these types of multisource reviews as part of maintenance of certification as well. These types of "360 degree" evaluations have been used in the business world for years but are increasingly becoming part of the culture in healthcare. Figure 5-4 presents the PAR Medical Colleague Questionnaire. The PAR program also produces a Co-Worker Questionnaire, Patient Questionnaire, and Self-Assessment Questionnaire. For full information, please visit http://www.par-program.org/information/survey-instruments.html

Many of the evaluation systems for multisource feedback incorporate patient satisfaction ratings, as seen above in the PAR. Another excellent example is the American Board of Internal Medicine's patient assessments of physicians' patient-centeredness, communication, accessibility, and other factors (see Chapter 4, Fostering Patient-Centered Care). Practicing internists who wish to maintain their board certification are required to collect patient ratings, and the Board provides collated feedback physicians can then use for quality improvement. Most hospitals participate in some type of program to collect patient feedback, but not all of them are used to give specific feedback to individual physicians.

Many physicians will be familiar with another, more informal source of patient feedback, in the form of "rate my doctor" types of Web sites. Opinions here are obviously less rigorously gathered; it is up to individual patients

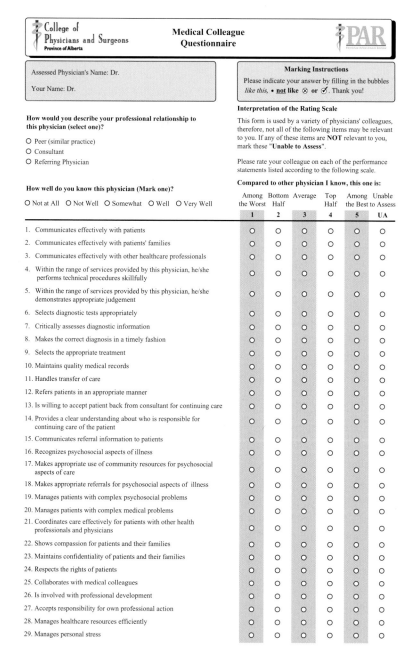

Figure 5-4 ▪ 360-degree feedback sample.

From Physician Achievement Review (PAR). PAR Survey Instruments. Available at:
http://www.par-program.org/information/survey-instruments.html

or family members to know about the sites, log on, and enter a rating and comments. Although physicians are often reluctant to view these sites, and discount them as unscientific, there is some evidence that these ratings may correlate with other outcomes, such as student ratings of faculty along similar dimensions (Young et al, 2012). Despite concerns that comments posted on such sites are predominantly from disgruntled patients, no evidence exists to support this. In fact, most ratings found on these web sites are fairly positive and physicians can learn something about themselves by seeing how they are perceived by patients (Jain, 2010; Gao et al, 2012). Even if comments are negative or critical, it is important for us as physicians to be aware of how we are perceived (even if just by a few patients) so that we can continue to improve our performance.

In summary, providing feedback to others, as well as soliciting and acting on feedback ourselves, is a professional responsibility. Through feedback we can reflect and improve upon our performance and simultaneously demonstrate our professionalism and accountability to the public.

Handoffs and Sign-Outs

In an era of reduced work hours for residents, handoffs of patient care have become more frequent, and reports of innovative methods for handoffs and sign-outs have proliferated. One might think this is a new issue, yet healthcare providers from all disciplines have always had to contend with issues around the transfer of care of their patients. Whether at change of shift, end of rotation, absences due to vacation, or simply the end of a normal working day, healthcare professionals are obligated to ensure a smooth transition of care for their patients. How we handle these transitions is an issue of accountability.

> *Ahmed is on his last day of a month-long hematology rotation, during which he has met all of the required learning objectives except for performing a bone marrow biopsy. He has seen several performed by others but has never done one himself. A patient he admitted overnight is suspected of having acute leukemia and requires an urgent biopsy. Recognizing that it's his last day, the senior resident offers the procedure to Ahmed, who is excited to finally have this opportunity. However, Ahmed is post-call and has been up most of the night. He really wants to do the procedure as he has gotten to know the patient and has a bond with him, and he feels he is capable, but technically he should be signing it out to someone else.*

What are Ahmed's options here, and who is he accountable to? He has not met all of his learning objectives for the rotation and is presented with an excellent learning opportunity that he would very much like to pursue. This speaks to his pursuit of excellence and perhaps accountability to his future patients. However, his first accountability should be to the patient, and Ahmed is fatigued. This may affect his cognitive as well as his motor skills and may add additional risk to the patient. Furthermore, he is not supposed to be working past scheduled hours, and is not sure how he would record this extra time if he were to stay. In this case, he is also accountable to his program. Let's also think about what the patient might want. If he is feeling scared about the procedure and the potential diagnosis, would he prefer to have the fatigued intern do it, as they have developed rapport and trust? Or would he prefer to have it done by someone who is more alert but a stranger? And even if someone else does the procedure, should Ahmed stay to help alleviate the patient's anxiety?

In residency education the topic of handoffs is now garnering much attention. In some education systems there is a cap imposed on the total number of hours that may be worked per week, whereas in others there are limits to the hours that may be worked consecutively (e.g., 16 hours for interns in the Accreditation Council for Graduate Medical Education (ACGME)-accredited programs and 24 hours in some Canadian programs). Yet residents are often put in difficult situations when sticking to these limits puts them at odds with educational or patient care needs. Consider the choices residents must make when a shift is over but they have an unstable patient under their care, or when a patient and family with whom they've developed strong rapport are in the midst of making end-of-life decisions, or when a pregnant woman who has been in difficult labor for hours is about to deliver. In one paper, aptly named "To leave or to lie," residents in internal medicine and surgery often expressed a tension between "blindly" obeying duty hour regulations and potentially staying longer without reporting it (Szymczak et al, 2010). Reasons for wanting to stay beyond shift limits include a desire to learn, to help their patients, and to not leave unfinished work for others. Residents also expressed many reasons why they sometimes lied when reporting their hours, such as not wanting to appear slow or inefficient, and wanting to protect their program from potentially losing funding.

In studies involving surgical training some researchers have suggested that a "new" professionalism is expected to develop, which emphasizes shared responsibility for patients and more reliance on teams and teamwork. However, recent studies find that surgical residents still often feel that working longer hours is "more professional," and only a minority feel it's acceptable to pass off work to night teams (Coverdill et al, 2010). In these and other studies, residents often note that they do not receive appropriate guidance or education around how to make these difficult decisions. There is also some concern that if they don't learn how to approach these situations during their residency, they will not know what to do once in practice, where no duty hour limits exist. This reinforces the need for education—for residents and for faculty—and for open discussion when these situations arise.

It is important to note that these tensions may be exacerbated by the fact that most attending physicians underwent training in a system without strict duty hour limits. This may result in misunderstandings or even resentment in some cases, if faculty do not understand or agree with the regulations. Faculty need education on this topic (Ginsburg, 2013).

THE ROLE OF THE HEALTHCARE SETTING

The healthcare setting has a key role to play in promoting integrity and accountability. For example, in the confidentiality section we noted that the institution could develop technology and strategies to maintain the privacy of patients' medical information, such as by imposing encryption standards for email and external storage devices and facing computer screens such that bystanders can't read them. But institutions can go much further to create cultures where integrity and accountability are embodied as core values. Institutional policies, both in documents and in practice, form a critical framework for physicians and other professionals working in those organizations and guide appropriate behaviors. The role of healthcare settings in supporting the disclosure and analysis of medical errors is a good example of how an institution can shape a culture of integrity and accountability.

Dr. Chow was sitting in his office in the dark, feeling sick to his stomach. His phone was ringing but he barely heard, as he was replaying over and over in his head the events of the last hour. He knew the case would be difficult but he never expected the patient to die on the table. He had done this surgery dozens of times without any difficulty. What was different this time? He was not overly tired, hungry, or ill. He was a bit distracted by a grant application due the next day, but that wasn't out of the ordinary. He started thinking maybe he was just a bad surgeon and had gotten lucky all those other times. Now he felt everyone would "know" and would not want him to operate on their patients. He felt guilty, embarrassed, and ashamed. If only he could go back and re-do the operation, avoiding that aberrant artery. How was he supposed to face the family and tell them what happened? He had really bonded with this patient and her family, and they trusted him completely. What if they sued him? How would he face his colleagues? What if they revoked his privileges, after he had worked so hard for so many years to be a surgeon? He couldn't even think about going home and facing his family.

Dr. Chow is devastated by the patient's outcome and the role he played in it, and now has the daunting task of disclosing the error he made to the patient's distraught family. Disclosing any error can be difficult, but this is especially true for those that lead to serious harm (or death), even for experienced physicians. There are many efforts to teach physicians how to disclose errors skillfully and sensitively following a clear set of communication steps (Stroud et al, 2013; Chan et al, 2005). However, it is not widely appreciated just how difficult this can be for clinicians. More than two decades ago researchers noted the crippling effects of making errors on healthcare workers themselves (Christensen, Levinson, & Dunn, 1992). Physicians and other healthcare professionals can be the "second victim" when they have made an error. Wu (2000) expressed it well: "Virtually every practitioner knows the sickening realisation of making a bad mistake. You feel singled out and exposed—seized by the instinct to see if anyone has noticed. You agonise about what to do, whether to tell anyone, what to say. Later, the event replays itself over and over in your mind. You question your competence but fear being discovered. You know you should confess, but dread the prospect of potential punishment and of the patient's anger."

The Institute of Medicine in the report, "To Err Is Human," published more than 10 years ago, brought the issue of medical errors to the attention of both the profession and the public. Since then there has been recognition of the role of individual healthcare professionals, teams, and healthcare settings in disclosing errors to patients and families and learning from the errors to prevent them from occurring to other patients in the future. Guidelines to help support disclosure have been published in countries throughout the world. Example documents are presented in Table 5-2.

All of these guidelines underscore the need to discuss the error among team members, disclose the error, and analyze the error. Healthcare institutions are key to helping to build the supportive environment to allow and facilitate these kinds of open discussions and to build an infrastructure to conduct the analysis of errors and build systems for prevention. Furthermore, regulatory bodies have created mechanisms to assess how an institution performs on handling medical errors. The National Quality Forum in the United States has articulated a "Safe Practice" guideline, which includes specific policies and procedures that healthcare settings should have in place to support disclosure of errors (see Table 5-2). The handling of medical errors, which years ago left an individual physician to hide the mistake and provided no opportunities to improve the system, has changed dramatically in the last decade. It is a perfect example of the value of integrity and accountability shared by all stakeholders in the system.

Table 5-2	MEDICAL DISCLOSURE AROUND THE GLOBE
Organization	Description
Canadian Patient Safety Institute	The Canadian Disclosure Guidelines, which were released in 2008 and revised in 2011, provide national guidelines for disclosure of adverse events. Its guidelines include guiding principles for disclosure, building an organizational foundation for disclosure, the stages of disclosures, and recommendations for special circumstances. (http://www.patientsafetyinstitute.ca/English/toolsResources /disclosure/Documents/CPSI%20Canadian%20Disclosure%20Guidelines.pdf)
Harvard-affiliated hospitals	In 2004–2005, A workgroup of risk managers and clinicians from Harvard-affiliated hospitals developed an evidence-based guide for its institutions to communicate about and manage adverse events. The guide covers the patient and family experience, the caregiver experience, and the institutional management of an adverse event. (http://www.macoalition.org/documents /respondingToAdverseEvents.pdf)
National Quality Forum	The "Safe Practices for Better Healthcare – 2009 Update" is a guideline for clinical settings (hospitals, ambulatory centers, emergency rooms, and so on) for supporting disclosure. The Safe Practice includes specifications for elements of the disclosure to patients, education of healthcare professionals, 24-hour advisory support, emotional support for providers, and suggested outcomes, process, structure, and patient-centered measures. (http://www.qualityforum.org /Publications/2009/03/Safe_Practices_2009_full(2).aspx)
National Health Service (U.K.)	The National Patient Safety Agency (NPSA) has developed best practices for creating an open and honest environment within healthcare organizations. (http://www.nrls.npsa.nhs.uk/resources/collections/being-open/?entryid45=83726)

LEARNING EXERCISE 5-3

1. Think of a recent incident where someone on your team made a mistake.
2. Describe what happened. How did you learn about it? What was your response? What, if anything, did you say to your colleague at the time or afterwards?
3. Did your colleague receive any support or counselling? If so, was it effective and sufficient? If not, what do you think might have helped?
4. If you had made the error, what supports or resources would you have found helpful?

THE ROLE OF ORGANIZATIONS

As we discussed at the beginning of this chapter, the medical profession has a social contract with society, which grants doctors, among other things, the right to self-regulation. Structures are in place to allow the profession to be autonomous while maintaining transparency. Patients, and society in general, place an enormous degree of trust in the profession. They assume that doctors are competent to practice and that they maintain our competency actively over time. Many members of the public assume that physicians take requalifying examinations to test their knowledge at time points throughout their careers, like airline pilots do, and they are surprised to learn that not all physicians are required to take examinations. In fact, patients largely assume that all is well and good with their physicians, until something happens to change their perceptions.

> *Amelia is a 32-year-old woman who underwent liposuction at a free-standing clinic that specialized in cosmetic procedures. Dr. Binden was the liposuction "specialist" at the clinic and had done many such procedures before. Tragically, the patient had immediate complications and while awaiting an ambulance she had a cardiac arrest. She was resuscitated successfully but spent many weeks in the intensive care unit (ICU) before finally being able to go home. As it turned out, Dr. Binden was not, as the family had assumed, a plastic surgeon—she was a general practitioner with some extra training in cosmetic procedures. On review, Dr. Binden's training consisted of a one-week course for which she received a certificate.*

This case, based on a real example, highlights the importance of transparency within the structure of self-regulation. Dr. Binden was a physician operating outside of an acceptable scope of practice. Saying she was "certified" to perform liposuction was misleading, but how would Amelia or her family know? She had a diploma and a certificate on her wall, and was registered in good standing with the state regulatory body. In fact, similar cases have arisen in many jurisdictions and have prompted change. In some jurisdictions regulatory bodies require physicians to formally apply to change their scope of practice, and for major changes they must provide evidence of new and relevant training, which is assessed by a committee before being approved. Processes such as this can help ensure accountability to the public.

Many licensing bodies for physicians have databases that are publicly searchable. Anyone can look up a doctor and see what their speciality and certifications are, along with information involving restrictions on their practice, complaints against them, and so on. Databases such as these have allowed for research to be conducted on the types of disciplinary actions physicians face in practice and what risk factors or "red flags" may be important. This information is important to feed back to medical school and residency curricula, as well as for faculty development and continuing education initiatives.

As described earlier in the Bristol case, physicians' contracts with society are fragile and can be revoked or rescinded, and the profession can lose its ability to self-regulate.

CONCLUSION

Integrity and accountability are critical to the public trust of physicians and the profession. The privilege of self-regulation is based on our commitment to be accountable to the public. This privilege is one that the profession must not take for granted as, once breached, physicians can lose it—in fact, this is the case in England.

CHALLENGE CASE

Dr. Shu is seeing one of her long-term patients, Mr. Habib, who has multiple medical problems for which he has had to be referred to several specialists. Mr. Habib is very organized and brings copies of all of his doctors' letters and test results to every visit. This time, he shows Dr. Shu a consult letter from Dr. Larkin, a very experienced senior pulmonologist who works down the hall. Mr. Habib had seen him for some shortness of breath, and was quite upset because the letter stated that Mr. Habib was a "malingerer" who was "abusing the healthcare system with his multiple hospital visits." Dr. Larkin did not think there was anything wrong with Mr. Habib, even though he had had asthma and previous pulmonary emboli. Dr. Shu was somewhat shocked at the tone of the consult letter, and reassured Mr. Habib that she would find him a better doctor, one who would not be so judgmental, and who would try to determine the true cause of the patient's dyspnea. Although Mr. Habib was relieved to hear that, he wondered if Dr. Shu was going to "do something" about the letter. Dr. Shu had unfortunately heard other complaints in the past about Dr. Larkin, from patients who thought he was "gruff" and unfriendly, but she had never seen something in writing like this.

What professional challenges exist in this encounter?
The most concerning issue here is the unprofessional language used by Dr. Larkin, not to mention the under-recognition of potentially serious

causes for the patient's shortness of breath. These issues had a negative impact on the patient, both clinically and emotionally. Furthermore, these actions might greatly undermine Mr. Habib's trust of physicians and of the healthcare system, especially if Dr. Larkin faces no accountability for his actions.

One challenge is to support Mr. Habib and reassure him that he is not abusing the system and has done nothing wrong. In fact, he should be commended for keeping such complete records of his own care.

Another challenge is the question posed by Mr. Habib—what should Dr. Shu do in this situation? She thought of talking to Dr. Larkin directly, but she was new on staff and he had been one of her attendings when she was a resident, so this option seemed too intimidating. She considered reporting Dr. Larkin to his chief at the hospital, as she was worried that this may represent a pattern of behavior and thus may be affecting other patients, who may not even be aware of what is contained in their records. However, because she works down the hall from Dr. Larkin, she was concerned that her actions could damage her collegial relationship with him and could even brand her as a whistleblower or tattle tale within his division.

What role does the system have in this situation?
The healthcare system may have played a role in enabling this situation. Dr. Larkin's division has not yet adopted an electronic health record (EHR), so consult letters are in hard copy form only and inaccessible to other members of the team. Dr. Shu feels that if there had been an EHR, Dr. Larkin could never get away with using such language in a patient letter. She also assumes that other physicians must have heard complaints from their patients as well, and wonders why they did nothing to intervene. Or perhaps they had, and nothing had changed. Dr. Shu realized she needed to learn more about her hospital's policies and procedures for dealing with physicians with professionalism issues.

What might Dr. Shu do?
As mentioned, Dr. Shu might speak to Dr. Larkin directly, letting him know that a patient showed her a letter that had some unprofessional language in it—although she may soften this by using a term other than "unprofessional," such as "questionable," so as not to begin in an accusatory manner. She could also say that the patient was upset by the letter and that it was likely that his other doctors had seen it. She also might consider going to the chief of Dr. Larkin's department and asking

for advice. Another option would be to simply stop referring patients to Dr. Larkin, but she realizes that although her patients would be spared, others would not be.

What should Dr. Shu do?

As difficult as it might be, Dr. Shu should not simply avoid the situation and stop sending patients to Dr. Larkin. One good option is to start with a conversation with Dr. Larkin. To prepare, Dr. Shu should identify the purpose of her conversation. That is, she should be clear in her mind what she hopes to achieve (apart from honoring her patient's request). Rather than being punitive or angry she hopes to draw attention to the issue and thereby prevent the behavior from recurring. Thus she should focus on the particular behavior (derogatory language) and its impact (on the patient but also on Dr. Larkin himself). Effects on Dr. Larkin include damage to his reputation among his colleagues, which could affect his practice and livelihood, but also might expose him to disciplinary action. Dr. Shu should make an appointment to see Dr. Larkin, in a one-on-one setting, and might bring the letter with her. She should be prepared for Dr. Larkin's potential reaction (he might be chastened and apologetic but he also might get angry and take it out on Dr. Shu). Finally, she should keep it brief and as nonjudgmental as possible.

A helpful template for working through dilemmas is found in Chapter 2, Resiliency in Facing Professionalism Challenges, Table 2-2. Following the template, this situation calls for:

Self-awareness (recognizing personal emotions or triggers, understanding personal limitations in skills and knowledge)

- Dr. Shu should be aware of her motivations and should recognize that she is upset on the patient's behalf but also feeling intimidated about having a difficult conversation with a colleague.

Self-regulation (managing strong emotions, accessing assistance for complex tasks)

- Dr. Shu should take time to reflect on her emotional state and should not just barge in to talk to Dr. Larkin (or to anyone) while she is still upset.

Social awareness (recognizing the importance of considering the needs and state of all participants)

- Although it might be hard to imagine, Dr. Shu should attempt to consider Dr. Larkin's perspective. Perhaps he was having a particularly bad day, or there is something else going on impairing his ability to provide compassionate care to his patients. Although that would not excuse his actions it would help put them in perspective.

Social regulation (seek to identify more than one option for action, assume positive intent to understand others' behaviors, develop crisis communication strategies and negotiation skills, be empowered to coach others)

- Dr. Shu may need to face the difficult truth that not everyone will walk away happy from this situation. She is already aware of the potential ramifications of either staying silent or of speaking up, and needs to make her decision based on what will do the most good for the most people in the end. She knows she needs to deescalate the emotions so she considered taking the approach of assuming Dr. Larkin may not know how he is perceived by others and may be ultimately grateful for the feedback.

Actions

At the time, after careful reflection, Dr. Shu still felt intimidated by Dr. Larkin, especially as a new faculty member, and was concerned about damaging otherwise collegial relationships. So she chose not to confront Dr. Larkin directly. Instead, she decided to utilize system resources already in place. She informed Mr. Habib that the hospital had a dedicated office for patient relations, where he could go with his letter and make a formal complaint. Dr. Shu reassured him that the process was meant to be educational and nonpunitive for the physician, and that he need not interact with Dr. Larkin directly at any time. The office takes all such issues seriously and aims for remediation of problematic behaviors, with a good track record. She also made an appointment to speak with the Chief of Staff at the hospital to discuss what to do. Although Dr. Shu felt guilty for taking the easy way out (and hoped to feel more empowered in the future), at the time she at least felt that if this lapse was part of a pattern of behavior, that she was at least doing something to get it to stop.

Dealing with systems issues

Dr. Shu learned a lot about the system and about herself during this incident. For one, she learned that she was not alone, as informal conversations with trusted colleagues brought up other issues related to professional practice that she had not been aware of. She decided to initiate a monthly gathering of these close colleagues where they could each raise concerns and get support from each other in dealing with difficult issues.

KEY LEARNING POINTS

1. Integrity and accountability are essential to maintaining the public's trust in the profession. Without them the profession may lose its ability to be self-regulating.
2. Individual students, residents, and physicians have a responsibility to behave in a way that is deserving of this trust by protecting patients' confidentiality; behaving responsibly in our professional, personal, and online lives; maintaining appropriate boundaries with patients; and avoiding and managing conflicts of interest.
3. Teams have a responsibility to be aware of and to report impaired or incompetent colleagues, to participate in peer review and multisource feedback, to disclose and investigate medical errors, and to ensure safe and effective transitions in care.
4. The healthcare setting has an important role to play in the prevention, detection, and investigation of errors, and in providing support to physicians in the aftermath of errors.
5. Professional organizations provide structures that allow the profession to remain autonomous while ensuring transparency and accountability to the public.

REFERENCES

1. Alam A, Klemensberg J, Griesman J, Bell CM. The characteristics of physicians disciplined by professional colleges in Canada. *Open Med*. 2011;5(4):e166–e172.
2. American Medical Association (AMA). *American College of Physicians—The Physician and the Patient*. 2013a. Available at: http://www.ama-assn.org/ama/pub/physician-resources/medical-ethics/about-ethics-group/ethics-resource-center/educational-resources/federation-repository-ethics-documents-online/american-college-physicians/acp-physician-and-patient.page#genetic
3. American Medical Association (AMA). *Opinion 9.031—Reporting Impaired, Incompetent, or Unethical Colleagues*. 2013b. Available at: http://www.ama-assn.org/ama/pub/physician-resources/medical-ethics/code-medical-ethics/opinion9031.page
4. American Medical Student Association (AMSA). *Conflict of Interest Policies at Academic Medical Centers*. 2012. Available at: http://www.amsascorecard.org/
5. Arnold L, Shue CK, Kalishman S, Prislin M, Pohl C, Pohl H, Stern DT. Can there be a single system for peer assessment of professionalism among medical students? A multi-institutional study. *Acad Med*. 2007 Jun;82(6):578–586.
6. Chan DK, Gallagher TH, Reznick R, Levinson W. How surgeons disclose medical errors to patients: a study using standardized patients. *Surgery*. 2005 Nov;138(5):851–858.

7. Chretien KC, Goldman EF, Beckman L, Kind T. It's your own risk: medical students' perspectives on online professionalism. *Acad Med.* 2010 Oct;85(10 Suppl):S68–S71.

8. Christensen JF, Levinson W, Dunn PM. The heart of darkness: the impact of perceived mistakes on physicians. *J Gen Intern Med.* 1992 Jul-Aug;7(4):424–431.

9. College of Physicians and Surgeons of Ontario. Members Dialogue: Maintaining Boundaries with Patients. September/October 2004. Available at: http://www.cpso.on.ca/uploadedFiles/downloads/cpsodocuments/members/Maintaining%20Boundaries.pdf

10. Coverdill JE, Carbonell AM, Fryer J, Fuhrman GM, Harold KL, Hiatt JR, Jarman BT, Moore RA, Nakayama DK, Nelson MT, Schlatter M, Sidwell RA, Tarpley JL, Termuhlen PM, Wohltmann C, Mellinger JD. A new professionalism? Surgical residents, duty hours restrictions, and shift transitions. *Acad Med.* 2010 Oct;85(10 Suppl):S72–S75.

11. DesRoches CM, Rao SR, Fromson JA, Birnbaum RJ, Iezzoni L, Vogeli C, Campbell EG. Physicians' perceptions, preparedness for reporting, and experiences related to impaired and incompetent colleagues. *JAMA.* 2010 Jul 14;304(2):187–193.

12. Ehringhaus SH, Weissman JS, Sears JL, Goold SD, Feibelmann S, Campbell EG. Responses of medical schools to institutional conflicts of interest. *JAMA.* 2008 Feb 13;299(6):665–671.

13. Ellaway R. Digital professionalism. *Med Teach.* 2010;32(8):705–707.

14. Farnan JM, Snyder Sulmasy L, Worster BK, Chaudhry HJ, Rhyne JA, Arora VM; for the American College of Physicians Ethics, Professionalism and Human Rights Committee; the American College of Physicians Council of Associates, the Federation of State Medical Boards Special Committee on Ethics and Professionalism. Online medical professionalism: patient and public relationships: policy statement from the American College of Physicians and the Federation of State Medical Boards. *Ann Intern Med.* 2013 Apr 16;158(8):620–622.

15. Finn G, Sawdon M, Clipsham L, McLachlan J. Peer estimation of lack of professionalism correlates with low Conscientiousness Index scores. *Med Educ.* 2009 Oct;43(10):960–967.

16. Gao GG, McCullough JS, Agarwal R, Jha AK. A changing landscape of physician quality reporting: analysis of patients' online ratings of their physicians over a 5-year period. *J Med Internet Res.* 2012 Feb 24;14(1):e38.

17. Ginsburg S. Duty hours as viewed through a professionalism lens. *BMC Med Educ.* 2013;(BMC Medical Education).

18. Ginsburg S, Bernabeo E, Ross KM, Holmboe ES. "It depends": results of a qualitative study investigating how practicing internists approach professional dilemmas. *Acad Med.* 2012 Dec;87(12):1685–1693.

19. Institute on Medicine as a Profession. *Conflicts of Interest Overview.* 2012. Available at: http://www.imapny.org/conflicts_of_interest/conflicts-of-interest-overview

20. Jain S. Googling ourselves—what physicians can learn from online rating sites. *N Engl J Med.* 2010 Jan 7;362(1):6–7.

21. Kesselheim AS, Robertson CT, Siri K, Batra P, Franklin JM. Distributions of industry payments to Massachusetts physicians. *N Engl J Med.* 2013 May 30;368(22):2049–2052.

22. King M, Essick C, Bearman P, Ross JS. Medical school gift restriction policies and physician prescribing of newly marketed psychotropic medications: difference-in-differences analysis. *BMJ.* 2013 Jan 30;346:f264.

23. Kovach RA, Resch DS, Verhulst SJ. Peer assessment of professionalism: a five-year experience in medical clerkship. *J Gen Intern Med*. 2009 Jun;24(6):742–746.

24. Lo B, Field MJ. *Conflict of Interest in Medical Research, Education and Practice*. 1st edition. Washington, DC: National Academies Press; 2009.

25. MacDonald J, Sohn S, Ellis P. Privacy, professionalism and Facebook: a dilemma for young doctors. *Med Educ*. 2010 Aug;44(8):805–813.

26. Miller-Keane, O'Toole M. *Miller-Keane Encyclopedia & Dictionary of Medicine, Nursing & Allied Health*. 7th edition. Philadelphia, PA: Saunders; 2003.

27. Nofziger AC, Naumburg EH, Davis BJ, Mooney CJ, Epstein RM. Impact of peer assessment on the professional development of medical students: a qualitative study. *Acad Med*. 2010 Jan;85(1):140–147.

28. Park J, Woodrow SI, Reznick RK, Beales J, MacRae HM. Patient care is a collective responsibility: perceptions of professional responsibility in surgery. *Surgery*. 2007 Jul;142(1):111–118.

29. Physician Achievement Review (PAR). 2011. Available at: http://www.par-program.org/

30. Physician Achievement Review (PAR). PAR Survey Instruments. Available at: http://www.par-program.org/information/survey-instruments.html

31. Regan S, Ferris TG, Campbell EG. Physician attitudes toward personal relationships with patients. *Med Care*. 2010 Jun;48(6):547–552.

32. Stroud L, Wong BM, Hollenberg E, Levinson W. Teaching medical error disclosure to physicians-in-training: a scoping review. *Acad Med*. 2013 Jun;88(6):884–892.

33. Szymczak JE, Brooks JV, Volpp KG, Bosk CL. To leave or to lie? Are concerns about a shift-work mentality and eroding professionalism as a result of duty-hour rules justified? *Milbank Q*. 2010 Sep;88(3):350–381.

34. Teherani A, Hodgson CS, Banach M, Papadakis MA. Domains of unprofessional behavior during medical school associated with future disciplinary action by a state medical board. *Acad Med*. 2005 Oct;80(10 Suppl):S17–S20.

35. Walshe K, Offen N. A very public failure: lessons for quality improvement in health care organisations from the Bristol Royal Infirmary. *Qual Health Care*. 2001 Dec;10(4):250–256.

36. Wazana A. Physicians and the pharmaceutical industry: is a gift ever just a gift? *JAMA*. 2000 Jan 19;283(3):373–380.

37. Woolliscroft JO, Howell JD, Patel BP, Swanson DB. resident-patient interactions: the humanistic qualities of internal medicine residents assessed by patients, attending physicians, program supervisors, and nurses. *Acad Med*. 1994 Mar;69(3):216–224.

38. Wu AW. Medical error: the second victim. The doctor who makes the mistake needs help too. *BMJ*. 2000 Mar 18;320(7237):726–727.

39. Young M, Cruess SR, Cruess RL, Steinert Y. Do students and patients agree? Is a good clinician teacher seen as a good clinician? *Med Educ*. 2012;46(Suppl. 1):61.

COMMITMENT TO EXCELLENCE

6

LEARNING OBJECTIVES

1. To describe the challenges that physicians face in maintaining excellence over the life of their professional career.
2. To identify best practices that physicians should follow to successfully engage in lifelong learning.
3. To communicate the role of physicians in leading and working within teams to achieve excellent patient outcomes.
4. To explain the roles that different organizations and accrediting bodies take to help ensure that physicians are achieving excellence in their practice.

Dr. Amineh finished a busy day in her primary care office. Although most of her patients had routine concerns, several patients raised questions that she needed to look up in the literature. There was a dermatologic problem she couldn't identify. One of her patients had been started on a new insulin regimen by her endocrinologist; Dr. Amineh had been to a continuing medical education (CME) program that mentioned this approach but couldn't remember the details of how to adjust it or potential drug interactions. She hoped to get a few minutes at the end of the day after completing her chart notes to address these questions.

Despite widespread access to medical information on the Internet, people who fear that they are ill still turn to their trusted physicians for knowledge and wisdom as well as compassion. The trust they place in us is based on an assumption that all physicians live up to their professional commitment to excellence: a commitment to maintain the up-to-date knowledge and skills needed to treat their patients. The public believes that the highly selective and rigorous educational journey that physicians undertake to earn their MD degree has imbued them with the ability and the drive to maintain excellence over the life of their career. Every physician aspires to live up to this commitment. No one wants to be a good enough physician—we all want to be the best physician possible for our patients.

A commitment to strive for excellence is a key component of professionalism. As discussed in Chapter 3, A Brief History of Medicine's Modern-Day Professionalism Movement, expertise in a body of knowledge is the core of a profession, and the social contract between the public and the profession requires that physicians maintain this competency. Fulfilling this obligation begins in medical school with the mastery of foundational social, biomedical, and behavioral science principles. It continues in practice with a commitment to continuously seek out, analyze, and apply the best available science and evidence to make patient care decisions, to continuously update procedural and clinical skills, and to acknowledge personal limitations. It is important to note that excellence today means demonstrating accountability by willingly participating in formal competency assessments as well as measurement of patient care process and outcome measurements throughout, not just at the start of, your career as a physician (Cassel & Holmboe, 2006; Weiss, 2010).

A commitment to excellence also means working with others to pursue improvements in safety, quality, patient satisfaction, and value in care delivery within your local care environment and within the larger institutions in which you practice (i.e., hospitals and integrated care systems). In appropriate settings, excellent physicians support research and education because they recognize that the biomedical advances that expand our capacity to reduce the burden of suffering and disease are the result of decades of carefully conducted scientific studies and the educational programs that have disseminated those results. Finally, excellence means understanding and working with the spectrum of organizations charged with ensuring the quality of physicians and healthcare institutions.

We know that excellence is an aspirational goal—the knowledge base of medicine is so large that we can only do our best to keep up to date with information in our field of practice. But striving to do so represents professionalism in action.

EXCELLENCE AND THE INDIVIDUAL PHYSICIAN

The Challenges of Maintaining Excellence

Physicians who enter practice today can expect to practice for three, four, or even five decades. Maintaining excellence for such an extended period is a tremendous challenge in today's dynamic scientific environment. Scientific

Table 6-1	A SNAPSHOT OF THE DRAMATIC CHANGES IN MEDICAL CARE OVER THE LAST 40 YEARS	
Condition	1973	2013
Rheumatoid arthritis	Gold and high dose aspirin	Biologic response modifiers
Peptic ulcer disease	Antacids and surgery	Antibiotics and proton pump inhibitors
Advanced heart failure	Digoxin and diuretics	Angiotensin-converting enzyme (ACE) inhibitors, angiotensin receptor blockers (ARBs) Ultrafiltration Left ventricle assist devices Transplantation
Acute cholecystitis	Open cholecystectomy after several weeks of "cooling off"	Laparoscopic cholecystectomy within days
Suspected appendicitis	Exploratory laparotomy	Diagnostic ultrasound
Early stage breast cancer	Modified radical mastectomy	Lumpectomy and radiation therapy with adjuvant chemotherapy
Diabetes in hospitalized patients	Sliding scale insulin	Basal control with pre-meal supplementation
Red blood cell transfusion	Liberal	Conservative
HIV	Not recognized	Highly active antiretroviral therapy

advances can dramatically change preventive, diagnostic, therapeutic, and procedural standards of care, requiring physicians to continuously update their practice. For example, in the 1980s, peptic ulcer disease was considered a mechanical problem and treated with antacids and surgery; in 2000 it was recognized as an infection treated with antibiotics. Table 6-1 outlines examples of dramatic changes in standards of care over the last 40 years.

In addition to advances in scientific understanding of disease and therapies, our understanding of how physicians develop and maintain expertise over the life of their careers has changed. In the past, physicians believed lifelong learning involved simply setting time aside each day to scan the latest journals. Given the pace of clinical advances, we now know that this alone will not lead to continued mastery. For example, remaining current in the field of internal medicine is estimated to require reading 33 publications a day (Sackett, 2002). The belief that expertise develops as function of time in practice appears to be an outdated notion as well. Recent literature has demonstrated that, in fact, the longer a physician is in practice, the less likely they are to incorporate new evidence-based guidelines in the care of their patients (Choudhry, Fletcher, & Soumerai, 2005). New literature even challenges the paradigm of self-directed learning (Davis et al, 2006; Eva & Regehr, 2005). Like many other people, physicians are notoriously poor at identifying gaps in their understanding or competence. We tend to focus on studying those aspects of medicine that we find most interesting, often subjects that we have already mastered. We are hard wired to avoid content that is difficult or uninteresting to us (Eva & Regehr, 2008).

Experts in continuing medical education have outlined a several-step process, described below, for designing and implementing comprehensive programs to help physicians update their medical knowledge (Hager et al, 2008). Physicians can use this framework to structure their own learning experiences. These steps include recognizing an opportunity or need for learning; searching for resources for learning; engaging in learning; trying out what was learned; and incorporating what was learned into routine practice.

LEARNING EXERCISE 6-1

Reflect on your approach to maintaining professional excellence in the domains of knowledge and clinical problem solving.

1. What journals do you routinely read? Why? Have they changed over the life of your career? Do you discuss articles with colleagues in a formal way (such as in a journal club)?

2. How do you decide which articles to read? If you read an article that outlines a different approach to a problem that you see in your practice, how do you decide whether to change your practice based on that study? If you do think that a change in your approach is needed, how would you find the patients in your practice who might benefit from this new approach?

3. When you are seeing patients during your workday, how often do you look up information while the patient is in the office? What resources do you use when you need to look up something? How do you know that these are trusted resources? What do you do when there are conflicting reports about a given approach?

4. How often do you read articles that detail new understandings in basic science, such as genomics or systems biology?

---

1. Recognizing Opportunities for Learning

Opportunities for learning present themselves when physicians scan journal articles or attend a formal CME course and recognize that new information is available on a clinical topic relevant to their practice. Physicians frequently recognize opportunities for learning in the course of patient care, such as when:

- a patient asks a question that the physician cannot answer or brings information from the Internet that the physician has not seen previously;
- a patient on usual treatment fails to improve;
- a consultant recommends a strategy previously unknown to them;
- a patient is doing poorly possibly because of an incorrect initial diagnosis.

An opportunity for learning may also present itself when a performance audit done by the physician on his or her own practice or by an external entity (e.g., a health plan or hospital) demonstrates outcomes that are less than optimal.

Dr. Kevan couldn't believe what he was seeing. He had passed his surgical boards with flying colors just 5 years ago and now was settled into a wonderful small group practice in a suburb of a large city. He worked hard to stay abreast of the medical literature and practiced diligently in the simulation center of a local medical school to perfect the latest surgical techniques. Despite his personal commitment to excellence, the most recent report on surgical site infections and 30-day readmission rates for his service at the hospital were terrible. His initial reaction was to disregard the results. After all, as one of the youngest surgeons, he took care of more emergency cases and his patients were sicker than everyone else's. There was really nothing he could do, was there?

Physician level performance data exist on outcome measures such as patient satisfaction, process measures such as frequency of performing diabetic foot exams, safety measures such as completion of surgical checklists, and complication measures such as wound infections and readmissions. In the preceding example, the surgeon could participate in the American College of Surgeons National Surgical Quality Improvement Program (NSQIP) (http://site.acsn-sqip.org/). Individual physicians and physician groups are receiving feedback on their performance regularly. For example, a report card for an individual doctor is presented in Figure 6-1. The goal of these report cards is to motivate physicians to work to improve quality.

Although data suggesting that our performance is not as good as we had hoped should be viewed as an opportunity to learn and improve, the reality is many physicians respond defensively at first. Like Dr. Kevan, they may criticize the collection of the data ("They must be including patients seen by residents—my records don't reflect this level of performance"), or the choice

Sample Physician Report Card

Physician Names:	John Doe, MD
Group Name:	ABC Family Medicine
Specialty:	Family Medicine

| Reporting Time Period: | 01/1/11–12/31/11 |
| Reporting Date: | 03/31/12 |

	Your Score	Your Specialty's Average Score	Organization's Average Score
Administrative Measures			
Meeting Attendance	90	50	60
EHR Usage	100	75	80
Clinical Measures			
Childhood Immunizations	80	95	9
Mammography Screening	70	80	55
Colorectal Cancer Screening	95	65	75
Depression Screening	45	55	40
Utilization Measures - for Commercial Patients			
Admits/1000	180	165	146
Readmits within 30 days	4	13	18
ALOS (acute care)	5.6	4.4	4.1
ED Visits/1000	538	477	420
Disease Management Program Support			
No. of Active DM Patients	15	25	19
% of Eligible Pts enrolled in DM	65%	80%	68%
Participation in DM	C	B	C
Case Management Program Support			
# of Active CM Patients	4	15	n.a.
Participation in CM	C	B	C

Figure 6-1 ■ Sample physician quality report card.
Reprinted with permission from Grauman DM, Graham CJ, Johnson MM. 5 pillars of clinical integration. *Health Finance Manage.* 2012 Aug;66(8):70–77. Copyright Healthcare Financial Management Association.

of benchmarks ("It didn't adjust appropriately for case mix, my patients are sicker"), or the appropriateness of the standards ("I don't agree with those guidelines") (Ofri, 2010). Still others warn that measuring and publicizing quality may have unintended consequences, such as encouraging physicians to avoid caring for the sickest patients in an effort to improve their report cards (Ofri, 2010; Werner & Asch, 2005). Although these are important considerations, physicians striving for excellence realize the value of periodic measurement of their performance to help them prioritize and focus on their greatest opportunity for learning.

It is clear that on a given day, there may be dozens of opportunities for physicians to update their knowledge in response to these learning cues. To avoid overlooking a learning opportunity, many now advocate that physicians track these learning cues in a portfolio and periodically check to ensure that they have followed up to learn, at least about some of the questions (D'Alessandro, 2011; Van Tartwijk & Driessen, 2009).

LEARNING EXERCISE 6-2

1. Have you received any data about your performance as a physician, other than the results of your latest licensing or certifying examination? (If you have not received any performance data, what data would you like to receive? Who should provide it? Can you seek out this information?)

2. If so, what aspects of your performance were measured? Compliance with administrative policies (such as billing)? Patient volume? Patient satisfaction? Patient access? Compliance with evidence-based guidelines for prevention? Rates of infection?

3. When you received these data, what surprised you most?

4. Did you know how to respond if your data were not as good as you hoped they would be?

---

2. Finding Resources for Learning

The widespread availability of web-based resources has made it easier to find resources for learning but more challenging to separate high quality from low quality information. Physicians need to develop a way to recognize the best available evidence for the patient in front of them. Sackett (2002) describes different ways that physicians can carry out this responsibility. Some may choose to identify and personally appraise the quality of the primary literature by conducting a literature review and applying evidence-based medicine quality criteria to the publication. Others may choose to seek out evidence that has been critically evaluated by others with more expertise in critical appraisal by searching for information in reliable evidence-based medicine journals or collections such as The Cochrane Collaboration (http://www.cochrane.org/), BMJ Evidence Centre (http://group.bmj.com/products/evidence-centre), ACP Clinical Practice Guidelines (http://www.acponline.org/clinical_information/guidelines/guidelines/), or UpToDate (http://www.uptodate.com/), or replicate the practice of experts by locating and applying clinical practice guidelines.

> *Dr. Sarah Parelly was skeptical about clinical practice guidelines until she joined a committee of the American College of Cardiology (ACC) charged with creating a guideline for ablation therapy for atrial fibrillation. She had always thought of guidelines as cookbook medicine or crutches for weak physicians who just didn't keep up with the literature. But the process the committee engaged in was amazing. They scoured the literature, debated which studies were sufficiently robust to include, and anticipated clinical situations for which the guidelines weren't appropriate. The process also made her reflect on which aspects of her practice were based on solid evidence and which were based on expert opinion without strong evidence. She thought it might be feasible to build some of the guidelines into her practice's newly implemented electronic medical record.*

In choosing to use literature that has been appraised by others as their strategy for identifying the best evidence, physicians must be sure that the experts upon whom they are relying are truly expert, as free from conflicts of interest as possible, and that the evidence they are recommending is relevant to the patient in front of them. Over the last decade, the Accreditation Council for Continuing Medical Education has worked to ensure that presentations for which CME credit is granted are free from commercial influence (Steinman, Landefeld, & Baron, 2012).

Sometimes the available evidence may not be appropriate for or effective in a given patient. This is when the physician must use his or her understanding of the foundational science to develop a reasoned approach to management. Knowledge of science and evidence also enables the physician to identify and assess or construct different options for care when patients are reluctant or unable to pursue standard treatment. When no conclusive evidence exists to guide the treatment for a particular patient's condition, physicians should encourage the patient to seek opinions from national experts and to consider participation in reputable clinical trials (Institute of Medicine, 2011).

3. Engaging in Learning

Engaging in learning is a key element of the continuing education paradigm. Research has consistently shown that interactive learning experiences are much more likely to result in behavior change than are passive experiences like the standard grand rounds lecture (Hager et al, 2008). There are many ways that individual physicians can make their learning interactive. A physician who translates his or her clinical uncertainty about a patient into an answerable evidence-based medicine question and then seeks the answer is creating an interactive learning experience. Other methods including reading material followed by doing multiple choice questions to assess learning, or participating in a webinar and an asynchronous chat group to discuss the application of the presented content. Another alternative is reading and discussing articles and how to apply them to practice with a group of colleagues. All of these methods require interactive learning.

> *Dr. Robiak has been a practicing gynecologist for 20 years. Over the past year, she has been reading about the advantages of robotic surgery in gynecology and urology. Two months ago, she saw a demonstration at one of the national meetings she regularly attends. The hospital that she admits to has recently purchased a robot for gynecologic procedures. Yesterday, she called her local medical school and found that they would be offering a simulation course in robotic surgery next month. It would require a full week out of the office, but Dr. Robiak feels that she should really practice in a low risk setting to begin to acquire these skills. She knows that one of her community colleagues had a serious complication when he first started using the equipment; she hopes the simulation teaching can help her prevent this.*

Excellence is not only relevant to a physician's knowledge. Physicians must also continuously update their skills as new instruments and techniques replace the clinical and procedural skills they learned as residents. Here, too, advances in education have changed the way we view procedural competency. Rather than relying on the old strategy of "see one, do one, teach one," we now seek opportunities for physicians to practice and refine new techniques in simulated environments before attempting them on patients. Simulation centers offer active learning opportunities in invasive procedural skills with task trainers and virtual reality programs, and clinical reasoning with sophisticated, physiologically realistic computer mannequins. Specialized centers can offer procedural training using unembalmed cadavers and carefully managed animals. Emerging literature has shown that physicians trained with use of simulation perform better with fewer complications than those trained in the traditional method of practice on patients (Barsuk et al, 2012; Buchs et al, 2013; McGaghie et al, 2011; Wayne et al, 2008). Simulation also offers the opportunity for assessing physician competence when they apply for credentials at a new hospital or for a new procedure. Standardized patients could also be used to help practicing physicians master new patient-centered communication techniques such as shared decision making; however, this is an underutilized strategy in continuing medical education.

4. Trying Out and Incorporating What was Learned

Medicine is an applied science. It is not sufficient for a physician to declare that they have learned a new concept—they must apply that new concept in their practice for the benefit of their patients. The first attempts by a physician or group of physicians to implement new information into practice are often challenging, since old habits must be changed. It can be helpful to use decision-support tools such as guidelines embedded into electronic medical records (Ebell, 2010) or cognitive tools such as checklists (Spector et al, 2012; Weiser et al, 2010) to remind physicians of the desired changes. Over time, the frequency of reminders can decrease, as the "new" information becomes the standard operating procedure. Many have found utility in continuing to use these strategies to reinforce critical information, even after the initial period of learning has been completed.

> *Dr. Smith-Barnes is a hospitalist who recently attended a CME program on basal-bolus management of insulin. When he returned to the hospital, he worked with a local endocrinologist to develop a training program for his colleagues, including the internists and family physicians, to update their knowledge on insulin strategy (many are still using sliding scale insulin). In addition to giving everyone pocket cards to remind them of what they learned, he has worked with the electronic medical records experts in his hospital to replace the old insulin sliding scale orders with a new basal-bolus insulin dose calculator for adult patients.*

5. Understanding Personal Limitations and Tolerating Uncertainty

> *Dr. Nakano hesitated. One of his long-term patients, Mrs. Johansen had just told him that her son, Jan, had recently been diagnosed with advanced HIV and was coming home to live with her. She asked Dr. Nakano if he would be Jan's doctor when he moved back. Dr. Nakano had last cared for a patient with HIV infection a decade ago and he hadn't kept up with the latest antiretroviral agents. He told Mrs. Johansen that he would be willing to continue to provide coordination of care but that it would be important for her son to have the expertise of an HIV specialist to assist. He also said that he would try to update his own knowledge in changes in HIV management so he could support the HIV specialist in implementing appropriate treatments.*

Excellence sometimes means admitting that you are not the right physician for a specific patient, even if you have worked hard to remain current in your field. You might be asked to care for a patient with a condition that you do not know how to manage. The patient may need a procedure that, while you could do, you know is done more effectively by one of your colleagues. Alternatively, the patient may need care after you have been up for 24 hours and, although you know the patient, someone who is more rested may make better decisions. It can be difficult to admit your limitation to your patients and let them know that you must refer them to someone with different expertise. Patients may even try to reassure you that you are "good enough" for them and dismiss your concerns that your knowledge and skills may not be ideal for this circumstance. In this situation, living the values of excellence, altruism, and prudence means staying involved with your patient's care but arranging for someone else to take the lead on directing the optimal care plan, as Dr. Nakano demonstrates in this case.

Striving for excellence also requires the ability to tolerate uncertainty. Rarely will patients present with textbook findings, where everything fits perfectly together. Far more common are situations in which information is incomplete or conflicting, yet one has to make treatment plans and communicate clearly nonetheless. For example, practicing physicians know well the uncertainties that surround prognosis (Smith, White, & Arnold 2013). Even when good data exists (e.g., a given malignancy might have a documented survival rate of 75% at 1 year), there is so much variation that it is often impossible to know if your patient will be in the 75% that lives or the 25% that does not. Even more often, prognostication is difficult as many patients have multiple diseases and conditions, each with their own effects on survival. This degree of uncertainty is very difficult for both patients and physicians to deal with.

This concept—tolerance of ambiguity and uncertainty—is now becoming recognized as distinct required dimension for physicians' competence (Smith, White, & Arnold, 2013; Epstein & Hundert, 2002). The ability to deal with this type of uncertainty can vary substantially from person to person—some people appear to be far more comfortable with the grey areas than others are. Greater tolerance for uncertainty was found in students who went into psychiatry when compared to those that chose surgery as a career (Geller, Faden, & Levine, 1990). Medical students who were more willing to disclose their own uncertainty to standardized patients were rated higher on humanism (Rogers & Coutts, 2000). Thus learning how to better tolerate and communicate uncertainty is important. Indeed, some think this capacity is so important that it should be considered by medical school selection committees (Geller, 2013).

Measuring one's own tolerance for uncertainty or ambiguity can help lead to greater self-awareness and help physicians develop capacity to tolerate uncertainty. The most frequently cited scale was published in 1962 and is still used by medical schools today (Budner, 1962). It is easy to administer and is amenable to self-scoring and reflection.

Maintenance of Certification: Supporting an Evidence-Based Approach to Physician Excellence

It was a great day. Dr. McNamara just received notice that she had passed her recertification exam. She was surprised that she was as thrilled today as she was when she passed her first exam 30 years ago. Although she was not required to participate in the maintenance of certification program, she decided that as the director of a medical practice group that required recertification for all the new physicians, she should set a good example. She had been nervous about the secure examination, but she found that she learned a lot while she prepared for the exam. In fact, she recognized that she needed to make changes in her treatment of some common conditions including congestive heart failure and diabetes; the studying was going to improve her patient care.

In past years, graduation from a reputable school, training in an accredited program, and passing a board certification exam meant that a physician was considered to be excellent for life. "Once in, good for life" was a common way of thinking about medical education (Klass, 2007). Excellence now demands measurement and continuous improvement over the duration of a physician's career. With an awareness of both the challenges and best practices for lifelong learning, the American Board of Medical Specialties and its member boards have created and implemented a comprehensive program for maintenance of certification. These programs motivate physicians to periodically update their knowledge in the breadth of areas that constitute their specialty.

Simply demonstrating that you have adequate knowledge is no longer considered to be sufficient evidence that you are an excellent physician. The components of the Maintenance of Certification (MOC) program, summarized in Table 6-2 reflect the steps required for high quality continuing education. The self-evaluation modules provide a mechanism for active learning, allowing physicians to select content that is most relevant to their practice and then providing them with questions to help them measure their mastery of the content. The secure examination provides a drive for learning across the breadth of a physician's discipline, thereby preventing them from focusing only on areas within their field that they find interesting. The performance improvement modules create a way for physicians to recognize an opportunity

Table 6-2   **COMPONENTS OF MAINTENANCE OF CERTIFICATION**
Part I —Licensure and professional standing Medical specialists must hold a valid, unrestricted medical license in at least one state or jurisdiction in the United States, its territories, or Canada.
Part II—Lifelong learning and self-assessment Physicians participate in educational and self-assessment programs that meet specialty-specific standards that are set by their specialty board.
Part III—Cognitive expertise They demonstrate, through formalized examination, that they have the fundamental, practice-related, and practice environment-related knowledge to provide quality care in their specialty.
Part IV—Practice performance assessment They are evaluated in their clinical practice according to specialty-specific standards for patient care. They are asked to demonstrate that they can assess the quality of care they provide compared to peers and national benchmarks and then apply the best evidence or consensus recommendations to improve that care through follow-up assessments.

From American Board of Medical Specialties (ABMS). MOC Competencies and Criteria. Available at: http://www.abms.org/Maintenance_of_Certification/MOC_competencies.aspx.

for learning, engage in active learning, and incorporate new strategies into their practice. Recent studies have shown that some patients of physicians who participate in these comprehensive programs have better health outcomes (Holmboe et al, 2008; Simpkins et al, 2007; Turchin et al, 2008). The dedication of physicians to continuous learning on behalf of their patients is a marker of their commitment to excellence.

EXCELLENCE AND TEAMS

Teams and the Pursuit of Excellence in Clinical Microsystems

Kendall Rivera, a 3rd-year medical student, was surprised at what she saw on her new clinical assignment. She was rotating through an ambulatory primary care practice. This practice started each day with a huddle—a meeting of all people involved in the practice, including the doctors, nurses, medical assistants, and even the phone triage staff. The practice nurse, not one of the physicians, led this meeting. They first reviewed the list of patients coming into the office that day to be certain that the physicians had all the information they needed for their visit with the patient. Then they reviewed the practice's patient satisfaction numbers and identified that improvement was necessary. The nurse led a quick brainstorming session to generate ideas on how to improve patient satisfaction. They settled on a strategy that gave the physicians more time to talk with the patients by having someone else manage the electronic medical record documentation. They finished by agreeing to review the data again in 2 weeks to see if they were on a path to improvement. Although Kendall had expected to see teamwork, this was really teamwork—everyone's opinions, regardless of their educational background, seemed to matter and everyone was committed to making this the best practice possible.

It is important to note that in the twenty-first century, a physician's excellence is dependent not only on his or her personal mastery of essential knowledge and skills, but also on her effectiveness in working within the complex systems required to deliver care. The increasing prevalence of chronic disease and the increasing options for prevention, diagnosis, and treatment have dramatically increased the complexity of medical practice. Experts have estimated that, using the traditional physician-centric model of practice, it would take more than 10 hours each workday to just implement the evidence-based prevention guidelines in a typical primary care panel of patients. It takes an additional 3.5 hours to care for all patients in that panel who have stable and controlled chronic disease and another 7 hours to manage patients with uncontrolled chronic disease (Østbye et al, 2005; Yarnall et al, 2003). Clearly, this is an unsustainable model. The unsuitability of this model in today's healthcare world probably accounts for the observation that adults and children with access to care still receive less than 50% of the evidence-based care interventions (McGlynn et al, 2003).

Excellence requires embracing new models of care along with new biomedical advances. Physicians must set up, lead, and participate in team-based activities directed at improving all relevant outcomes in patient care, including those related to patients' experience of care. Practices are known as clinical microsystems that include healthcare professionals, processes, technology, and the patients they serve. Highly functional microsystems, like the one in which Kendall is learning, follow best practice guidelines for continuous quality improvement. They integrate quality improvement activities into the daily activities (Mohr & Batalden, 2002; Nelson, Batalden, & Godfrey, 2007). They expect everyone to take ownership of identifying problems, suggesting solutions, and participating in implementing strategies that may help improve the practice. Data are critically important in these clinical microsystems. Ideal practices have figured out how to use technology to collect, analyze, and compare data on practice and individual performance for use in the continuous improvement of care. Using data and ensuring that all on the team are working to the height of their competency to solve important problems requires new skills for many physicians. The benefit of learning these new skills is that the work done to serve patients can be shared among many. The literature suggests that the patient outcomes in these highly functioning clinical microsystems are better and the satisfaction of the members of the team is high.

Teams and the Work of Improving Patient Safety

Dr. Gorgas was scrubbing in on a case with the chief of surgery. A 4th-year resident, she was interested in staying on for a fellowship in hepatobiliary surgery once her residency was completed. It was important that she make a good impression on Dr. Laver. Twenty minutes into the liver transplant surgery, she saw the medical student accidentally contaminate Dr. Laver's sleeve. Dr. Gorgas was nervous about speaking up but she remembered that during the time out at the beginning of the procedure, Dr. Laver had encouraged all of them to speak up if they saw something unsafe. Somewhat tentatively, she said, "Dr. Laver, your sleeve has been contaminated, you'll need to re-gown." Dr. Laver grimaced behind her mask but then stepped away from the table and removed her gown. "Thanks!" she said. "This patient can't afford anything that increases his risk of infection. I want all of you to be as vigilant and direct as Dr. Gorgas."

The 1999 Institute of Medicine report, *To Err is Human*, called attention to the significant problem of errors in medical practice (Institute of Medicine, 2000) (see Chapter 5, Integrity and Accountability). They urged that the profession take a systems-based approach to preventing errors, recognizing that all humans (even physicians) are fallible and that we have a collective responsibility to protect our vulnerable patients from this fallibility. Teams play an essential role in ensuring that physicians deliver the safest care possible to their patients—one of the aims of excellence.

To be maximally effective in supporting safety, teams need to have a good culture of safety (Halligan & Zecevic, 2011; Pronovost et al, 2003). Characteristics of strong cultures of safety include stable team membership, respect for all roles, effective communication, and a flattened team hierarchy, which allow everyone to make recommendations for the benefit of the patient. Dr. Laver's team is exhibiting one behavior seen in a flattened hierarchy: a subordinate is praised for challenging or correcting the team leader. In a study done by the Harvard Business School, teams with a flattened hierarchy, as opposed to a traditional vertical hierarchy with a "big boss surgeon" at the top, learned how to do a new surgical procedure much more quickly and with fewer errors (Gawande, 2010).

Teamwork extends to people who collaborate outside of the operating room as well. Studies have assessed the "relational coordination" in practice groups and the association of this quality of the group with outcomes. Relational coordination is the extent to which professionals in the different roles have shared goals, shared knowledge, mutual respect, and communicate in a frequent timely and accurate matter (Gittell, Seidner, & Wimbush, 2010). Groups with high relational coordination solve problems together and share responsibility for errors or gaps in care. Recent studies on relational coordination have shown that patients cared for in settings where there was a high degree of relational coordination between all involved with a given patient throughout that patient's hospitalization (physicians, nurses, pharmacists, physical therapists, social workers, and others) had higher patient satisfaction and lower wound infection and readmission rates. Team-based excellence in today's world requires physicians who commit to learning and practicing skills in crisis communication, team development, and relationship coordination (Mitchell et al, 2012).

Teamwork in Support of Education and Research

Dr. Halima was thinking about how to respond to the phone call she had just received. A physician from the medical school near her practice called looking for preceptors for a new longitudinal clerkship model, as opposed to the traditional 1-month block, for 3rd-year medical students. They wanted her to take a student for one-half day a week for a year and help connect that student with a small panel of patients that the student could follow over the year. Dr. Halima loved to teach, but her practice productivity had suffered when she had a different medical student every month. Perhaps this new model would allow her to keep teaching.

Since the time of Hippocrates, physicians as a profession have accepted the responsibility to educate the next generation of physicians. The breadth and complexity of the content we must master and the substantial amount of judgment required to apply science in the human context make it difficult for anyone who is not already a physician to understand when someone has developed the necessary competencies to practice independently. Indeed, a key difference between a profession and trade is that the body of knowledge that must be mastered by a profession is so specialized that only those who are already within the profession can determine if mastery has been accomplished. Part of our commitment to excellence is the expectation that all physicians will work to provide educational opportunities for the next generation of physicians. Although the primary responsibility for education lies within our medical schools and academic medical centers, community-based physicians also play a key role. Community-based preceptorships enable students and residents to benefit from the practical wisdom of the practicing physician and to see a wider variety of patients than would be the case if their education was limited to the academic medical centers that coordinate educational programs. This is not a minor obligation. Agreeing to supervise a learner in a clinical workplace learning experience means agreeing to allow students to interact with your patients and staff, to find time to observe and coach them for improvement, and to evaluate their performance at the end of a rotation. All of these activities take time. Longitudinal rotations like the one in which Dr. Halima has been asked to participate, appear to provide better learning opportunities for the students because they form strong relationships with patients, staff, and physicians. Because the practice gets to know the student and their capabilities well, they can find ways for the student to contribute, rather than interfere, with the smooth functioning of the office (Poncelet et al, 2011; Teherani et al, 2009).

> *Dr. Kiminyo was a practicing oncologist working with several colleagues in a community practice. He belongs to a large National Institutes of Health (NIH)—supported community-based research collaborative that works to enroll patients with cancer into well-constructed clinical trials when there is no evidence-based treatment available for their particular clinical situation. He recently referred a patient with multiple myeloma to a clinical trial after standard chemotherapy had produced no improvement. He thinks it would be good for his partners to all participate in these trials but they are concerned about the "hassle" and overhead costs. He asks the group if they could dedicate one of their monthly meetings to a discussion on the topic so that they can collectively consider joining the research effort. Because they have a very busy practice, it might benefit some of their patients who fit into the subgroup of myeloma patients likely to benefit from this experimental treatment and might also contribute to addressing gaps in the literature.*

With the tremendous diagnostic and therapeutic strategies available to physicians today, it is sometimes easy to be lulled into a false sense that we know all there is to be known about medicine. However, in just the last 30 years, clinical research has been instrumental in extending the lives of patients infected with the HIV virus, minimizing disability in patients with rheumatoid arthritis, preventing cancer in patients infected with human papilloma virus, and achieving cures in leukemia and lymphoma, to name a few successes. At the same time, we continue to struggle to know how best to prevent or optimally treat many patients with acute and chronic diseases. It is clear that continued advances in medicine will require continued basic science and clinical trials to elucidate the mechanisms of disease and treatment and to propose and test new strategies for prevention, care, and cure. Physician scientists will undoubtedly serve as leaders in this area of excellence. Clinicians must be willing to collaborate with physician scientist colleagues to identify problems that need to be solved, participate in the ethical conduct of clinical trials, and advocate for community and governmental support of health-related research (Institute of Medicine, 2011).

EXCELLENCE AND HEALTH SYSTEMS

Systems Solutions to Enhance Safety and Quality of Care

When Dr. Bartok began working at the Manassett Valley Hospital as a hospitalist 3 months ago, he asked to join the Quality Council. During his residency program, he had participated in an educational program through the Institute for Healthcare Improvement (IHI). At his first Council meeting, he was assigned to participate in a root cause analysis of a serious transfusion error. Using tools from the IHI, Dr. Bartok and the rest of the root cause analysis team identified multiple problems that would require institutional investment to remedy. Today, he was scheduled to present their findings and advocate for a barcoding system. It was expensive but critically important.

LEARNING EXERCISE 6-3

1. Can you name a key quality initiative within your institution? Do you know how your institution is doing in terms of compliance with hand washing, decreasing central line infections, minimizing readmissions?

2. How involved are you in the development and implementation of care protocols in your practice or hospital?

3. How would you describe the culture of your institution? Would your peers welcome standardization of care processes?

Striving for excellent patient care demands physician expertise, high functioning teams, and institutional systems to support those physicians and teams (Bodenheimer, 1999). The literature on medical errors identifies two categories of errors: active errors, which are the result of human mistakes; and latent errors, which are management or administrative decisions that either precipitate human error or fail to protect patients from human error (Reason, 2000). Institutions across the country are using lessons learned from systems engineering and human factors science to retool their care delivery processes with a goal of minimizing latent error to achieve the highest quality care. Pioneering physicians, and the institutions in which they work, are using tools like Hardwiring Excellence, LEAN/Six Sigma, and Baldrige to tackle problems like hospital acquired infections (Mazzocato et al, 2010). As a result, many institutions have shown a dramatic decrease in these life-threatening complications (Shannon, 2011). For example, Intermountain Health System in Utah has reduced readmissions, improved quality and decreased costs by identifying best practices, evaluated local performance, employed principles of standardization, and provided feedback to physicians who are outliers (James & Savitz, 2011). This strategy, coupled with a culture that prioritizes engagement of physicians in front-line care in improvement initiatives, successfully decreased elective deliveries prior to 39 weeks (Oshiro et al, 2009). Systems strategies can be low cost, such as standardization of human performance, using checklists to prevent ventilator associated pneumonia, or timeouts before surgery to prevent wrong patient and wrong-sided procedures (Weiser et al, 2010). They can also be resource intensive, such as barcoding, implementation of electronic medical records, and extra staffing. Physicians committed to excellence understand the importance of seeking out, advocating for, and participating in systems strategies to enhance safety.

The Role of Accreditation, Licensing and Specialty Boards, and Organized Medicine in Advancing Excellence

There is a complex network of organizations that is working to support and assess physicians and institutions as they work to live their commitment to excellence, diagrammed in Figure 6-2.

Accrediting bodies, such as the Liaison Committee on Medical Education (responsible for overseeing undergraduate medical education programs) and the Accreditation Council for Graduate Medical Education (responsible for overseeing graduate medical education programs) set minimal standards for the conduct of training programs. Their role is to optimize the safety and

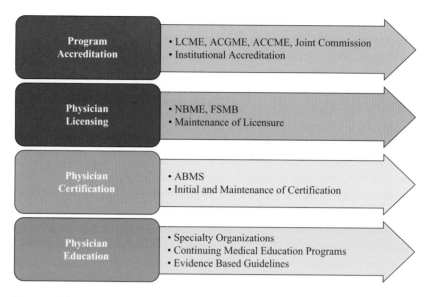

Figure 6-2 ▪ Complex collaborative of organizations supporting and assessing excellence in physician practice and healthcare delivery.

*LCME = Liaison Committee on Medical Education; ACGME = Accreditation Council for Graduate Medical Education; ACCME = Accreditation Council for Continuing Medical Education; NBME = National Board of Medical Examiners; FSMB = Federation of State Medical Boards; ABMS = American Board of Medical Specialties

effectiveness of the training environments. Led by physicians and expert administrative staff, these organizations have implemented many new standards, such as work hour restrictions and mandates on particular curricular themes, such as quality and safety (Nasca et al, 2010; Nasca et al, 2012; Swing et al, 2013). The Accreditation Council for Graduate Medical Education has implemented standards for educational programs offered to physicians (Steinman, Landefeld, & Baron, 2012). They have implemented stringent requirements to guard against inappropriate commercial support of educational offerings and to ensure that the programs for which physicians earn continuing education credit are educationally sound and effective. Systematic reviews have assessed the impact of continuing medical education (CME) in improving physician knowledge, attitudes, skills, performance, and patient outcomes (Mansouri & Lockyer, 2007; Marinopoulos et al, 2007; Satterlee, Eggers, & Grimes, 2008).

The Joint Commission is responsible for overseeing the quality of hospitals. They establish institutional requirements for safe and effective care. Their pioneering use of core measures has contributed to improved care for patients with myocardial infarction and ventilator-associated pneumonia, and other important conditions (Schmaltz, 2011).

State licensing boards have long been responsible for responding to complaints about physicians and setting minimum standards for lifelong learning by requiring licensing exams (provided by the National Board of Medical Examiners) and continuing medical education credits as a condition of licensure. The Federation of State Medical Boards is currently working to increase the rigor of lifelong learning for non–board certified physicians by developing a program known as maintenance of licensure (MOL) (Chaudhry et al, 2012).

The unified Boards of the American Board of Medical Specialties (ABMS) set the cognitive and procedural requirements for board certification, a marker of clinical expertise in a specific discipline. Physician experts work with evaluation experts to ensure that certified physicians—called diplomates—are appropriately assessed in the breadth and depth of their fields. ABMS Boards now all require diplomates to participate in maintenance of certification as a condition of retaining the credential of board certification. Increasingly, integrated health groups and hospitals are using board certification as a marker of excellence, requiring new physicians to remain board certified to remain employed or retain hospital privileges.

Physician specialty organizations have a long history of supporting excellence by establishing practice guidelines to support evidence-based care and presenting robust educational programs to assist their members in achieving and maintaining clinical excellence.The American College of Physicians Medical Knowledge Self-Assessment Program (MKSAP®) has been used by many generations of physicians to help them prepare for their certification exams. The American College of Radiology has established appropriate use guidelines for different radiologic imaging studies, and has recently led work to standardize radiation dosing during diagnostic imaging. The American College of Cardiology and the American Society of Clinical Oncology have developed extensive clinical practice guidelines to facilitate the evidence-based practice of the profession. Recently, dozens of physician specialty organizations have come together to support the Choosing Wisely campaign, aimed at reducing waste and harm to patients that results when physicians use unnecessary tests and treatments (Cassel, 2012) (see Chapter 7, Fair and Ethical Stewardship of Healthcare Resources). Table 6-3 summarizes additional examples in which physician-led specialty organizations work to support the professionalism value of excellence.

Table 6-3	**EXAMPLES OF PROJECTS AND PRODUCTS OF SPECIALTY ORGANIZATIONS THAT SUPPORT PHYSICIAN EXCELLENCE**
Specialty society	**Project or product description**
American Academy of Orthopaedic Surgeons	In the TeamSTEPPS Training Program, selected orthopaedic surgeons will serve as TeamSTEPPS trainers and will conduct workshops comprising orthopaedic surgeons, other physicians, and allied health professionals on effective team communication. (http://www.aaos.org/education/TeamSTEPPS/teamtraining.asp)
American College of Cardiology	The Hospital to Home (H2H) initiative is a national quality improvement campaign to reduce cardiovascular-related hospital readmissions and improve transitions from hospital to home. The program provides toolkits, webinars, and surveys. (http://www.h2hquality.org/)
American College of Physicians	The Medical Knowledge Self-Assessment Program (MKSAP®) provides up-to-date content on internal medicine and its subspecialties and self-assessment tools. (http://www.acponline.org/products_services/mksap/16/letter.htm)
American College of Radiology	The ACR Appropriateness Criteria® are evidence-based guidelines to enable referring physicians and others to make the most appropriate imaging or treatment decision for a specific clinical condition. They currently cover 186 topics. (http://www.acr.org/Quality-Safety/Appropriateness-Criteria)
American College of Surgeons	The ACS National Surgical Quality Improvement Program (ACS NSQIP®) provides a database of pre-operative to 30-day postoperative surgical outcomes based on clinical data. Participating institutions can access outcomes reports to assess and improve the quality and cost of surgical care. (http://inspiringquality.facs.org/about/acs-nsqip/)
American Society of Clinical Oncology	The ASCO Virtual Learning Collaborative will create a technology platform and learning network to disseminate evidence-based palliative care approaches in oncology. Participating medical oncology practices will participate in quality improvement projects and share best practices and resources. (http://www.asco.org/institute-quality/asco-virtual-learning-collaborative)

CONCLUSION

A commitment to strive for excellence is at the heart of professionalism. The behaviors of professionalism include a commitment to remain knowledgeable across a lifetime of practice, willingness to use evidence-based guidelines in the care of patients, recognition of the importance of scientific reasoning in situations for which evidence does not exist, acceptance of measurement of personal abilities and patient outcomes, acceptance of the importance of data-driven continuous improvement, and an understanding that excellence in today's health-care environment requires teams of professionals. Supporting the profession's commitment to excellence requires intense collaborative efforts on the part of individual physicians, the teams of which they are a part, the institutions in which they work, and the robust network of accreditation, licensing, certification, and educational organizations with which they come in contact.

CHALLENGE CASE

Dr. Wong is a 2nd-year resident in internal medicine who has been struggling on some of her rotations. Although she has passed all of them, her in-training evaluations put her in the bottom 10th percentile on a fairly consistent basis. She has received feedback and offers of coaching and tutoring, but since she hasn't failed anything she is not obligated to participate in extra work. Last week all the residents took part in a formative Objective Structured Clinical Examination (OSCE) and although it "doesn't count" toward a final grade, she did quite poorly and failed two stations. Her program director has called her in for another meeting. Dr. Wong seemed surprised that she didn't do well on the OSCE, but didn't think it mattered because it didn't count. She again reminded her program director, Dr. Gandhi, that she had passed all her rotations and she didn't see what all the fuss was about. Dr. Gandhi is concerned that this is a professionalism issue and is also worried about Dr. Wong's apathetic response. He wonders if there may be an underlying issue such as personal or family illness, or other stressors. He broaches this, but Dr. Wong states that she does not wish to talk about her personal life. At this point she starts getting defensive and asks if she can leave.

What professional challenges exist in this encounter?
There are several professional challenges here. Dr. Wong has not been doing well in terms of both clinical and academic performance, yet she has been resistant to remediation because she has technically passed all required elements. She doesn't seem to appreciate that barely passing—and being fine with it—runs counter to the profession's call to continually strive for excellence. She doesn't seem recognize that her knowledge and performance gaps can have real effects on patients, especially as she is entering her senior year, which includes less oversight and supervision. The program director also faces a challenge, in that it is true that technically she is passing required elements and he has no mandate to enforce remediation.

What role does the system have in this situation?
The evaluation system currently in place unfortunately allows for residents to squeak by, barely passing their rotations, and only mandates

remediation if there is a failure recorded. In fact, Dr. Gandhi wonders if this sends a hidden message to the residents that passing is all that matters. Furthermore, the formative nature of the OSCE makes it difficult for the program director to use it as an impetus to get Dr. Wong into remediation. These issues have made it difficult to convince the resident that there is a problem.

What might the program director do?
He might try again to appeal to Dr. Wong and try to convince her of the need for remediation. He could show her where she stands in relation to the rest of the class, so she might see more clearly that she is an outlier in need of improvement. He also might remind her of her future life as a professional and the effect that her knowledge and skill gaps might have on her future patients. It is also important for Dr. Wong to understand that all professionals need to have a plan to continually improve their skills throughout their career, no matter what their level is. Dr. Gandhi sharing his own strategies for keeping up to date could be a powerful teaching moment. He might even acknowledge that the current system does not support this message, but that it is a key concept of professionalism nonetheless. This may not be successful given her previous reluctance, but it is worth repeating the messages as they are so important. He also might try a different approach, such as asking a trusted colleague or the chief resident (perhaps of the same gender or background as Dr. Wong) to see if there are underlying issues that perhaps she would disclose to someone other than her program director.

Situational analysis: Dr. Wong is a resident who is struggling academically and who declines offers of assistance.

A helpful template for working through dilemmas is found in Chapter 2, Resilience in Facing Professionalism Challenges, Table 2-2.

Regarding Dr. Wong, this situation calls for:

Self-awareness (**recognizing personal emotions or triggers, understanding personal limitations in skills and knowledge**)
- Dr. Wong should realize that she is not performing to an acceptable standard, even though she is technically passing. She should also recognize by now that this issue has persisted and is unlikely to go away without something needing to change.

Self-regulation (**managing strong emotions, accessing assistance for complex tasks**)
- Dr. Wong is likely feeling vulnerable and exposed. She should ask for a moment to reflect and consider her situation and her options. This

would help avoid her instincts of "flight" and perhaps avoid her urge to "fight."

Social awareness **(recognizing the importance of considering the needs and state of all participants)**

- Dr. Wong will hopefully come to realize that Dr. Gandhi is really trying to help and has her best interests at heart. She realizes that he is concerned for good reason and that he is on her side.

Social regulation **(seek to identify more than one option for action, assume positive intent to understand others' behaviors, develop crisis communication strategies and negotiation skills, be empowered to coach others)**

- Dr. Wong should try to remain calm and really listen to Dr. Gandhi's concerns without resorting to defiance and anger. She should recognize that others' views of her abilities do not match up to her own, and she should respect their expert assessments. Ideally she should also come to realize that they are not trying to punish her but to help her improve—assuming this positive intent will help her accept their recommendations.

Actions

Both Dr. Wong and Dr. Gandhi take a few minutes to reflect on their own and then they restart the conversation. Dr. Gandhi says, "I know you have passed all of your rotations, but there have been persistent concerns about your performance both clinically and on the OSCE. I am concerned that you will continue to struggle and may not pass your board exams. Can you tell me what you think about what I've told you?" At this point Dr. Wong opens up and acknowledges that she has been concerned as well but has been too embarrassed to acknowledge her problems. She knows she's at risk of failing but thought she could remedy the situation on her own, by studying harder. This worked for her in medical school but doesn't seem to be cutting it these days. She just doesn't seem to know what to study and at what depth because the amount of material is so vast. She is also concerned about having "remediation" appear on her transcripts. Dr. Gandhi now presents an option—instead of framing it as remediation, he suggests that Dr. Wong receive "tutoring" from the chief resident who she gets along well with. They could work on the practical issues of how best to study and learn while working on a busy clinical rotation. Dr. Wong agrees to meet with the chief resident on a weekly basis, with progress reports going back to the program director. She will retake the OSCE in 3 months to assess her learning and improvement. She agrees that if she does not improve she will accept formal remediation. Dr. Gandhi thinks that this is an indication that Dr. Wong is learning that bare competence is not adequate and that our profession strives to achieve excellence.

Dealing with systems issues

As program director, Dr. Gandhi realizes that the system in place is inadequate. He decides to get involved in the program's remediation committee and helps to draft new guidelines for borderline but passing residents. These new guidelines state that residents who are passing but consistently in the bottom 10% of their cohort (e.g., over more than two rotations) can be mandated to receive an official remediation plan.

KEY LEARNING POINTS

1. Keeping up to date is a lifelong process that requires recognizing opportunities for learning, finding learning resources, actively engaging in learning, incorporating the new learning into practice, and tolerating personal limitations and uncertainty.
2. Participation in certification and maintenance of certification is a structured program that supports excellence and is widely viewed as part of physicians' accountability to the public.
3. Healthcare professionals work in teams, embedded in clinical microsystems. These teams are critically important to seeking the use of best evidence and striving for the best outcomes for patients.
4. Healthcare systems can implement systems solutions through information technology, quality improvement strategies, and so on, to support best practices.

REFERENCES

1. American Board of Medical Specialties (ABMS). MOC Competencies and Criteria. Available at: http://www.abms.org/Maintenance_of_Certification/MOC_competencies.aspx
2. Barsuk JH, Cohen ER, Vozenilek JA, O'Connor LM, McGaghie WC, Wayne DB. Simulation-based education with mastery learning improves paracentesis skills. *J Grad Med Educ*. 2012 Mar;4(1):23–27.
3. Bodenheimer T. The American health care system—the movement for improved quality in health care. *N Engl J Med*. 1999 Feb 11;340(6):488–492.

4. Buchs NC, Pugin F, Volonté F, Morel P. Learning tools and simulation in robotic surgery: state of the art. *World J Surg.* 2013 May 3 [Epub ahead of print].

5. Budner S. Intolerance of ambiguity as a personality variable. *J Pers.* 1962 Mar;30:29–50.

6. Cassel CK, Guest JA. Choosing wisely: helping physicians and patients make smart decisions about their care. *JAMA.* 2012 May 2;307(17):1801–1802.

7. Cassel CK, Holmboe ES. Credentialing and public accountability: a central role for board certification. *JAMA.* 2006 Feb 22;295(8):939–940.

8. Chaudhry HJ, Talmage LA, Alguire PC, Cain FE, Waters S, Rhyne JA. Maintenance of licensure: supporting a physician's commitment to lifelong learning. *Ann Intern Med.* 2012 Aug 21;157(4):287–289.

9. Choudhry NK, Fletcher RH, Soumerai SB. Systematic review: the relationship between clinical experience and quality of health care. *Ann Intern Med.* 2005 Feb 15;142(4):260–273.

10. D'Alessandro MP. Connecting your radiology learning to your clinical practice: using personal learning environments, learning portfolios and communities of practice. *Pediatr Radiol.* 2011;41(Suppl 1):S245–S246.

11. Davis DA, Mazmanian PE, Fordis M, Van Harrison R, Thorpe KE, Perrier L. Accuracy of physician self-assessment compared with observed measures of competence: a systematic review. *JAMA.* 2006 Sep 6;296(9):1094–1102.

12. Ebell M. AHRQ White Paper: use of clinical decision rules for point-of-care decision support. *Med Decis Making.* 2010 Nov-Dec;30(6):712–721.

13. Epstein RM, Hundert EM. Defining and assessing professional competence. *JAMA.* 2002 Jan 9;287(2):226–235.

14. Eva KW, Regehr G. Self-assessment in the health professions: a reformulation and research agenda. *Acad Med.* 2005 Oct;80(10 Suppl):S46–S54.

15. Eva KW, Regehr G. "I'll never play professional football" and other fallacies of self-assessment. *J Contin Educ Health Prof.* 2008 Winter;28(1):14–19.

16. Gawande A. *Complications: A Surgeon's Notes on an Imperfect Science.* London, UK: Profile Books; 2010.

17. Geller G. Tolerance for ambiguity: an ethics-based criterion for medical student selection. *Acad Med.* 2013 May;88(5):581–584.

18. Geller G, Faden RR, Levine DM. Tolerance for ambiguity among medical students: implications for their selection, training and practice. *Soc Sci Med.* 1990;31(5):619–624.

19. Gittell JH, Seidner R, Wimbush J. A relational model of how high-performance work systems work. *Organization Science.* 2010 March-April;21(2):490–506.

20. Grauman DM, Graham CJ, Johnson MM. 5 pillars of clinical integration. *Healthc Financ Manage.* 2012 Aug;66(8):70–77.

21. Hager M, Russell S, Fletcher SW, Macy J Jr. *Continuing Education in the Health Professions: Improving Healthcare Through Lifelong Learning.* New York, NY: Josiah Macy, Jr. Foundation; 2008.

22. Halligan M, Zecevic A. Safety culture in healthcare: a review of concepts, dimensions, measures and progress. *BMJ Qual Saf.* 2011 Apr;20(4):338–343.

23. Holmboe ES, Wang Y, Meehan TP, Tate JP, Ho SY, Starkey KS, Lipner RS. Association between maintenance of certification examination scores and quality of care for Medicare beneficiaries. *Arch Intern Med.* 2008 Jul 14;168(13):1396–1403.

24. Institute of Medicine. *Public Engagement and Clinical Trials: New Models and Disruptive Technologies: Workshop Summary.* Washington, DC: National Academies Press; 2011.

25. Institute of Medicine. *To Err is Human: Building A Safer Health System.* Washington, DC: National Academy Press; 2000.

26. James BC, Savitz LA. How Intermountain trimmed health care costs through robust quality improvement efforts. *Health Aff (Millwood).* 2011 Jun;30(6):1185–1191.

27. Klass D. A performance-based conception of competence is changing the regulation of physicians' professional behavior. *Acad Med.* 2007 Jun;82(6):529–535.

28. Mansouri M, Lockyer J. A meta-analysis of continuing medical education effectiveness. *J Contin Educ Health Prof.* 2007 Winter;27(1):6–15.

29. Marinopoulos SS, Dorman T, Ratanawongsa N, Wilson LM, Ashar BH, Magaziner JL, Miller RG, Thomas PA, Prokopowicz GP, Qayyum R, Bass EB. Effectiveness of continuing medical education. *Evid Rep Technol Assess (Full Rep).* 2007 Jan;(149):1–69.

30. Mazzocato P, Savage C, Brommels M, Aronsson H, Thor J. Lean thinking in healthcare: a realist review of the literature. *Qual Saf Health Care.* 2010 Oct;19(5):376–382.

31. McGaghie WC, Issenberg SB, Cohen ER, Barsuk JH, Wayne DB. Does simulation-based medical education with deliberate practice yield better results than traditional clinical education? A meta-analytic comparative review of the evidence. *Acad Med.* 2011 Jun;86(6):706–711.

32. McGlynn EA, Asch SM, Adams J, Keesey J, Hicks J, DeCristofaro A, Kerr EA. The quality of health care delivered to adults in the United States. *N Engl J Med.* 2003 Jun 26;348(26):2635–2645.

33. Mitchell P, Wynia M, Golden R, McNellis B, Okun S, Webb CE, Rohrbach V, Von Kohorn I. *Core Principles & Values of Effective Team-Based Health Care. Discussion Paper.* Washington, DC: Institute of Medicine; 2012. Available at: www.iom.edu/tbc

34. Mohr JJ, Batalden PB. Improving safety on the front lines: the role of clinical microsystems. *Qual Saf Health Care.* 2002 Mar;11(1):45–50.

35. Nasca TJ, Day SH, Amis ES Jr; ACGME Duty Hour Task Force. The new recommendations on duty hours from the ACGME Task Force. *N Engl J Med.* 2010 Jul 8;363(2):e3.

36. Nasca TJ, Philibert I, Brigham T, Flynn TC. The next GME accreditation system—rationale and benefits. *N Engl J Med.* 2012 Mar 15;366(11):1051–1056.

37. Nelson EC, Batalden PB, Godfrey MM. *Quality By Design: A Clinical Microsystems Approach.* San Francisco, CA: John Wiley & Sons; 2007.

38. Ofri D. Quality measures and the individual physician. *N Engl J Med.* 2010 Aug 12;363(7):606–607.

39. Oshiro BT, Henry E, Wilson J, Branch DW, Varner MW; Women and Newborn Clinical Integration Program. Decreasing elective deliveries before 39 weeks of gestation in an integrated health care system. *Obstet Gynecol.* 2009 Apr;113(4):804–811.

40. Østbye T, Yarnall KS, Krause KM, Pollak KI, Gradison M, Michener JL. Is there time for management of patients with chronic diseases in primary care? *Ann Fam Med.* 2005 May-Jun;3(3):209–214.

41. Poncelet A, Bokser S, Calton B, Hauer KE, Kirsch H, Jones T, Lai CJ, Mazotti L, Shore W, Teherani A, Tong L, Wamsley M, Robertson P. Development of a longitudinal integrated clerkship at an academic medical center. *Med Educ Online.* 2011 Apr 4;16.

42. Pronovost PJ, Weast B, Holzmueller CG, Rosenstein BJ, Kidwell RP, Haller KB, Feroli ER, Sexton JB, Rubin HR. Evaluation of the culture of safety: survey of clinicians and managers in an academic medical center. *Qual Saf Health Care.* 2003 Dec;12(6):405–410.

43. Reason J. Human error: models and management. *BMJ.* 2000 Mar 18;320(7237): 768–770.

44. Rogers JC, Coutts L. Do students' attitudes during preclinical years predict their humanism as clerkship students? *Acad Med.* 2000 Oct;75(10 Suppl):S74–S77.

45. Sackett DL. Clinical epidemiology: what, who, and whither. *J Clin Epidemiol.* 2002 Dec;55(12):1161–1166.

46. Satterlee WG, Eggers RG, Grimes DA. Effective medical education: insights from the Cochrane Library. *Obstet Gynecol Surv.* 2008 May;63(5):329–333.

47. Schmaltz SP, Williams SC, Chassin MR, Loeb JM, Wachter RM. Hospital performance trends on national quality measures and the association with Joint Commission accreditation. *J Hosp Med.* 2011 Oct;6(8):454–461.

48. Shannon RP. Eliminating hospital acquired infections: is it possible? Is it sustainable? Is it worth it? *Trans Am Clin Climatol Assoc.* 2011;122:103–114.

49. Simpkins J, Divine G, Wang M, Holmboe E, Pladevall M, Williams LK. Improving asthma care through recertification: a cluster randomized trial. *Arch Intern Med.* 2007 Nov 12;167(20):2240–2248.

50. Smith AK, White DB, Arnold RM. Uncertainty--the other side of prognosis. *N Engl J Med.* 2013 Jun 27;368(26):2448–2450.

51. Spector JM, Agrawal P, Kodkany B, Lipsitz S, Lashoher A, Dziekan G, Bahl R, Merialdi M, Mathai M, Lemer C, Gawande A. Improving quality of care for maternal and newborn health: prospective pilot study of the WHO safe childbirth checklist program. *PLoS One.* 2012;7(5):e35151.

52. Steinman MA, Landefeld CS, Baron RB. Industry support of CME—are we at the tipping point? *N Engl J Med.* 2012 Mar 22;366(12):1069–1071.

53. Swing SR, Beeson MS, Carraccio C, Coburn M, Iobst W, Selden NR, Stern PJ, Vydareny K. Educational milestone development in the first 7 specialties to enter the next accreditation system. *J Grad Med Educ.* 2013 Mar;5(1):98–106.

54. Teherani A, O'Brien BC, Masters DE, Poncelet AN, Robertson PA, Hauer KE. Burden, responsibility, and reward: preceptor experiences with the continuity of teaching in a longitudinal integrated clerkship. *Acad Med.* 2009 Oct;84(10 Suppl):S50–S53.

55. Turchin A, Shubina M, Chodos AH, Einbinder JS, Pendergrass ML. Effect of board certification on antihypertensive treatment intensification in patients with diabetes mellitus. *Circulation.* 2008 Feb 5;117(5):623–628.

56. Van Tartwijk J, Driessen EW. Portfolios for assessment and learning: AMEE Guide no. 45. *Med Teach.* 2009 Sep;31(9):790–801.

57. Wayne DB, Didwania A, Feinglass J, Fudala MJ, Barsuk JH, McGaghie WC. Simulation-based education improves quality of care during cardiac arrest team responses at an academic teaching hospital: a case-control study. *Chest.* 2008 Jan;133(1):56–61.

58. Weiser TG, Haynes AB, Lashoher A, Dziekan G, Boorman DJ, Berry WR, Gawande AA. Perspectives in quality: designing the WHO Surgical Safety Checklist. *Int J Qual Health Care.* 2010 Oct;22(5):365–370.

59. Weiss KB. Future of board certification in a new era of public accountability. *J Am Board Fam Med.* 2010 Mar-Apr;23 Suppl 1:S32–S39.

60. Werner RM, Asch DA. The unintended consequences of publicly reporting quality information. *JAMA.* 2005 Mar 9;293(10):1239–1244.

61. Yarnall KS, Pollak KI, Østbye T, Krause KM, Michener JL. Primary care: is there enough time for prevention? *Am J Public Health.* 2003 Apr;93(4):635–641.

FAIR AND ETHICAL STEWARDSHIP OF HEALTHCARE RESOURCES

7

LEARNING OBJECTIVES

1. To understand the rationale for physicians to address the stewardship of finite resources.
2. To understand the dilemma physicians experience in caring for individual patients and simultaneously considering the use of resources.
3. To learn specific communication skills for conducting conversations with patients about unnecessary tests or treatments.
4. To learn the roles of teams, healthcare systems, and professional organizations in stewardship of finite resources.

Donna Johnson is a 40-year-old woman who is the CEO of a small manufacturing company. Her job is stressful and she has a long history of headaches, but recently she feels the headaches are increasingly frequent despite her efforts to manage them with stress reduction. She has a neighbor who recently was diagnosed with a malignant brain tumor who also had headaches, and she is asking her family doctor, Dr. Hernandez, to order a computerized tomography (CT) scan to be sure she does not have a tumor.

Dr. Hernandez takes a detailed history and rules out any other neurologic symptoms. Her complete physical examination, including a careful neurologic examination, is all normal. Dr. Hernandez concludes that these are tension headaches and discusses this with the patient. Ms. Johnson would like a CT scan just to be 100% sure, but

Dr. Hernandez does not think it is clinically indicated. Furthermore, the test is expensive, even though the patient has insurance that would cover it. Dr. Hernandez thinks to herself that it is just easier to order the test than try to explain the risks and benefits to a worried patient.

Every day physicians make many decisions about whether to order, or not to order, laboratory tests and imaging procedures. This scenario and similar scenarios are very common in daily practice. Patients with symptoms are worried and want their physicians to use the best of medical science to quickly diagnose and treat a problem or to reassure them that nothing serious is wrong. Some believe that tests and x-rays are perfectly accurate and humans are not, so they equate an order for a test as better care than a careful clinical examination. Consumer advertising and Internet sites recommending non–evidence-based tests and treatments reinforce these beliefs.

Physicians worry as well. Test ordering can be driven by a physician's concern that they might miss an important diagnosis and cause their patient unnecessary suffering. Worry that declining to order an unnecessary test might negatively affect their patient's satisfaction may also prompt decisions to obtain tests that are not truly indicated. Belief that test ordering represents the standard of care and thus is a defense against malpractice claims also drives this behavior. It is safe to say that we have a "more is better" view of medical testing, even when we know that these tests do not add value to patients' care and when these tests may even have some risks for patients. Even more concerning is the reality that current strategies in healthcare financing often make it more lucrative for some physicians, and the institutions that employ them, to order tests of marginal or no benefit than to guard against this approach.

Stewardship of valuable resources is a complex topic in professionalism. It is clearly unprofessional to order tests that are unnecessary simply because the physician will earn more money if they do so and probably unprofessional to routinely order tests as a strategy to protect against personal injury from a malpractice claim. Yet, ordering tests of marginal or no benefit to allay concerns, avoid missed diagnoses, and comply with patient requests (or demands) may seem compatible with professionalism values of prudence, and respect for patient autonomy. However, ordering unnecessary tests and treatments that are unlikely to yield benefits and may cause physical harm to patients (such as radiation exposure or antibiotic-associated diarrhea) or adverse financial consequences for patients (such as out-of-pocket expenses) is counter to the professionalism values of excellence and nonmaleficence. In addition, spending valuable national resources on unnecessary tests and treatment, leaving less money for improving quality, increasing access for the underserved, and targeting complex problems of the social determinants of health is contrary to our professional commitment to social justice.

In this chapter, we tackle the complex professionalism decisions that physicians need to make in their day-to-day work with patients. We discuss the rationale for physicians to care about the use of finite resources. We use the professionalism framework to illustrate behaviors that can be demonstrated by individual physicians, the healthcare team, the healthcare setting, and professional organizations in order to manage limited resources wisely.

WHY SHOULD WE CARE ABOUT HEALTHCARE SPENDING?

The problem of the rising and unsustainable cost of healthcare is a pressing issue in all developed countries. The total healthcare expenditure as a percentage of the gross domestic product (GDP) has been rising in many countries over the last decades; the United States spent 7.4% of GDP on health in 1970, 11.9% in 1990, and 16.0% in 2008. Estimates are that this will rise to 20% by 2020 (Keehan et al, 2011; Shatto & Clemens, 2011)—a figure that is unacceptable if society hopes to have resources for other social goods including education, environmental issues, and public safety. Part of this relentless increase in expenditures is a consequence of the tremendous biomedical advances of the last century; the availability of new diagnostic and therapeutic options has increased the number of people who live longer. However, some of the drivers of healthcare expenditures relate to the administrative complexity and fragmentation of care that characterize our healthcare system. Countries with more coordinated care, better primary care services, and financial mechanisms to control cost (Figure 7-1) spend a lower percentage of GDP on healthcare than the United States does. For example, in 2008 Canada spent 10.4% of GNP on healthcare and the United Kingdom spent 8.7%, compared to 16% in the United States.

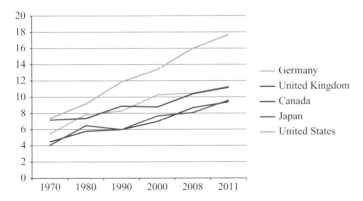

Figure 7-1 ■ Total health expenditures as a percentage of gross domestic product (GDP), 1970–2008.

From Organisation for Economic Co-operation and Development (OECD). Health expenditure: Total expenditure on health, % gross domestic product, 2013. http://www.oecd.org/els/healthsystems/oecdhealthdata2013frequentlyrequesteddata.htm.

	Infant mortality, Per 1000 live births[a]	Life expectancy at birth (years)[a]		Life expectancy at age 65 (years)[a]		Mortality amendable to healthcare, 2002-3, deaths per 100,000 population[b]
		Men	Women	Men	Women	
Germany	3.6	78.4	83.2	18.2	21.2	90
United Kingdom	4.7	79.1	83.1	18.6	21.2	103
Canada	4.9	78.7	83.3	18.5	21.6	77
Japan	2.3	79.4	85.9	18.7	23.7	71
United States	6.1	76.3	81.1	17.8	20.4	110

Table 7-1   **HEALTHCARE OUTCOMES**

From (a) Organisation for Economic Co-operation and Development (OECD). Health expenditure: Total expenditure on health, % gross domestic product, 2013. http://www.oecd.org/els/health-systems/oecdhealthdata2013-frequentlyrequesteddata.htm.
(b) Nolte E, McKee CM. Measuring the health of nations: updating an earlier analysis. Health Aff (Millwood). 2008 Jan-Feb;27(1):58–71.

What makes this high spending in the United States even more unacceptable is that health outcomes are not better but actually worse than in the countries that spend less. Measures used to assess quality of care by the Organisation for Economic Co-operation and Development (OECD) include infant mortality rates, life expectancy at birth, life expectancy at age 65 years, and mortality amenable to healthcare (a measure intended to assess the functioning of the healthcare system). On many of these measures the United States performs least well (Table 7-1). For example, infant mortality rates are 6.7 per 1000 live births in the United States, compared to 5.1 in Canada and 3.5 in Germany in 2008. Life expectancy for a man is 3 years lower in the United States compared to Canada. Simply stated, we spend more, but do not have better outcomes for the population.

Despite the high expenditures on healthcare in the United States, many Americans do not have access to medical care. Surveys demonstrate that approximately 25% of Americans did not get a prescribed medication, test, or treatment due to their lack of ability to pay for it. In 2009, 51 million Americans were lacking any form of health insurance (U.S. Census Bureau, 2010, page 22); a number that has been steadily rising over the last three decades. Poorer Americans are less likely to have health insurance than wealthy Americans. In addition, 62% of all people filing for personal bankruptcy cite high healthcare costs and 25% of citizens over 65 who file for bankruptcy identify out-of-pocket healthcare expenses as a major cause for their financial problems, despite the fact that they are enrolled in Medicare (Bodenheimer & Grumbach, 2012).

Of great concern is the observation that much of the vast amount of money poured into the U.S. healthcare system is not well spent and does not add value to care. Studies estimate that 30% of our healthcare expenditures can be attributed to waste; duplicative, non–evidenced-based or harmful tests or treatments (Berwick & Hackbarth, 2012). The aphorism that the most expensive medical device is the physician's pen (or keyboard in today's environment) is true: 80% of all healthcare expenditures are driven by physician decisions. Economists estimate that if we could increase the value of our healthcare expenditures to rival our world peers, our expenses would go down by 15% to 30% and we could use those dollars to achieve better healthcare and better social conditions for all.

One way of dealing with rising healthcare costs would be to have payers and regulators simply cut reimbursement rates and deny expenditures. This approach, initiated by stakeholders outside of the profession, could result in rationing by denying people needed care. Instead, ethicists and physician leaders have suggested that the profession should solve the problem of high costs and low values, using the values of professionalism. Instead of worrying about rationing, we should be focusing on reducing waste—eliminating care that does not confer a benefit and, in some circumstances, may result in harm. Diverting the dollars spent on waste to improving our society's access to care that is reliably safe, effective, and high quality is an aspirational goal that should be motivating to all physicians.

IS STEWARDSHIP OF VALUABLE RESOURCES A WAY OF JUSTIFYING RATIONING AT THE BEDSIDE?

Dr. Green is a 3rd-year internal medicine resident. At morning rounds, he presents a case of an 83-year old patient admitted the previous night with a recurrent episode of congestive heart failure due to ischemic cardiomyopathy. Dr. Green presents the details of the history, physical examination, and the results of initial investigations, including cardiac magnetic resonance imaging (MRI). The attending cardiologist inquires about why Dr. Green ordered the MRI and whether it was helpful to the care.

Training shapes professional practice patterns. Studies show that physicians who are trained in high-quality environments learn patterns of care that influence their future practice in positive ways. For example, Asch and colleagues (2009) found that the obstetrical training program where a physician trained was associated with the physician's maternal complication rates in practice. Women treated by obstetricians trained in residency programs in the bottom quintile for risk-standardized major maternal complication rates had an adjusted complication rate of 13.6%, approximately one third higher than the 10.3% adjusted rate for women treated by obstetricians from programs in the top quintile. The Dartmouth Atlas, which describes variations in the quality of care between hospitals, has recently published a report entitled, "What kind of physician will you be? Variation in healthcare and its importance for residency training" (Arora & True, 2012). This report emphasizes that residents shape their ideas about what it means to be a good physician by emulating the behavior of the supervising attending physicians and by responding to cues in the environment. Dr. Green's decision to order an MRI may be prompted by a specific diagnostic question (perhaps there were findings suspicious of amyloidosis on the patient's exam). Alternatively, he may be ordering the test because her prior attending physicians included it in their "usual" workup of cardiomyopathy patients and did not convey to him what constituted a "usual" case that justified the MRI. Hospital reimbursement may favor rapid discharge of patients, and hence residents are counseled to pay attention to length of stay. Dr. Green may believe that ordering the test now, before he discusses the case with the attending physician, may shorten the patient's time in the hospital. He may also be ordering the MRI because he is interested in learning more about cardiac MRI and doesn't realize the cost that the patient will bear because of his curiosity. In fact, the reason the indirect medical education component of Medicare payment to hospitals exists is because of the assumption that care provided by residents includes some waste in the form of excess tests and treatment delays. In short, the culture in many medical training programs encourages trainees to order unnecessary tests, and the patterns learned in residency training may influence future practice of physicians.

IF PROFESSIONALISM INCLUDES STEWARDSHIP OF VALUABLE RESOURCES, WHY IS THE TOPIC SO RARELY DISCUSSED IN EDUCATION AND IN PRACTICE?

One simple answer is that the actual costs of care are often hidden from the view of the physicians and their patients. Even less transparent is how much a specific patient will be charged for care, what part of that charge their insurer will pay, and how much they will personally be required to pay. Some experts in cost-conscious care have urged physicians to manage this problem of cost confusion by taking the approach of "universal financial precautions." Modeled on the same principles as universal precautions for blood-borne illness, universal financial precautions urge physicians to assume that each patient in front of them is one major diagnostic test away from bankruptcy. A recent randomized trial demonstrated that physicians who saw the cost of tests as they ordered them (with no other intervention) decreased their ordering resulting in a 10% saving (Feldman et al, 2013).

More difficult to navigate is the perceived conflict between the professionalism values of patient welfare and social justice. Some physicians believe that even a negative test provides useful information, and that discussions of cost in the care of individual patients is contrary to the primacy of patient welfare. They argue that considering social justice while caring for an individual patient may be construed as rationing at the bedside. A resolution of this perceived conflict between patient-centered professionalism values and society-centered professionalism values can be achieved, if one considers the reality of diagnostic testing and treatment decisions. Commitment to care for the individual patient can be fulfilled if the physician is equally concerned with avoiding errors of commission (those that result from ordering diagnostic tests or treatments of questionable value) and simultaneously errors of omission (those that result from not ordering indicated tests and treatments). The decision to order only evidence-based tests and treatments protects patients from the harm that may result when false-positive results lead to additional, often more invasive, tests (e.g., when cumulative radiation exposure increases the risk of cancer; and when seemingly benign antibiotics and corticosteroids cause rare, but disabling complications).

Some physicians also express concern about patient autonomy, as many patients may wish us to order certain tests and request that we do so. Ethicists tell us that, in contrast to liberty, autonomy is not absolute. Autonomy must be exercised with information and understanding. Supporting the principle of respect for patient autonomy means that the physician educates, informs, and counsels patients about the evidence-based choices available to them. It does not mean complying with patient demands for non–evidenced-based care. With these frames, the physician can maintain patient-centered professionalism, while they address their society-centered commitments to steward valuable resources.

In fact, we believe that we are at a time of a significant shift from a prior culture of caring for just one patient to a newer view of concurrent broader societal perspective. Below, we discuss the roles that each part of the system—individual patient and physician, the team, the healthcare setting, and professional organizations—can play in shepherding finite resources to provide the highest quality of care for the greatest number of patients. We also provide specific strategies for conducting conversations with patients about the choice of ordering (or not ordering) tests and procedures.

LEARNING EXERCISE 7-1

1. Think of a recent time when a patient asked you to order a test that you thought was not indicated medically.
2. What were your thoughts about ordering or not ordering the test?
3. What factors did you consider? Were there factors favoring and opposing ordering the test?
4. Did you discuss the issues with the patient? Was the outcome of that conversation satisfactory?

PHYSICIAN–PATIENT INTERACTION

John King is a 36-year-old man who works as a contractor. He comes in to see his family doctor with a 1-week history of low back pain, which is interfering with his ability to work; in fact, he has missed 5 days from work. The pain started after Mr. King lifted a heavy pail and twisted his back. He is frustrated because he does not get paid if he is not at work, but he is very uncomfortable, especially when he bends forward. The pain is disturbing his sleep; he wakes when he rolls over in bed. He has no radiation of the pain into his legs. He has not had any change in his bowel or bladder function. He requests a CT of his back so that he can "figure out the problem and get back to work sooner."

Dr. Deyo examines Mr. King and finds no evidence of any neurologic signs in his legs. He is aware of the literature indicating that imaging is not indicated in the absence of neurologic symptoms or signs, particularly with a short (less than 6-week) history of pain. Although he knows that the CT is not indicated, he also knows from experience that it takes time to explain the reason the test is not indicated and sometimes patients leave his office unhappy when they didn't get the test they requested. He is already behind in his schedule and the office staff has encouraged him to hurry up if he can.

This is a very common situation for practicing physicians in all specialties. Patients request treatments and tests that are not indicated—antibiotics for an upper respiratory tract infection, stress electrocardiography to check for coronary disease, and so on. Dr. Deyo's reflection on this situation is also common: Is it worth the effort to explain the rationale for not ordering the test? Is it just more expedient to order the CT despite the lack of necessity? He knows the conversation will take some time and that not all patients accept the explanation. Furthermore, Dr. Deyo may think that if he does not order the test now, the patient will just go to another doctor to get the CT, making the whole exercise futile. Even worse, they might complain about him on a public Web site, like Angie's List or Yelp, and that may make other patient's doubt his competency and compassion (Ginsburg, Bernabeo, & Holmboe, 2013; Ginsburg et al, 2012).

Explaining the rationale for not ordering the imaging study can be done efficiently using specific communication skills. We use the situation above to illustrate the communication steps involved in explaining that a requested test is not necessary, accompanied by sample words a physician might use. Obviously these words are embedded in a longer back and forth conversation between the physician and patient.

1. After listening carefully to the patient's concern, specifically state an understanding of the patient's situation and validate his feelings (i.e., express empathy).
   Example: *"I can understand why the back pain is really frustrating to you. Not only is it painful, but your income depends on getting back to work. Do I have that right?"*
2. State the goal that the physician and patient share in common.
   Example: *"We both want to try to get your pain under control and get you back to work as quickly as possible."*
3. Provide clear recommendations in lay language and without jargon.
   Example: *"Usually low back pain improves in a few weeks with the muscles recovering and that is what will likely happen for you. In the meantime, it is good to keep moving, rather than staying in bed, and we can try to control the pain with safe and effective medication. You will likely be able to go back to work soon with this approach."*
4. Explain why the requested test is not useful or even harmful if applicable.
   Example: *"Back x-rays, like a CT scan, don't help in this situation. Studies show that patients with acute back pain and no abnormalities on physical examination, like you, don't benefit from x-rays and, in fact, there is some risk from unnecessary radiation from CT scans. It is best to avoid that risk if possible."*
5. Check to see what the patient thinks or what concerns remain.
   Example: *"What do you think of this approach? What remaining concerns do you have?"*

This approach will inevitably not be effective with every patient, but since this type of request is so common, it is important for physicians to be skilled in conducting this type of conversation. Researchers from the Drexel University College of Medicine have developed instructional videos to teach physicians how to communicate in these challenging situations. The videos are based on lists of medical tests and procedures that physicians and patients should question, lists that specialty societies developed for the Choosing Wisely campaign (further information on the campaign will follow). The video modules include a generic scenario and others (Table 7-2) tailored to different specialties, using illustrative examples of common situations encountered in the field. A sample instructional tape can be found at www.modules.choosingwisely.org.

However, the learning of effective communication skills is best done by practice and preferably observed by a colleague who can provide feedback.

Table 7-2	COMMON TOPICS IN DISCUSSING TESTS AND TREATMENTS WITH PATIENTS
Specialty	Module topics
Allergy, asthma, and immunology	• Patient seeking antibiotics to treat viral sinusitis • Patient seeking gamma globulin treatment to boost immune system • Patient seeking further tests on chronic urticaria
Cardiology	• Patient seeking preoperative stress test • Patient seeking stress test years after coronary bypass surgery • Low-risk patient seeking stress test
Family medicine	• A patient with sinusitis who requests antibiotics • Exercise stress test in low-risk patient • Imaging for a patient who suffers back pain
Generic scenarios	• Headache sufferer requests imaging study • Patient with back pain who requests an MRI
Internal medicine	• Patient requests check-up with ECG stress test • Patient requests chest x-ray for preoperative evaluation • Patient with vasovagal syncope requests brain CT • Resident requests from Attending to do a CT angiogram to exclude pulmonary embolism
Nephrology	• Pros and cons of dialysis • Patient request for routine cancer screening while on dialysis • Discussion about PICC line with residents
Pediatrics	• Call with mother who is asking for antibiotics for her child with an upper respiratory infection • Mother requests CT after her child has a head injury
Radiology	• Radiologists discuss best imaging study in a child • Radiologists discuss imaging in low risk pulmonary embolism • Radiologists discuss proceedings for small ovarian cyst

From ABIM Foundation. Choosing Wisely. Available at: http://www.choosingwisely.org/.

Alternatively, communication skills can be practiced with simulated patients. Similar to other procedural skills, learning of communication skills requires repeated use, as well as reflection on what worked well and what aspects need modification.

An additional resource that can be helpful to physicians and patients has been developed by *Consumer Reports*. *Consumer Reports* has produced materials, in collaboration with medical specialty societies, that physicians can give to patients who request tests or treatments that are not necessary, such as imaging studies for uncomplicated low back pain. These materials are designed for patients and written in lay language. They present a variety of topics explaining the evidence, or lack thereof, for tests, and the alternative treatments that may be useful. The materials explain the potential side effects of treatments and procedures and provide specific information about when these tests are indicated. For example, the materials on low back pain explain why imaging is often not required, but also what signs and symptoms would indicate the need for the MRI. A sample patient information sheet is presented in Figure 7-2. All of the patient information material is available at http://consumerhealthchoices.org/.

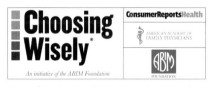

Choosing Wisely®
An initiative of the ABIM Foundation

ConsumerReportsHealth

AMERICAN ACADEMY OF FAMILY PHYSICIANS

ABIM FOUNDATION

Imaging tests for lower-back pain
When you need them—and when you don't

Back pain can be excruciating. So it seems that getting an X-ray, CT scan, or MRI to find the cause would be a good idea. But that's usually not the case, at least at first. Here's why.

They don't help you get better faster.
Most people with lower back pain feel better in about a month whether they get an imaging test or not. In fact, those tests can lead to additional procedures that complicate recovery. For example, a study that looked at 1,800 people with back pain found that those who had imaging tests soon after reporting the problem fared no better and sometimes did worse than people who took simple steps like applying heat, staying active, and taking an OTC pain reliever. Another study found that back-pain sufferers who had an MRI in the first month were eight times more likely to have surgery, and had a five fold increase in medical expenses—but didn't recover faster.

They can pose risks.
X-rays and CT scans expose you to radiation, which can increase cancer risk. One study projected 1,200 new cancers based on the 2.2 million CT scans of the lower back performed in

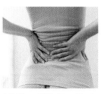

the U.S. in 2007. While back X-rays deliver less radiation, they're still 75 times stronger than a chest X-ray. That's especially worrisome to men and women of childbearing age, because X-rays and CT scans of the lower back can expose testicles and ovaries to radiation. And the tests often reveal spinal abnormalities that could be completely unrelated to the pain. For example, one study found that 90 percent of older people who reported no back pain still had spinal abnormalities that showed up on MRIs. Those findings can cause needless worry and lead to

unnecessary follow-up tests and procedures such as injections or sometimes even surgery.

They're often a waste of money.
An X-ray of the lower back ranges from about $200 to $290, an MRI from $880 to $1,230, and a CT scan from $1,080 to $1,520, according to HealthcareBluebook.com. Imaging also accounts for a big chunk of the billions Americans spend on lower back pain each year, not only for the tests themselves, but also the unnecessary interventions they trigger.

When do imaging tests make sense?
It can be a good idea to get an imaging test right away if you have signs of severe or worsening nerve damage, or a serious underlying problem such as cancer or a spinal infection. Red flags that can make such testing worthwhile include a history of cancer, unexplained weight loss, fever, recent infection, loss of bowel or bladder control, abnormal reflexes, or loss of muscle power or feeling in the legs. In other cases, you probably don't need an imaging test for at least several weeks after the onset of your back pain, and only after you've tried the self-care measures described at right.

USING THIS INFORMATION
[small print block]

Published by Consumer Reports © 2012 Consumers Union of U.S., Inc., 101 Truman Ave., Yonkers, NY 10703-1057. Developed in cooperation with AAFP. [...]

Consumer Reports Advice
How should you treat lower-back pain?

Most people get over back pain in a few weeks, and these simple steps might help.

• **Stay active.** Resting in bed for more than a day or so can cause stiffness, weakness, depression, and slow recovery.

• **Apply heat.** A heating pad, electric blanket, or warm bath or shower relaxes muscles.

• **Consider over-the-counter medicines.** Good options include painrelievers such as acetaminophen (Tylenol and generic) or anti-inflammatory drugs such as ibuprofen (Advil and generic) and naproxen (Aleve or generic).

• **Sleep comfortably.** Lying on your side with a pillow between your knees or on your back with a few beneath them might help.

• **Talk with your doctor.** If symptoms don't improve after a few days, consider seeing a doctor to make sure that the problem doesn't stem from a serious underlying health problem. If the pain is severe, ask about prescription painrelievers.

• **Consider alternatives.** If you don't feel better after four weeks or so, it might be worth talking with your doctor about other options, including physical therapy, chiropractic care, yoga, massage, acupuncture, cognitive-behavioral therapy, and progressive muscle relaxation. More invasive choices, such as surgery, should be considered only if those other treatments don't help.

Figure 7-2 ■ Patient-friendly resource from specialty societies and consumer reports sample.

TEAMS AND STEWARDSHIP OF RESOURCES

Dr. Shah is a dermatologist who is seeing a 32-year-old woman referred by her family doctor because of diffuse hair loss on her head over the last 4 months. The woman notices that hair is coming out more than it used to when she showers, and she finds hair on her pillow in the morning. Dr. Shah suspects that this may be due to one of the common causes for hair loss—either low total body iron stores or hypothyroidism. He wants to order a thyroid-stimulating hormone (TSH) and serum ferritin, but the patient says that her family doctor did a number of blood tests and thinks these were included. Dr. Shah asks the patient to wait while his office staff tries to reach the family doctor to get the results of the tests. Although it might be faster to order them again at the local laboratory, he thinks this is wasteful.

In addition to individuals, teams also have a major role to play in the stewardship of finite resources. Although the costs of a few relatively inexpensive blood tests may seem inconsequential, the redundancy does cause waste. Dr. Shah's solution is the correct one at the moment, but it can be difficult to implement because it takes precious time for office staff to make a phone call and try to find laboratory results. Often family physicians and specialists care for patients together, but lack the infrastructure to make communication efficient and reliable for the team of caregivers. In the long term, Dr. Shah and her colleagues should work to identify ways to improve the system, so that a patient's test results, problem lists, and medication lists are available to all physicians who might need them—and hence avoid duplicative and wasteful care. Physicians who work in integrated healthcare systems may find it easier to orchestrate strategies, like shared electronic medical records. Physicians who are practicing independently may need to work with their referring and referral colleagues to create new models of communicating important information, either by ensuring that the patient carries his or her information with them, or by standardizing referral forms within a community.

In 2001, the report entitled "Crossing the Quality Chasm," by the Institute of Medicine, compared the U.S. healthcare delivery system to a railroad whose tracks change gauge every few miles. "Healthcare is composed of a large set of integrating systems—paramedic, emergency, ambulatory, inpatient, and home healthcare; testing and laboratories, pharmacies and so forth" (Institute of Medicine, 2001). It is not surprising that it is nearly impossible to coordinate care across all these locations and that chasms in quality of care occur in these transitions. There has been increasing attention paid to the transitions in care between hospitals and outpatient settings where gaps are well documented. In addition, in any particular healthcare setting, patients are managed by a variety of providers, but frequently there are gaps in communication between members of the team. For example, hospital teams "hand off" care between shifts. Each of these transitions is high-risk for patients—often one provider does not know what the last provider knew or what they did for the patient. The patient safety movement has helped to highlight the importance of good hand-offs between sites and between providers, and tools have been developed to optimize these transitions. For example, checklists can be useful to ensure full transfer of information, particularly at the time of discharge from the hospital (Table 7-3).

Not only do these discontinuities between sites and between providers lead to gaps in the quality of care, but they also lead to increased financial costs and wasted resources. Physicians may order certain medications not realizing that the prior team changed or stopped those drugs. They may repeat tests not knowing that the test was already done or that the results are pending. Lack

Table 7-3 **A CAREGIVER DISCHARGE CHECKLIST**
Discharge medications
Review with patient
Highlight changes from hospital
Specifically inform patient about side effects
Discharge summaries
Dictate in a timely fashion
Include discharge medical (highlight changes from admission)
List outstanding test and reports that need follow-up
Give copies to all providers involved in the patient's care
Communication with patient/family
Provide patient with medication instructions, follow-up details, and clear instructions on warning signs and what to do if things are not going well
Confirm that patient comprehends your instructions
Include a family member in these discussions if possible
Communication with the primary physician
Make telephone contact with primary care physician prior to discharge
Follow–up plans
Discharge clinic
Follow-up phone calls
Appointments or access to primary providers

From Wachter RM. *Understanding Patient Safety*. 2nd ed. New York, NY: McGraw Hill Professional; 2012, p. 136.

of computerized linkages between sites makes good communication difficult. However, a particularly costly consequence is readmission to the hospital after a recent discharge. A study by Jencks, Williams, and Coleman (2009) found that 20% of Medicare patients are readmitted within a month of discharge and one-third return within 90 days. These authors estimate that the cost of preventable readmissions is $17 billion per year. Additional studies find gaps in quality at discharge: 45% of patients have tests pending and many of these are never completed; 15% have significant discrepancies in their medication lists; and discharge summarizes rarely reach the primary care provider by the time of the first post-discharge visit. Increasing attention to preventing readmissions, and financial penalties in some settings, is leading to efforts to share best practices to prevent readmission. Novel and creative approaches range from discharge checklists, to special teams of providers to provide intensive management post-discharge. Although the more intensive approaches can be expensive to implement owing to the human resources needed to create these new coordinating teams, the hope is that they will prevent expensive return emergency department visits and readmissions. There is some emerging evidence of their effectiveness (Hansen et al, 2011; Epstein, Jha, & Orav, 2011).

Specialists at a large urban hospital are trying to reduce avoidable visits to the emergency department (ED). They are frustrated by some family doctors who seem to send their patients to the ED frequently. In order to explore the reasons for this, they ask the hospital to help them do a needs assessment and visit the offices of these family doctors. What they learn surprises them. The family doctors are also frustrated, because they don't want to send patients to the ED. However, patients with multiple problems come to their office late in the day with symptoms that need relatively urgent investigation or care from specialists. Because the specialists' phone lines are closed by 4:30 or 5:00 pm, they can't get the advice they need for urgent patient problems and so they send patients to the ED to get urgent care. If they could talk to a specialist and make an alternative plan for the next day, they could avoid the ED visit. The specialists agree to create ONE phone number that their family doctor colleagues can call to get urgent advice. The hospital agreed to collect data to assess the number and sources of ED referrals before and after the implementation of the new program.

This is another example of a team of physicians taking leadership to solve a problem and develop a local strategy to prevent ED visits. The solution required the physicians to consider the care of patients beyond their own offices and to reach out to the family doctors to find out how they saw the issue. With this information, they created a new approach that was cost-effective and feasible. In this case, the solution can both improve the quality of care for patients and simultaneously avoid wasted ED visits and cost.

> *Dr. Hopper-Jones is a 3rd-year resident in neurology. She took part in a novel quality improvement elective working with physicians, nurses, and administrators of the neurology intensive care unit. They identified that the use of intravenous nicardipine for management of blood pressure following hemorrhagic hypertensive strokes was much greater in one of the hospitals they rotated through than in all of the other hospitals. The team reviewed the latest evidence on post-stroke blood pressure management, mapped the process of blood pressure management, and analyzed patient characteristics in each hospital. They found that the high-nicardipine-use hospital only changed blood pressure medications once a day. They implemented a rapid cycle quality improvement project where blood pressure was assessed and medications were adjusted twice a day. Within 2 months, the use of nicardipine trended down, patient outcomes were improved, and the hospital was on target to saving $500,000 a year from reduced drug costs.*

The use of structured quality improvement processes that involve interprofessional teams is critically important to the success of this project. Benchmarking of care metrics, reviewing the published literature, and measuring all important outcomes (quality, satisfaction, and cost) help ensure that changes in care processes are offered as a way to improve care, not just reduce costs. We believe that it is important for teams to gear their efforts toward improving quality of care, a component of which is the efficiency of care. In our experience, healthcare professionals are most likely to engage in efficiency when evidence-based measures of quality of care are central to the considerations—cost savings alone are less likely to engage their efforts. The illustration of the neurology resident is important for another reason;

LEARNING EXERCISE 7-2

1. Think of one process that you and your team colleagues do frequently and that you think is inefficient and wasting resources (human or financial resources).

2. What do you need to measure to assess the extent of the problem?

3. Who would need to be involved in the discussion to consider the data and potential approaches to improve it?

4. What would the barriers to change be in your setting and how could they be ameliorated?

residents are well-positioned to lead, with the support of hospital administrators, quality improvement efforts that improve efficiency. Residents are well aware of the inefficiencies in the system, and often learn to use "work-arounds" to handle them. We find that residents are often enthusiastic about participating in solutions to these inefficiencies.

THE ROLE OF HEALTHCARE SYSTEMS IN FAIR AND ETHICAL USE OF RESOURCES

Healthcare systems can demonstrate their commitment to professionalism in the domain of the fair and ethical use of resources in a variety of ways. Several of the prior examples related to managing finite resources are systems problems. For example, the lack of shared electronic health records (EHRs) across different settings in a region is a systems issue best solved by a regional health unit, hospital, and the affiliated physician offices, or by an integrated delivery system. The implementation of one EHR, while difficult in any setting, is easier in a single integrated healthcare system. However, the Centers for Medicare & Medicaid Services recently created an Office of the National Coordinator for Health Information Technology that provides financial incentives for healthcare systems to implement effective information technology. They set standards for elements of an information technology solution, like an EHR, that meet their criteria for financial federal support. Evidence suggests that use of an EHR can improve the quality of care; for example, care for diabetes was significantly higher quality at community practices with EHRs compared to sites using paper records (Cebul et al, 2011). However, whether there are truly cost savings from implementing these information systems is still unclear. The implementation on an EHR is one example of how a healthcare system can demonstrate its commitment to professionalism—both in the value of "pursuit of excellence" and in the use of finite resources. There are many other examples of healthcare system professionalism in this domain; for example, providing data on variation in outcomes and cost of care to providers, implementing incentives that support integration of care across settings and providers, or adopting clinical decision support that includes information about value and costs of tests and procedures.

PHYSICIAN ADVOCACY AND PROFESSIONAL ORGANIZATIONS

The CEO of the American College of Cardiology is asked to participate in an Institute of Medicine panel discussion on the rising cost of care and "waste" in the medical system. Each medical society, like the American College of Cardiology, is asked to consider the tests or procedures that its members do frequently or routinely that may not add value to the care of patients, and that add unnecessary cost. The CEO realizes that cardiologists do many tests, often as part of routine practice, that may be unwarranted. Yet, he also knows that these tests may generate significant revenue for the cardiologists. How can he raise this issue without his own society members feeling that he is undermining their financial best interest? Who is his primary responsibility—patients, cardiologists, or broader society? Whose interest comes first if they are in conflict?

Leaders have a particular responsibility to use the power of their organizations to encourage and support physicians to do the right thing. These organizations have the respect of their members and a long tradition of providing continuing medical education. This positive track record allows the societies to provide leadership in educating physicians about both evidence-based standards for care and issues of value in care.

The Choosing Wisely campaign, launched in 2012 by the ABIM Foundation, leverages and builds on the professionalism and leadership of physician organizations and their members. The campaign is based on the ideas of ethicist and physician Dr. Howard Brody, who encourages physicians to shift the conversation from the highly controversial use of the term "rationing" (making choices about how to limit care even if that care is appropriate) to the more accurate and appropriate language of "avoiding waste" (Brody, 2012). In this view, each patient should receive what is best evidence-based care for their condition based on his or her own values and choices, but should not receive tests or procedures where evidence shows they don't add benefits and may even harm patients. Unnecessary procedures, especially invasive procedures, can harm patients by side effects or complications. Savings from such unnecessary procedures can, theoretically and hopefully in practice, be directed to benefit services for a larger number of patients.

The goal of the Choosing Wisely campaign was to catalyze conversations between patients and their physicians about the overuse of tests, procedures, and treatments. As part of the campaign, physician specialty societies (n = 50) were asked to identify a list of "Five Things Physicians and Patients Should Question" based on specific, evidence-based data. As mentioned earlier in the chapter, *Consumer Reports* partnered with Choosing Wisely and developed materials designed to help patients engage in these conversations. Lists focused on commonly performed tests or procedures that are often used, but that do not benefit patients and may even cause harm. Each of the lists is simple and succinct. The list of the American Academy of Family Physicians is presented in Figure 7-3.

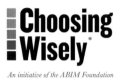

American Academy of Family Physicians

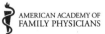

Five Things Physicians and Patients Should Question

Don't do imaging for low back pain within the first six weeks, unless red flags are present.

Red flags include, but are not limited to, severe or progressive neurological deficits or when serious underlying conditions such as osteomyelitis are suspected. Imaging of the lower spine before six weeks does not improve outcomes, but does increase costs. Low back pain is the fifth most common reason for all physician visits.

Don't routinely prescribe antibiotics for acute mild-to-moderate sinusitis unless symptoms last for seven or more days, or symptoms worsen after initial clinical improvement.

Symptoms must include discolored nasal secretions and facial or dental tenderness when touched. Most sinusitis in the ambulatory setting is due to a viral infection that will resolve on its own. Despite consistent recommendations to the contrary, antibiotics are prescribed in more than 80 percent of outpatient visits for acute sinusitis. Sinusitis accounts for 16 million office visits and $5.8 billion in annual health care costs.

Don't use dual-energy x-ray absorptiometry (DEXA) screening for osteoporosis in women younger than 65 or men younger than 70 with no risk factors.

DEXA is not cost effective in younger, low-risk patients, but is cost effective in older patients.

Don't order annual electrocardiograms (EKGs) or any other cardiac screening for low-risk patients without symptoms.

There is little evidence that detection of coronary artery stenosis in asymptomatic patients at low risk for coronary heart disease improves health outcomes. False-positive tests are likely to lead to harm through unnecessary invasive procedures, over-treatment and misdiagnosis. Potential harms of this routine annual screening exceed the potential benefit.

Don't perform Pap smears on women younger than 21 or who have had a hysterectomy for non-cancer disease.

Most observed abnormalities in adolescents regress spontaneously, therefore Pap smears for this age group can lead to unnecessary anxiety, additional testing and cost. Pap smears are not helpful in women after hysterectomy (for non-cancer disease) and there is little evidence for improved outcomes.

Figure 7-3 ▪ Specialty society list of five things physicians and patients should question (for physicians) sample.

From Copyright Consumers Union of U.S., Inc. Yonkers, NY 10703-1057, a nonprofit organization. Reprinted with permission of Consumer Reports® for educational purposes only. www.ConsumerReports.org

For example, both the American College of Physicians (internists) and the American Academy of Family Physicians listed the use of imaging tests for the investigation of low back pain. Both organizations said that in the absence of "red flags" in the history or physical examination, imaging (plain radiography or CT) should not be done, as these tests do not improve patient outcomes, but do expose patients to unneeded x-ray radiation.

This is a clear example of leadership from the medical profession, using the professionalism of its members and their commitment to provide evidence-based care tailored to the needs of patients to address the important responsibility to steward finite resources.

ETHICAL USE OF RESOURCES

In this chapter, we have focused on the stewardship of finite resources to illustrate professionalism in the value of "fair and ethical use of resources." However, we could also have explored the roles of individual physicians, teams, healthcare settings, and professional organizations in improving the *fairness* of the use of resources. The Agency for Healthcare Research and Quality (2012) regularly publishes a "National Healthcare Disparities Report." The reports document the disparities in quality of care based on ethnic and racial groups—consistently demonstrating lower quality in minority and low-income patients. Figure 7-4 presents key results from 2011.

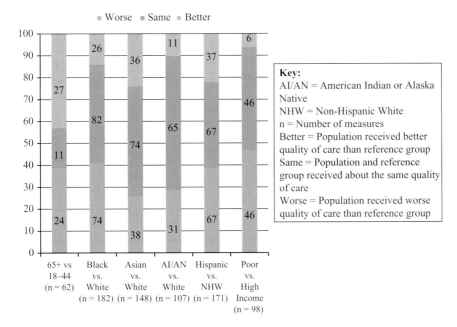

Figure 7-4 ■ Number and proportion of all quality measures for which members of selected groups experienced better, same, or worse quality of care compared with reference group.

Credit: Agency for Healthcare Research and Quality. National Healthcare Disparities Report 2011. Rockville (MD); 2012. Available at: www.ahrq.gov/qual/qrdr11.htm.

In the framework for professionalism, each player in the system (medical students, residents, practicing physicians, nurse practitioners, physician assistants, teams, the healthcare setting, and the professional organization) can demonstrate their commitment to improve these disparities. Physicians and teams can ensure that they have the ability to meet the needs of their non–English-speaking minority patients. Healthcare settings can develop programs to identify people in their communities who may not seek needed care due to language and financial barriers, and develop ways to facilitate needed care. Although a full discussion on "fair care" is beyond the scope of this chapter, the principles are similar to the previous discussion related to the use of finite resources.

LEARNING EXERCISE 7-3

1. Is there a group of patients in your practice, or in your community, that may be receiving lower quality of care than other groups? Think of differences based on race, ethnicity, income, gender, or age.
2. What data can you feasibly collect to examine potential differences?
3. Whose help do you need to collect this data?
4. Based on the data, what stakeholders could work together to address the findings to both understand the barriers and develop plans for improvement?

| CONCLUSION

Traditionally, physicians have considered their responsibility as caring for the individual patients they see and have not considered their role to be stewards of just distribution of finite resources. In 2002, the *Physician Charter* articulated the responsibilities of physicians to *both* the individual and to society more broadly. We observe a real and significant change in the attention of physicians and medical organizations to the principle of social justice and the use of finite resources in a fair and ethical way. The Choosing Wisely campaign, and the very large number of medical societies participating, seems to us to be a major and favorable change in the views and actions of physicians in this domain. However, the challenges are still large, both in the need for medicine to address the unsustainable cost of care and to address the persistent and troublesome disparities in care based on race and income. These challenges truly require a commitment all stakeholders to shape a fair and sustainable future.

CHALLENGE CASE

Dr. Garcia recently completed her cardiology fellowship and joined a large group of cardiologists practicing in a midsize city about 30 miles from the medical school where she did her training. She is training in interventional cardiology and recently passed her certification examination in both cardiology and interventional cardiology. After a month in the new practice, she is noticing that several of her partners are doing invasive procedures more than she would have expected. When she cross-covered for one of them recently, she thought that a particular patient had undergone a relatively risky procedure without the indications supported by the existing literature. Furthermore, at a recent group meeting, one of the senior cardiologists presented some of the financial data on the performance of the group that showed that the practice had produced less revenue over the last 6 months than prior. He encouraged the cardiologist to try to improve this situation so that they did not need to lay off staff.

What professionalism challenge exists in this case?
The cardiologist faces several professionalism challenges. Although she does not have systematic data about the patients in the practice, she thinks that the practice patterns of her colleagues may be outside of "best practices" for invasive procedures. She wants to ensure high quality of care for the patients cared for by the group (they could be exposed to unnecessary harm from risky procedures), but she also wants to be seen as a "good colleague" and she doesn't know if the culture in the group welcomes (or might discourage) questioning each other regarding their clinical practices. At her previous medical center, difficult patient cases were discussed at case conferences, but this is not the practice in the group. In addition, she wonders whether there is a subtle pressure on the cardiologists to "produce" by doing procedures that bring in revenue for themselves or the hospital. But then, who is she to judge—she just joined the practice and they have been there a long time. Should she try to raise these issues or just let it be? If so, how can she raise them in a way that does not appear judgmental (although she is feeling critical of them)?

A helpful template for working through dilemmas is found in Chapter 2, Resilience in Facing Professionalism Challenges, Table 2-2. Following the template, this situation calls for:

What role does the system have in this case?
The clinic does not participate in a systematic review of cases or any registry to assess outcomes of patients. The team of cardiologists, nurses,

and technicians have not set up practice improvement strategies based on measuring their team outcomes, in comparison to their prior performance, nor have they developed any quality improvement process. Absent data from outside the group, it is difficult for the individual cardiologists to assess how they are performing.

Self-awareness (recognizing personal emotions or triggers, understanding personal limitations in skills and knowledge)

- Dr. Garcia recognizes that this situation makes her uncomfortable. She should also realize that at the moment she does not have all the necessary information to judge whether "best practices" are being followed. She might remember being told once—"when in doubt, be curious."

Self-regulation (managing strong emotions, accessing assistance for complex tasks)

- Dr. Garcia should try to remain calm and nonjudgmental, despite her concerns. She should realize that in addition to needing more information, she also needs help to determine the best way to approach the group, especially since she is new.

Social awareness (recognizing the importance of considering the needs and state of all participants)

- Dr. Garcia should remind herself that people feel defensive if criticized or confronted, and if she is too critical, they might be less open to exploring the issues. But Dr. Garcia also knows her most important responsibility is to the patients, to ensure that they are receiving safe, high-quality care.

Social regulation (seek to identify more than one option for action, assume positive intent to understand others' behaviors, develop crisis communication strategies and negotiation skills, be empowered to coach others)

- Dr. Garcia needs to resist her impulse to judge the other physicians negatively. Although that might be her first instinct, she should try to come up with alternative courses of action. She could try assuming a positive intent, by considering the possibility that her colleagues are most likely working hard and doing their best for their patients. They may think that they are practicing in accordance with guidelines, and in fact, that may be true. She needs to consider how to raise the issues in an open minded and nonjudgmental way, and create a "win-win" situation by valuing their hard work while seeking to improve outcomes. It is possible that making them aware of their outcomes, and how they may stack up against other units, might be motivational.

Actions

Dr. Garcia decides to raise the issue in a monthly meeting. "During my training, we had a database to review all the invasive procedures done by the group to understand our indications, technical challenges during the procedures, and patient outcomes at 1 week and 30 days. We compared our own data to a national register of the American College of Cardiology. We all found it very helpful and informative and I was wondering if the group might want to consider doing something like this."

The cardiologists thought this was a reasonable idea and decided to invite one of the academic cardiologists from the medical center, who was responsible for their database, to come to the practice and present their data.

KEY LEARNING POINTS

1. The United States spends a greater proportion of its gross national product (GNP) on healthcare than any other industrialized country and yet many indicators of quality of healthcare are poorer. It is estimated that 30% of healthcare spending may be "waste" as it does not add value in care.
2. The culture in many medical training programs encourages trainees to order unnecessary tests, and the patterns learned in residency training may influence future practice of physicians.
3. Physicians can maintain patient-centered professionalism while addressing their commitments to steward valuable resources as a strategy to achieve social justice.
4. Physicians can learn specific communication skills to discuss with patients whether tests or procedures are unnecessary or even harmful.
5. Interprofessional teams can eliminate wasteful use of resources by improving care coordination between team members, particularly at times of patient transition between sites.
6. Professional organizations can play an important role in stewardship of finite resources. The Choosing Wisely campaign is an example.

REFERENCES

1. ABIM Foundation. Choosing Wisely. Available at: http://www.choosingwisely.org/
2. ABIM Foundation. Choosing Wisely Lists. Available at: http://www.choosingwisely.org/doctor-patient-lists/
3. Agency for Healthcare Research and Quality. National Healthcare Disparities Report 2011. Rockville (MD); 2012. Available at: www.ahrq.gov/qual/qrdr11.htm
4. Arora A, True A. What kind of physician will you be? Variation in health care and its importance for residency training. Hanover, NH: The Dartmouth Institute for Health Policy and Clinical Practice; 2012.
5. Asch DA, Nicholson S, Srinivas S, Herrin J, Epstein AJ. Evaluating obstetrical residency programs using patient outcomes. *JAMA*. 2009 Sep 23;302(12):1277–1283.
6. Berwick DM, Hackbarth AD. Eliminating waste in US health care. *JAMA*. 2012 Apr 11; 307(14):1513–1516.
7. Bodenheimer T, Grumbach K. *Understanding Health Policy: A Clinical Approach*, 6th ed. New York, NY: McGraw Hill Professional; 2012.
8. Brody H. From an ethics of rationing to an ethics of waste avoidance. *N Engl J Med*. 2012 May 24;366(21):1949–1951.
9. Cebul RD, Love TE, Jain AK, Hebert CJ. Electronic health records and quality of diabetes care. *N Engl J Med*. 2011 Sep 1;365(9):825–833.
10. Epstein AM, Jha AK, Orav EJ. The relationship between hospital admission rates and rehospitalizations. *N Engl J Med*. 2011 Dec 15;365(24):2287–2295.
11. Feldman LS, Shihab HM, Thiemann D, Yeh HC, Ardolino M, Mandell S, Brotman DJ. Impact of providing fee data on laboratory test ordering: a controlled clinical trial. *JAMA Intern Med*. 2013 May 27;173(10):903–908.
12. Ginsburg S, Bernabeo E, Holmboe ES. Doing what might be "wrong": Internists' struggles in response to professional challenges. 2013. In press.
13. Ginsburg S, Bernabeo E, Ross KM, Holmboe ES. "It depends": results of a qualitative study investigating how practicing internists approach professional dilemmas. *Acad Med*. 2012 Dec;87(12):1685–1693.
14. Hansen LO, Strater A, Smith L, Lee J, Press R, Ward N, Weigelt JA, Boling P, Williams MV. Hospital discharge documentation and risk of rehospitalisation. *BMJ Qual Saf*. 2011 Sep;20(9):773–778.
15. Institute of Medicine. *Crossing the Quality Chasm: A New Health System for the 21st Century*. Washington, DC: National Academies Press; 2001.
16. Jencks SF, Williams MV, Coleman EA. Rehospitalizations among patients in the Medicare fee-for-service program. *N Engl J Med*. 2009 Apr 2;360(14):1418–1428.
17. Keehan SP, Sisko AM, Truffer CJ, Poisal JA, Cuckler GA, Madison AJ, Lizonitz JM, Smith SD. National health spending projections through 2020: economic recovery and reform drive faster spending growth. *Health Aff (Millwood)*. 2011;30(8):1594–1605.
18. Nolte E, McKee CM. Measuring the health of nations: updating an earlier analysis. *Health Aff (Millwood)*. 2008 Jan-Feb;27(1):58–71.
19. Organisation for Economic Co-operation and Development (OECD). Health expenditure: Total expenditure on health, % gross domestic product, 2012. Available at: http://www.oecd.org/els/health-systems/oecdhealthdata2012-frequentlyrequesteddata.htm

20. Shatto JD, Clemens MK. Projected Medicare Expenditures Under an Illustrative Scenario with Alternative Payment Updates to Medicare Providers. Washington, DC: Centers for Medicare & Medicaid Services, Office of the Actuary; 2011. Available at: https://www.cms.gov/ReportsTrustFunds/Downloads/2011TRAlternativeScenario.pdf

21. U.S. Census Bureau. Income, Poverty, and Health Insurance Coverage in the United States: 2009. Washington, DC: U.S. Government Printing Office; 2010. Available at: http://www.census.gov/prod/2010pubs/p60–238.pdf

22. Wachter RM. *Understanding Patient Safety*. 2nd ed. New York, NY: McGraw Hill Professional; 2012.

THE HIDDEN CURRICULUM AND PROFESSIONALISM

8

LEARNING OBJECTIVES

1. To describe how medical learning environments are composed of a complex interplay of the formal curriculum, informal curriculum, and the hidden curriculum.
2. To explain how the hidden curriculum of a medical school or health-care organization influences professionalism in trainees and practicing physicians.
3. To demonstrate how to assess and address these hidden rules in a learning environment.

It was the first day of orientation for new residents and fellows. Following a series of welcoming remarks from the school's dean and the vice president for health sciences, trainees were scheduled for a 2-hour block on professionalism. The lead individual responsible for this block had persistently lobbied the orientation planning committee to have professionalism assigned to a prominent place within the overall 2-day program. She, therefore, was pleased to find that the professionalism segment was to be "first up" and to directly follow the dean's and vice-president's opening remarks.

During the first break in this session, two incoming residents stopped by to say hello to one of the professionalism program faculty. "You know," said the first, "none of this is going to matter all that much," followed by the second, "Except to make us even more cynical." Although the faculty member had a suspicion about where this conversation was headed, she responded, "How so?" The second resident continued, "What <u>really</u> matters is what we are going to see on Wednesday when we have our first clinic rotation. You taught us *the bottom line in medical school—namely to pay attention to what you do rather than what you say. What you <u>really</u> mean by professionalism is shown in how you act."*

In this example, these two residents are articulating a key message about professionalism they acquired during undergraduate medical education via the hidden curriculum. The residents are describing the gap between what they were taught during their professionalism lectures and what they saw their role models do in practice—the latter of which, they also came to learn, signaled the real lesson. Obviously, faculty members do not intend to undermine the curriculum, and training programs expect the faculty to model the lessons taught in the lectures. So, how has this hidden curriculum evolved, what are the implications, and how can it be improved?

Over the last decades, professionalism has evolved (see Chapter 3, A Brief History of Medicine's Modern-Day Professionalism Movement). Numerous definitions have been created; curricula, codes, and charters have been developed; and educators have articulated competencies and milestones in professionalism. Despite all of this hard work and good intentions, there is a tension in the teaching of professionalism. Faculty may be impassioned in their commitment to improving student and resident education, but the creation of curricula or assessment tools has taken a path of least resistance. Finding 2 hours during resident orientation is operationally far easier and more readily justifiable (e.g., "See, we *are* doing something"), than undertaking the extensive work necessary to do the following: (1) change the actual practice behaviors of the physician role models that trainees will encounter during their clinical experiences; and (2) alter the conditions under which these physicians carry out their work. In short, codes and curricula are easier to create than new models of practice. The consequence has been a perfect storm of contradictions experienced by students. Students will receive a morning conflict-of-interest lecture stressing the importance of curbing bias in clinical decision-making, only to later find themselves following a preceptor who will meet with three drug representatives, belong to an industry sponsored speaker's bureau, and work for a contract research organization to enroll patients in clinical trials—all of which generate revenue for the physician. To make the messages even more confusing for students, this preceptor may explain why his work with pharmaceutical companies is good for patients because the company provides much needed free samples for the clinic and, ultimately, the research will improve patient care.

Today's trainees are finding themselves exposed to two sets of curricula—a formal and often more ideal "classroom" version, and a more pragmatic "real life" clinical version. In some instances, the messages students receive are synergistic and reinforcing. In other instances, however, trainees hear some set of ideal professionalism messages in class and then see contradictory messages in action.

LEARNING EXERCISE 8-1

1. Identify an instance in your present work environment where the formal professionalism message is "DO THIS" and the actual practice you observe is "PEOPLE DO THAT."
2. What is the formal message? How is it communicated?
3. Conversely, how do people learn about these other and more informal "rules of the road?"
4. Is there a difference between the two?
5. If there is a difference, how might it be reconciled?

WHAT IS THE HIDDEN CURRICULUM?

The term, "hidden curriculum" (HC), is a concept to help understand the potentially conflicting messages of complex medical learning environments. Using the HC, we can biopsy the range of different messages that individuals receive as they go about their daily routines of interacting with faculty, peers, staff, and patients, as well as the organization itself. As is true for social life in general, the messages students receive can be divided into two broad categories—formal and informal. Some of the rules that govern our daily lives

DEFINITIONS

1. **Formal curriculum:** The formal curriculum of each teaching institution is contained in its mission statement, course objectives, and course materials. It contains what the faculty believes they are teaching and what they hope students will learn.
2. **Informal curriculum:** Teaching and learning that occurs outside of the formal curriculum in variety of settings (i.e., ward rounds and bedside) that is unscripted and predominantly ad hoc. This learning can be consistent or inconsistent with the formal curriculum.
3. **Hidden curriculum:** Lessons that are learned, but are not explicitly intended. These lessons may be contrary to the formal curriculum. The hidden curriculum is embedded in the organizational structure and culture and influences the norms and values that students learn.

are formal in nature. Examples include laws or other types of formally written policies. These more formal rules can be learned by formal training and reinforced by a variety of rewards or punishments. However, we also organize our social and work lives around ways of doing things that are more tacit and informal in nature. These more informal rules are not codified in any formal way, but their power over human and/or organizational behavior can be just as strong. Oftentimes, the only way we learn about their existence is by watching others go about their daily routines—and then being observant when these informal norms are violated.

There are innumerable examples of these informal rules and how they govern our daily lives, with most flying beneath our perceptual radar because of their highly taken-for-granted nature. One example is getting on a bus or train; no formal rules govern such behaviors, but informal rules exist. Consider City A and City B. In City A, bus riders may mill about on a platform waiting for the bus to arrive—each staking out turf where they thought the bus door would open. As the bus arrives, riders surge forward, jockeying for position as they tightly bunch on either side of the bus door, forcing disembarking riders to move through a narrow gauntlet of bodies. The actual boarding is an every-man-for-himself scene. Even people who are naturally timid, and do not like to be pushy, will soon realize that they need to push like others or they will be left behind. In City B, riders form a queue with later arrivals adding themselves to the end of the line. When the bus arrives, debarking is easier for exiting riders, since the line was on only one side of the door. In turn, new riders enter the bus in the order they arrived at the bus stop. City A behaviors in City B would violate City B's informal rules for bus lines.

Driving an automobile is another example of the intersection of formal and informal "rules of the road." On the one hand, drivers must be licensed and insured (each by a different type of organization). Your "right" to drive is also subject to a myriad of restrictions. You must pass a driving test, and a

---

Imagine that this is your first day in either city and you needed to take a bus. How would you know which behavior to adopt?

Answer: You watch, learn, and act accordingly.

To shove your way to the front in a queue-normed city would be unthinkable to those waiting in line, and might invite public rebuke. Conversely, to "line-up" in a mob-boarding milieu might subject you to ridicule, or at minimum leave you perpetually stranded on the platform as others rushed by you to board.

thriving industry provides classes to teach you driving skills, as well as the formal rules of the road. Those not following these rules are subject to an array of sanctions, including arrest and detainment. Highways are littered with signs telling you how fast you can drive and where you can or cannot turn, and so on. However, drivers also learn that these formal rules of the road are not the entire story. For example, sooner or later, most drivers "figure out" that while there is a posted (i.e., formal) speed limit, the "real" limit is somewhat higher—often you can drive 10 miles per hour faster than the speed limit without getting a ticket. Some formal rules can be broken without consequences.

The same range, and mingling, of messages also is true for medical education. Students come to medical school knowing (and if they do not know, they quickly learn) that much of what transpires in medical school will be determined not by the rules contained in the student handbook or in course syllabi, but in the way "things are done around here" at their medical school. Furthermore, they also know that there will be different rules depending on the teacher and/or setting. As such, students spend a considerable amount of time and mental energy "figuring out" the rules governing each new course and/or clinical setting as they transition between and among the hundreds of settings and situations in their medical training journey. In addition to considerable *transition* costs associated with moving in and out of new learning environments, trainees also encounter significant *translation* costs as they figure out how the informal rules in their newest class, clinical service, or even specialty area differ from the formal rules (Hirsh, 2013). Students even come to know that individual faculty within a given setting may have different "styles" of communication or informal rules, thus requiring learners to master an even broader range of styles and preferences. Becoming a good medical student is not only about mastering the formal curriculum. It also is about mastering the space between the formal and the more hidden dimensions of student learning (Snyder, 1971).

What do students learn when they master this "other" curriculum? If they are successful navigators of that space between the formal and the hidden curriculum, they learn not only that such a space exists, but, more importantly, that their "survival" is *highly* dependent on their ability to decode that space. The "best" students are often not the most academically brilliant, but rather the ones who are able to understand the prevailing culture of their current learning environment and act accordingly—and do so regardless of the formal rules. What students learn is to give faculty what faculty expect from good students; the "right" answer to an exam or to attending questions during rounds; the "right" deportment in front of patients versus away from patients, or the right (and wrong) way to log duty hours (Brainard & Brislen, 2007; Prentice, 2012). Students learn to "play the game" and to become experts

A SAMPLE HIDDEN CURRICULUM EXERCISE

At medical school X, 4th-year students were asked to compile "Rules of the House of X"—rules they had "picked up" during their 4 years at this school, and rules that could be passed on to the next class of incoming students. These students identified 103 rules, 8 of which appear below.

- Learn how to act like you know everything, whether or not you do.
- Ask for expectations from evaluations on day 1.
- It's about surviving, not excelling.
- Be good at getting people to like you and know what that means on different rotations.
- Never ask to go home, but if you are told to go home, ask once if there is anything you can do, then leave.
- Politics matter—spend the most time with the most powerful person.
- The attending is right, even when the attending is wrong.
- Every attending will have different expectations about how to write a note and orders.

at what sociologists call "impression management" (Giacalone & Rosenfeld, 1989). Perhaps most insidious, students learn to play knowing that faculty recognize (if only on an implicit level) that gamesmanship is the prevailing order of the day—for faculty too were once students. What students learn, in a most fundamental sense, is the strategic importance of becoming "situational chameleons" (Dalfen, 1999; Hafferty & Hafler, 2011).

WHERE DO YOU FIND THE HIDDEN CURRICULUM?

It was the first day of class, directly following 2 days of orientation. Students were organized into small groups, each with two faculty preceptors and a patient visitor. The intent of the class, as formally stated to faculty, was to have students listen to "the patient's story" and then to ask the patient questions. Faculty were there "as facilitators." The patients were told to speak about their medical history to whatever degree they felt comfortable and to answer student questions likewise.

In one group, the two-person faculty team was made up of a physician and a PhD faculty member. An overview of the class and its format was provided by the physician, and introductions were made around the table (somehow skipping over the PhD faculty – Hidden Curriculum [HC] lesson 1). Next, the patient was invited to speak by the physician. Almost directly after the patient began her narrative, the physician "surreptitiously" palmed his iPhone below the level of the table and began checking messages (HC lesson 2, 3). This continued for the duration (15 minutes) of the patient's narration. At no point during the class did the PhD speak to the physician about this behavior or attempt to bring the physician back into the class (HC lesson 4). Finally, at no point during or following the class did either facilitator ask students about their thoughts or reactions regarding the patient-contact experience (HC lesson 5, 6, 7).

HIDDEN "LESSONS" FROM THE ABOVE EXAMPLE

1. PhD faculty are less important than MD faculty.
2. MDs are busy people—and need not explain, or apologize, for the demands on their time.
3. Whatever faculty are attending to in the moment is more important than what either students or patients may require.
4. PhD faculty recognize (and acquiesce to) this hierarchy of importance.
5. Clinical faculty have "heard it all before," and therefore do not need to be "fully present" when patients (or students) speak.
6. Student feedback is neither necessary nor encouraged.
7. Students should not say anything about unprofessional behavior of faculty.

We are sure that the physician in the scenario above did not go to the teaching session with a plan to communicate these hidden lessons. However, unfortunately, the HC potentially operates within any educational milieu ranging from the classroom on the first day of medical school described above to all clinical settings. Virtually every learning environment contains some interplay of formal and informal rules, and thus, the potential for inconsistent or incompatible messages about what is expected of participants. These expectations not only cover behavior (what to do), but also what one should think regarding what is going on (the norms behind the behaviors). Although the classic HC distinction is between lessons taught "in the classroom" versus those that happen "in the clinic," it is important to recognize that each and every setting contains its own set of formal/explicit versus informal/implicit rules and messages. The HC can even be present in student examinations. For example, a faculty member noticed that the scenarios in a student multiple choice examination were likely to portray female patients, as opposed to male patients, as having psychosomatic ailments.

Another common HC example is that students quickly learn that what is formally taught about "good communication skills" may not be what they actually see when it comes to interactions between faculty role models and their patients (Browning et al, 2007). Students may learn that poor communication styles are acceptable, including not expressing empathy when it is called for or hurrying through informed decision making conversations. If a clerkship director states that one of the key objectives of her clerkship is to learn the principles of patient-centered care, then this is the formal curriculum. At the same time, trainees will be monitoring how the faculty role-model patient-centered care, and depending on what they see, may decide that the formal curriculum is being supported or undercut by what is being played out in these more informal learning environments. Students may decide that what they see being role modeled as representing "patient-centered care" is the "real deal," even if it is not exactly what they were formally taught.

Because of this duality, students constantly are engaged in what we might think of as "gap analysis"—and thus actively monitor the space between what they formally have been told to expect and what actually unfolds on the shop floor of their daily experiences. The smaller the gap, the more reassured students are about "getting it." The larger the gap, the more anxious students become about their learning, their ability to "figure out" what is going on, and thus their long-term survivability.

ARE MEDICAL SCHOOLS REQUIRED TO ADDRESS HC AND PROFESSIONALISM ISSUES?

In terms of accreditation, medical schools are required to operate under a series of formal rules governing the types of information they must present to the Liaison Committee on Medical Education (LCME). This compendium of standards and requirements (a veritable formal curriculum) lists in great detail how medical schools are supposed to conduct the business of medical education with respect to issues of governance, curriculum delivery, structure, management, student and curriculum evaluation, admissions, student services, student life, faculty requirements, and educational resources. Within this gaggle of standards, the LCME has one reporting requirement (MS-31-A) that indirectly addresses the HC. This standard, located in a section of the document labeled, "The Learning Environment," calls upon schools to address the following:

"MS-31-A: A medical education program must ensure that its learning environment promotes the development of explicit and appropriate professional attributes in its medical students (i.e., attitudes, behaviors, and identity).ʺ The standard goes on to specify that the learning environment, "includes both formal learning activities and the attitudes, values, and informal 'lessons' conveyed by individuals who interact with the medical student. The medical education program and its faculty, staff, medical students, and residents should also regularly evaluate the learning environment to identify positive and negative influences on the maintenance of professional standards and conduct and develop appropriate strategies to enhance the positive and mitigate the negative influences" (Liaison Committee on Medical Education, 2012).

The standard acknowledges that there are vehicles of learning beyond the formal curriculum, and it formally links these to issues of professionalism. It can be difficult to notice the learning environment because it becomes our norm. The exercise below presents one way to study the learning environment in a medical school through recording the use of awards. Awards are a concrete and public way to indicate what is valued and lauded.

It is important to realize that MS-31-A is a relatively new standard (2009) and thus lacks the institutional track record necessary to discern how MS-31-A actually is being interpreted by medical schools and, in turn, by the LCME. For example, how does the LCME address a medical school that measures these positive and negative influences but does not remediate problems identified? There is insufficient experience with the standard to date.

LEARNING EXERCISE 8-2

1. Record all the awards handed out by your medical school that are announced via plaques, etc.

2. Note the name and purpose of the award, including from whom (awarder) to whom (awardee).

3. Also record the "visibility" of this award, including its location (e.g., is the award hung in the student lounge or in a back hallway).

4. Next, try and identify when and where this award is bestowed (e.g., privately versus a major ceremony such as graduation), along with how the award otherwise is publicized (e.g., newsletters, school wide emails, faculty assembly).

5. Check your list against the awards the medical school says it is awarding to try and identify those awards that are conferred, but not recognized via an announcement.

6. Finally, brainstorm with colleagues (including students) about awards they feel should or should not be given, with a particular eye toward identifying awards that should be awarded but are not.

THE CONSEQUENCE OF THE HIDDEN CURRICULUM ON STUDENTS

It is in the early spring of year three and a group of students are about to begin the sixth of seven required clerkships they are required to take for that year. During the morning orientation session, the department chair comes in, welcomes the students, and explicitly mentions that she considers issues of patient safety and quality-of-care to be paramount on her service. She expects students to "speak up" when they see things that may negatively impact on patient safety and/or quality. The chair also explicitly links quality, safety, and speaking up to professionalism to the "professional responsibility" students have as "members of the healthcare team."

While inspired by these words, students are also filled by a modicum of confusion and dread, since one of the core implicit rules they have learned on her last rotation was that "the attending is always right, even when the attending is wrong."

As the 3rd years file out of the room, one mutters to another, "Great! Now all I have to do is figure out who is going to be thrilled when I speak up and who is not going to be so happy."

Clearly, the chair did not wish to leave the students with this sense of confusion. One solution for the students might be to meet with the chair, perhaps after the lecture, and ask for some guidance on how to bring up these sensitive issues related to quality and safety. Also they might ask how students should speak up when they are not certain about whether quality or safety issues are present, since they are inexperienced. This conversation might help students address their HC concerns.

Medical schools, as social and psychological environments, often are characterized as extraordinarily stressful, traumatic, and angst-ridden places for trainees, requiring intense amounts of memorization and time commitments, along with isolation from family and past circles of support (Roberts, 2009). As a consequence, medical students have high levels of depression, burnout, and other measures of psychological anxiety (Dyrbye et al, 2006). Perhaps not surprisingly, both clinical medicine and medical education make frequent use of military metaphors, including those of war and carnage to characterize the experience (Fuks, 2009; Harrington, 2012). If we assume that faculty members are not striving to create a pedagogical chamber of horrors, then much of what we have is a series of unintended consequences. The greater the gap between the formal and HC, the more students will experience stress and the more compromised learning via the intended curriculum will become. Meanwhile, faculty will find themselves teaching "against the current," as students develop their own "readings" for what they consider important and their own "work-arounds" to battle the ambiguities they encounter.

In short, students figure out how to work around the formal rules and do what is needed in the situation in order to "survive." However, this dance has a personal cost for students, requiring a significant amount of mental energy and leading to stress.

IS THERE A HIDDEN CURRICULUM FOR FACULTY?

Dr. Martens was delighted to receive an email announcing an upcoming event at which her colleagues would be presenting the latest research and findings from the annual national meeting of their professional society. She felt bad for not being able to go to the conference itself, but she had just come off clinical service and needed to spend some more time with her young children. Thus, this looked like a great way for her to catch up on the cutting edge scientific developments while being able to interact with her peers. She was about to hit the RSVP button when she realized that in small print, at the bottom of the notice, it said the event was sponsored by XYZ Pharmaceuticals, and would be held in an expensive restaurant nearby. This surprised her, as her university has a strict policy governing physicians' relationships with industry representatives. She checked the policy, which is prominently posted on the faculty Web-page, and it clearly states that industry-sponsored dinners, even for purposes of education, are not allowed. Dr. Martens felt conflicted—on the one hand, the policy said these dinners should not exist, but on the other, this invitation came from the office of her division head. She really did want to get caught up on the latest research, and not feel out of the loop, but it just didn't feel right.

We think there are some alternative approaches Dr. Martens could use to reconcile this dilemma. She could talk to her division head and find out if she perhaps misunderstood the policy, or talk to another more experienced member of her division and find out what other people do to manage this problem. Alternatively, she could consider attending the talk but paying for her own meal. If she felt that the practice was not consistent with university policies, she could ask her division head to bring this up for discussion at a division meeting. If other methods failed, she could consider "reporting" the violation to the dean's office.

Although not as well explored or elucidated as is the case for students, faculty members also have their own HC issues. In fact, faculty form an interesting subgroup when it comes to the HC in that faculty are both agents for the HC (in the case of students) and objects of their own HC (Hafler et al, 2011). Like students, faculty are not born knowing how to be faculty—including how to act and think like faculty. They must learn to be faculty and with much of that learning taking place "on the job." Some of this learning is the result of a formal faculty development curriculum, whereas the majority is more tacit in nature.

CAN INDIVIDUALS DO ANYTHING ABOUT THE HIDDEN CURRICULUM?

There are no easy answers when it comes to working with and within the HC. Not to turn a phrase, but much of the HC is, after all, hidden. Much of the HC is tied to serendipitous, happenstance, and unscripted social interactions; trying to uncover the HC is hard work. At the same time, pretending that you can run a formal curriculum without accounting for the learning that takes place within the HC is futility.

The opportunities to address the HC, when they occur, must be pursued. Some of these actions can be implemented by an individual faculty member while others will require a group effort on the part of a department or medical school. Here are some examples:

Example 1

Objective Structured Clinical Examinations (OSCEs) or case studies used in class need to be vetted not only for any underlying messages that may be embedded within the various scripts, but also for variations in how faculty are conforming to the "letter" of those scripts.

Example 2

Faculty should be careful about counseling students about their career choice. Statements like, "Why would you want to go into family medicine when you could get into a competitive subspecialty?" are clearly inappropriate.

Example 3

When one faculty finds (via a student's questions, and so on) that he is at odds with what another faculty has said about a basic science or clinical matter, it serves no good purpose to "trash talk" that other faculty in front of students. Conversely, it serves every good learning purpose to speak to that other faculty person, find out what they in fact did say, and finally try to reconcile the two positions in class and with students.

The collective of faculty members can address other key areas that relate to the HC—for example, the evaluation system. Examinations can function as an important source of messages to students about "what is really important," including the fact that these messages often trump the more official statements about course objectives and grading policies contained in documents such as course syllabi. Including questions related to professionalism on an examination can signal that this domain is important and that mastery of the content is required. Course evaluations also offer an opportunity to learn about the HC. Asking students to rate their satisfaction with a course is less helpful than probing their specific experiences during the course. Asking questions like, "Describe how you saw the principles of patient-centered care demonstrated (or not demonstrated) during this rotation?" or "Provide an example of a respectful (or disrespectful interaction) you observed during the rotation?" allows an opportunity to biopsy the HC.

The Medical School Graduation Questionnaire, which is administered and analyzed by the Association of American Medical Colleges (AAMC), has a strong experience-thrust in its questions. At present, the questionnaire does not ask any questions about the HC, but questions are being considered. This would allow medical schools to compare results on HC questions and to learn from one another about "best practices."

LEARNING EXERCISE 8-3

1. Think of a situation where you hear one faculty member say something disparaging about the care provided by another physician or nurse.
2. Who heard this disparaging comment? What were they likely to think?
3. How did you feel at the time? Did you address the issue directly? Why or why not?
4. What is the HC that was being communicated and to whom?
5. What is the implication for the learning climate?
6. What are your options for addressing a similar situation in the future?

GOLD FOUNDATION

This chapter has thus far shown many examples of the hidden curriculum in action, at the pre-clerkship, clerkship, residency, and practicing physician levels. Together, these examples may paint a picture of a pervasive negative culture acting against the ideals of developing professionals. However, this picture is incomplete, because it neglects some very positive and successful attempts to improve the culture and counteract the negative effects of the HC. Perhaps the best known example of this is the Arnold P. Gold Foundation's "Gold Humanism Honor Society (GHHS)." The Gold Foundation has dedicated itself to supporting and promoting excellence in humanistic care of patients. In 2002, it established the GHHS as an "international association of individuals and medical school Chapters whose members are selected as exemplars of empathy, compassion, altruism, integrity and service in working with patients and others in the field of medicine." The GHHS was created to "elevate the values of humanism and professionalism in medicine." By creating a Chapter of the GHHS, an institution signifies to its students and faculty that it highly values the skills and attitudes essential for compassionate patient care.

Students, residents, and faculty can be nominated to be GHHS members, usually by peer-nomination or similar processes. It is a highly prestigious distinction, making up no more than about 10% to 15% of a graduating class, and a few select faculty and residents. Similar to the well-established Alpha Omega Alpha Honor Medical Society, induction into the GHHS is noted on a medical student's dean's letter.

A medical school can apply to become a "Chapter" by filling out an application form and outlining how the GHHS will fit within the structure and culture of the school, by proposing ideas for humanistic projects, as well as a plan for sustainability. Once a Chapter has been approved it becomes part of the network of existing Chapters and is eligible for grants and support to promote humanism in patient care. One look at the GHHS website illustrates the wealth of Chapter activities that have been supported by the foundation, all focusing on improving humanistic, patient-centered care. This year the Gold Foundation held their third annual "Solidarity Day for Compassionate Patient Care," during which Chapters across the country (and even internationally) hosted simultaneous events to "celebrate the power of compassion" (The Arnold P. Gold Foundation, 2010). The Gold Foundation presents one, well-established example of how to change a school's culture and reduce (at least somewhat) the hidden curriculum. Further examples are provided in Chapter 12, Organizational Professionalism.

CONCLUSION

Given the sheer volume of work that has taken place over the last 20 years on the HC and medical education, it is no longer justifiable to frame medical training as adequately captured by "what faculty teach." Instead, the focus rightly has shifted to what students (and faculty) learn about what it means to be a good medical student, a good faculty member, and/or a good physician. This shift in focus has helped to fuel a new appreciation for the medical school as a "learning environment" and the role of professional formation in that environment.

KEY LEARNING POINTS

1. The term hidden curriculum (HC) allows us to understand the lessons being delivered via the formal curriculum *versus* lessons being delivered (and not necessarily intended) by the more tacit dimensions of medical education.
2. The HC can be conveyed by observed interpersonal interactions and through the organizational practices and culture.
3. Teaching is not the same thing as learning.
4. Students are constantly trying to "make sense" of their medical training and to reconcile the various pieces of that experience—many of which are not readily reconcilable. Medical education thus becomes a highly difficult environment to negotiate.
5. Individual faculty members, and the collective of faculty, can identify and address the HC when it is opposed to the formal curriculum.

REFERENCES

1. Brainard AH, Brislen HC. Viewpoint: learning professionalism: a view from the trenches. *Acad Med.* 2007 Nov;82(11):1010–1014.
2. Browning DM, Meyer EC, Truog RD, Solomon MZ. Difficult conversations in health care: cultivating relational learning to address the hidden curriculum. *Acad Med.* 2007 Sep;82(9):905–913.
3. Dalfen AK. Med students as emotional chameleons. *CMAJ.* 1999 Jan 26;160(2):182–183.
4. Dyrbye LN, Thomas MR, Huntington JL, Lawson KL, Novotny PJ, Sloan JA, Shanafelt TD. Personal life events and medical student burnout: a multicenter study. *Acad Med.* 2006 Apr;81(4):374–384.
5. Fuks, A. The Military Metaphors of Modern Medicine. Available at: http://www.inter-disciplinary.net/wp-content/uploads/2009/06/hid_fuks.pdf
6. Giacalone R A, Rosenfeld P. *Impression Management in the Organization.* Hillsdale, NJ: Lawrence Erlbaum; 1989.
7. Hafferty FW, Hafler JP. The hidden curriculum, structural disconnects, and socialization of new professionals, in extraordinary learning in the workplace. In Hafler JP

(Ed.), *Innovation and Change in Professional Education (Volume 6)*. New York, NY: Springer; 2011.

8. Hafler JP, Ownby AR, Thompson BM, Fasser CE, Grigsby K, Haidet P, Kahn MJ, Hafferty FW. Decoding the learning environment of medical education: a hidden curriculum perspective for faculty development. *Acad Med*. 2011 Apr;86(4):440–444.

9. Harrington KJ. The use of metaphor in discourse about cancer: a review of the literature. *Clin J Oncol Nurs*. 2012 Aug;16(4):408–412.

10. Hirsh, D. Longitudinal integrated clerkships: embracing the hidden curriculum, stemming ethical erosion, transforming medical education. In Hafferty FW, O'Donnell JE (Eds.), *The Hidden Curriculum in Health Professions Education*. Hanover, NH: Dartmouth College Press; 2013. (In press)

11. Liaison Committee on Medical Education (LCME). *Functions and Structure of a Medical School*: *Standards for Accreditation of Medical Education Programs Leading to the MD Degree*. May, 2012. Available at: http://www.lcme.org/functions.pdf.

12. Prentice, R. *Bodies in Formation: An Ethnography of Anatomy and Surgery Education*. Durham NC: Duke University Press; 2012.

13. Roberts LW. Hard duty. *Acad Psychiatry*. 2009 Jul-Aug;33(4):274–277.

14. Snyder BR. *The Hidden Curriculum*. New York, NY: Alfred A. Knopf; 1971.

15. The Arnold P. Gold Foundation. *Gold Humanism Honor Society (GHHS)*. 2010. Available at: http://www.humanism-in-medicine.org

EDUCATING FOR PROFESSIONALISM | 9

LEARNING OBJECTIVES

1. To provide an overview of educational theories and best practices that can be leveraged to create a comprehensive educational program in professionalism.
2. To describe elements of a formal curriculum for teaching professionalism.
3. To explain the relationship between the formal and informal curriculum within professionalism education.
4. To analyze the primary components of the informal curriculum related to professionalism.

Dr. Fraser, a senior faculty member, was frustrated by his latest teaching assignment. For years he has taught clinical skills to medical students in small group sessions, but this year they added on a module on professionalism, which all preceptors were required to teach. It includes definitions of professionalism along with expected behaviors for students. Dr. Fraser felt that these did not belong in a "skills" workshop, because, in his view, "You can't teach this stuff—students will either be professional or they won't. Besides, they should already know how to behave appropriately, by watching their attending physicians and residents."

Dr. Fraser does not consider professionalism a competency or skill that can be learned—rather, he thinks of it as a trait that one possesses (or fails to possess). The evidence does not support this view, and one goal of this book is to demonstrate that if professionalism is properly viewed as a competency, it follows that it can be taught, learned, and developed over time. Dr. Fraser also mistakenly assumes that professionalism is easily learned by watching more senior physicians. This is partly true, in that excellent positive (and unfortunate negative) role models can certainly imprint on learners and affect their behavior. But it is also clear that relying on passive observation is insufficient at best, and potentially harmful at worst (also see Chapter 8, The Hidden Curriculum and Professionalism).

Of interest, there is some suggestion that students are also unhappy with current educational approaches to professionalism. One school reported on their experience in teaching professionalism and found that a large portion of students felt the word professionalism itself was overused, and that the course content felt like "a collection of excessive directives, lectures, rules, and moral pronouncements that they found repetitive and patronizing" (Goldstein et al, 2006). Some educators focus heavily on evaluation and espouse a zero tolerance policy for transgressions. This leads students to be fearful of admitting difficulty. Students also frequently describe a disconnect between lessons learned in the classroom and lessons based on (and behavior modeled in) the clinical environment. This can be disorienting and confusing, and may lead to cynicism and a sense of futility (e.g., why learn about it if it doesn't occur in practice?). Another reason for the backlash is that professionalism is often taught in a negative manner, focusing on "lapses" and when things go wrong—medical errors, disruptive physicians, impairment, intimidation and harassment, and so on. This may set students up to expect the worst rather than the best from their preceptors and colleagues. It also may carry the presumption that everyone is susceptible to displaying unprofessional behavior. Although this may in fact be true, it is disquieting to young students, who can't imagine that doctors can be anything but exemplars of altruism, compassion, and excellence.

A comprehensive overview of educational strategies relevant to professionalism is beyond the scope of this book. In this chapter, we provide an overview of educational theories and best practices that can be leveraged to create a comprehensive educational program in professionalism. Although the literature suggests that there is no one best single approach to teaching professionalism, there are a number of emerging strategies based on accepted pedagogy that can help educators develop and implement a strong program in professionalism. Dominant themes identified in a recent Best Evidence in Medical Education (BEME) review included the importance of selecting students with well-developed capacity for humanism, attending to their moral development, including professionalism as a major theme through the formal medical education process, using experiential learning supported by guided critical reflection as a best practice, and optimizing the culture and values of the institutions in which education occurs (Birden, Glass, & Wilson, 2013).

EDUCATIONAL THEORIES THAT CAN GUIDE OUR WORK

Being an outstanding physician is a complex task. Not only are physicians expected to sustain their mastery of a conceptually difficult body of knowledge and to behave in a manner that is compatible with the tenets of professionalism, but they are expected to be able to demonstrate these abilities while interacting with an increasingly diverse set of patients in a very dynamic healthcare delivery environment. Given the complexity of the tasks in front of physicians, it is not surprising that teaching professionalism as a set of inviolate rules has not been a successful educational strategy. As Huddle (2005) describes, teaching professionalism requires strategies that bring about "a personal transformation—the shaping of the moral identity of the learner." Achieving this transformation requires more than just a will to behave professionally. It requires knowledge, attitudes, judgment, and skills. Physicians and physicians in training need to *know* the values of professionalism, they need to *commit* (or profess) to following those values, they need *judgment* to understand the complexity of the situations in which professionalism must be lived, and they must have *skills* to apply their knowledge, attitudes, and judgment in the sometimes chaotic real world of medicine. Cooke, O'Brien, and Irby (2011) as well as others (Cruess & Cruess, 2009) have argued for the explicit teaching of professionalism and professional identity formation.

Educational theories that describe how young doctors learn and how expertise develops underpin the most successful strategies in educating for professionalism (Yardley, Teunissen, & Dornan, 2012). Piaget's (1985) constructivist theory states that we "construct" new learning during the intersection of ideas with experience. New experiences are either assimilated or adapted to fit our current schemas. Kolb (1984) further refines this thought by describing a cycle of learning in which a learner participates in an experience, reflects on that experience, works to develop abstract rules they can use in future situations, and then plans to experiment with these rules before repeating the experience again. This cycle of learning (Figure 9-1) is launched when the learner, comparing his or her current experience to past experiences, realizes that something is different.

Mezirow (2009) has called this the "disorienting dilemma," wherein something is amiss and the learner will seek to understand the differences and decide whether his or her existing approach should be changed based on this new experience. Experts in the education of adults and professionals realize that the experiences most likely to result in these high-impact disorienting dilemmas occur in the workplace and then only if the student is engaged in work that they, and the others in the environment, view as authentic and valued—this is referred to as "legitimate peripheral participation" (Lave & Wenger, 1991). Learning lessons in the workplace requires

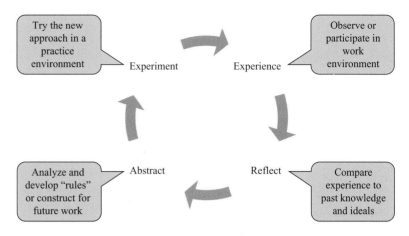

Figure 9-1 ▪ Learning occurs in a series of iterative reflective cycles.

the skilled guidance of workplace professionals with more experience than the learner in question. This learning is thought to occur best in the "zone of proximal development," which is described by Vygotsky (1978) as the difference between what a learner can do with assistance and what they can do alone. In the zone of proximal development, the learner is encouraged to practice skills beyond their current capability with support from experts within the workplace. In a process known as scaffolding, faculty initially provide substantial support and then gradually withdraw that support and guidance as the learner demonstrates greater proficiency with their assigned work. Table 9-1 summarizes important educational theories that guide the construction of a professional curriculum.

Educational theorists who study the development of expertise reinforce the importance of authentic workplace experience. The foundational work of Dreyfus and Dreyfus (1980) on the stages of skill acquisition is highly relevant to the work of educating for professionalism (Batalden et al, 2002). Medical students are *novices*, capable of reciting the "rules" of professionalism (be altruistic, be respectful, be honest), yet they may stumble when asked to apply these values in a busy clinical environment. Interns and residents are capable of performance described as *competent*. They are able to apply standard rules in standard circumstances but may struggle with complex or novel situations. *Proficiency* is a more advanced level of performance, found in residents and practicing physicians early in their careers. The proficient physician is able to view every situation holistically and to balance multiple competing demands. When proficient physicians recognize a professionalism problem, they can craft a work-around that generally fits the situations at hand. *Expert* performance is developed only after extensive experience. At this level, the

Table 9-1	**EDUCATIONAL THEORIES THAT GUIDE THE CONSTRUCTION OF A PROFESSIONALISM CURRICULUM**	
Piaget	Constructivist theory	Learning is constructed at the intersection of new ideas with the mental models (schema) formed from past experience.
Kolb	Experiential learning	Learning progresses through a cycle of adaptive learning; experience is followed by reflection, then abstraction, then experimentation.
Knowles	Adult learning theory	Adults bring past experience to learning and learn best when they participate in selection of learning goals, see immediate relevance in lessons, and are engaged in problem solving activities.
Mezirow	Transformative learning	Learning and transformation occur when learners experience disorienting dilemmas that suggest their past knowledge is inadequate and then work to construct new mental models.
Lave and Wenger	Situated learning theory	Learning occurs when learners are engage in legitimate peripheral participation in the workplace communities of practice.
Vygotsky	Socio-cultural learning theory	The zone of proximal development is the difference between what a learner can do independently and what a learner can do with the assistance of more experienced members of the community or practice.
Dreyfus & Dreyfus	Model of skill acquisition	Learners develop skills in a predictable sequence, starting with learning context-free rules and culminating in practical wisdom that allows them to function in almost any context.
Ericsson	Development of expertise	The development of expertise, as opposed to experience, requires deliberate practice with coaching.

physician acts instinctively and correctly in a wide variety of circumstances, drawing on vast stores of experientially acquired knowledge and skills. Many call this intuitive performance phronesis, or practical wisdom. Ericsson (2004) has added an important construct to the work of Dreyfus and Dreyfus. He recognized that routine practice, described as simply doing the same activity over and over, does not help one develop skills to master new circumstances. To successfully navigate the Dreyfus stages of skill acquisition, physicians and physicians in training must engage in ***deliberate practice,*** meaning they should be encouraged to take on increasingly complex challenges in the workplace with direct observation, debriefing, and coaching by a more expert individual (Figure 9-2).

Putting these theories into action means that professionalism education cannot end in the classroom and it cannot be left to chance in the clinical environment. In an ideal approach to learning professionalism, learners at all stages

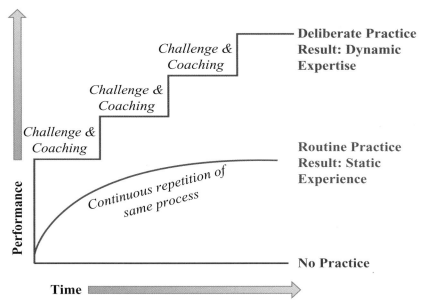

Figure 9-2 ▪ Practice and expertise development.

From Ericsson KA. Deliberate practice and the acquisition and maintenance of expert performance in medicine and related domains. *Acad Med.* 2004 Oct;79(10 Suppl):S70–S81.

need to be prepared to participate in authentic workplace experiences using classroom and simulated activities and then be assigned to work in the patient care environment under the guidance of expert clinical faculty. The faculty must be prepared to welcome the learner into the clinical community of practice, offer authentic but developmentally appropriate roles in that community, provide role modeling and supervision with coaching, and guide critical reflection of the inevitable disquieting dilemmas learners will experience.

DEVELOPING A FORMAL CURRICULUM FOR PROFESSIONALISM

The formal curriculum describes what faculty believe the students need to learn, methods they will use to help students learn, and tools and strategies faculty will employ to assess the learner and evaluate the curriculum. Like any other curriculum, the development of a formal professionalism curriculum must proceed in a structured way, using a model such as Kern's (2009) six-step model for curriculum. Unlike other curricula that focus on discrete biomedical science disciplines, formal curricula in professionalism are highly affected by the culture and the climate of the educational and clinical arena in which learners learn. The informal curriculum, including teaching that occurs outside in a variety of settings (i.e., ward rounds, bedside, and so on) that are unscripted and predominantly ad hoc, and the hidden curriculum, including lessons that are learned, but are not explicitly intended or embedded in the organizational structure and culture, can either reinforce or negate the impact of the formal curriculum. Experts in professionalism education have outlined a set of principles that must be addressed to ensure that the formal, informal, and hidden curricula are all aligned and synergistic in their impact on learners (Table 9-2). Chapter 12, Organizational Professionalism, illustrates examples of institutions that have worked to ensure that their institutional values resonate with the professionalism curriculum.

Planning for a formal curriculum in professionalism begins with the end in mind: the description of the behaviors and responsibilities of a physician who is successfully living the values of professionalism in the workplace. Educators must then work to identify or develop a series of developmentally appropriate educational activities to move the learner from classroom learning (aspiring to be a professional) to simulated and early authentic workplace learning (acting as a professional) to successful workplace performance (being a professional).

Content of the Formal Curriculum

The cognitive base of professionalism includes the enduring virtues, values, and behaviors of professionalism, the rationale for their existence, and the

Table 9-2 **PRINCIPLES TO GUIDE CURRICULA DEVELOPMENT**	
Curricular element	Guideline
Definition of professionalism	Should be consistent throughout the institution and be prominently displayed and promoted.
Institutional support	Should be strong and publicly expressed.
Allocation of responsibility	Directors of curricula/courses should be highly respected, with clear and direct lines to senior administration and leadership.
The environment	Should be consistent with professional values and the institution's mission statement.
The "cognitive" base (knowledge)	Should be explicitly taught at every level, including professional values, attributes, history, and the role of organizations.
Faculty development	All faculty should be educated in the content of professionalism and given strategies for how to teach and evaluate it in their own settings.

Adapted from Cruess RL, Cruess SR. Principles for designing a program for the teaching and learning of professionalism at the undergraduate level. In: Cruess RL, Cruess SR, Steinert Y, editors. Teaching Medical Professionalism. 1st ed. New York, NY: Cambridge University Press; 2009. p. 73–93.

consequences to individuals and to the profession when lapses occur (Cruess & Cruess, 2009). Learners must be continuously reminded that the driving force for professionalism is our moral responsibility to our patients.

In addition to understanding professionalism values in the abstract, students must learn how these values are translated into behaviors. In a systematic review of the literature, Wilkinson, Wade, & Knock (2009) summarized thematic categories of behavioral competencies relevant to professionalism (Figure 9-3).

In addition to teachings in ethics and doctor-patient communication, lessons from social, behavioral, and engineering sciences can be used to ensure that the curriculum embraces the complexity of professionalism and prepares learners to face a multitude of different and challenging circumstances. Mindfulness training can help learners attend to their thoughts and emotions in the moment and to decrease likelihood that they will overreact to challenging professional situations (Epstein, 1999). Managing and communicating uncertainty can help physicians remain honest and avoid arrogance (Smith, White, & Arnold, 2013). Lessons on boundaries, commonly found in psychiatry programs but rare in

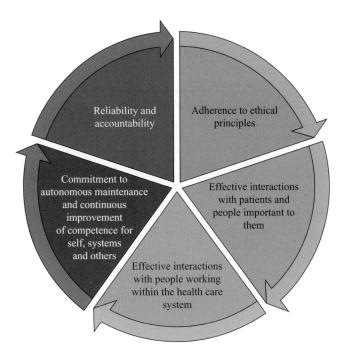

Figure 9-3 ■ Competencies relevant to professionalism.

Adapted from Wilkinson TJ, Wade WB, Knock LD. A blueprint to assess professionalism: results of a systematic review. Acad Med. 2009 May;84(5):551–558.

other training environments, can be used to prepare students and residents to recognize and manage requests for inappropriate favors or relationships. Wellness awareness programs can remind learners and practicing physicians of the importance of attending to personal health and wellbeing as a requisite for sustaining energy and enthusiasm for high-quality patient care. Information from cognitive psychology and organizational development can help physicians-in-training learn about embedded cognitive biases and inferential thinking that explain how all people (including physicians and their patients) react in stressful situations (Senge, 2006; Croskerry, 2013). Leadership and change management instruction can help learners develop skills in leading, working within, and continuously improving the work of teams and systems. Conflict resolution skills can help physicians learn to navigate disagreements with peers, physicians from other disciplines, other professionals, patients, families, and administrators. "Crucial Conversations" training can provide physicians with tools to engage in difficult conversations in a respectful but direct manner (Patterson et al, 2002). Feedback skills can empower students and residents to engage in peer coaching when professionalism lapses occur.

There are numerous case studies about instructional methods for the formal professionalism curriculum. Early in the curriculum, context for professionalism education must be provided to students so they understand professionalism as a living construct. Successful interventions include those that help students focus on the personal needs and perspectives of real patients (Kumagai, 2008; Stern et al, 2008). In the classroom, films, poetry, and prose can supplement case studies to provide students with a reminder of the ideals to which they aspire (Coulehan, 2004; Kumagai, 2008). As they progress through the curriculum into authentic workplace experiences, students will be able to provide their own context. Regardless of the stimulus provided, critical reflection has been recognized as an essential tool for learning. For it to be maximally effective, reflections must be reviewed and critiqued by faculty with whom the learner has a trusting relationship (Wear & Zarconi, 2008; Hatem & Ferrara, 2001; Goldie et al, 2007). Some evidence suggests that verbal debriefing of reflection is more effective than written commentary by faculty (Baernstein & Fryer-Edwards, 2003). A more extensive discussion of reflection follows later in this chapter.

The way in which the curriculum is structured can affect the success of professionalism education. Consensus is emerging that engaging students in working relationships with patients and clinical faculty early in the course of their medical school career significantly enhances their understanding of professionalism (Monrouxe, Rees, & Hu, 2011; Kumagai, 2008; Hatem, 2003). The importance of embedding formal educational activities for professionalism across the continuum of medical education is undisputed. Although structured learning activities during the intense clinical years are necessary, they are not sufficient. A truly successful formal curriculum must be coupled with attention to the informal curriculum.

OPTIMIZING THE INFORMAL CURRICULUM: STRATEGIES FOR EFFECTIVE WORKPLACE LEARNING

A 3rd-year student, Suzanne, was more than a little unnerved. For several days, she and her team had been caring for Anita, a 26-year-old woman with asthma, and she was much better. This was Anita's 3rd hospitalization for asthma this year. When the team entered the room during attending rounds, Anita's father was there and he was furious with the team. He raged at them for not bringing in a pulmonary consultant and accused them of not giving Anita the best available care because she was poor. Suzanne didn't know what to do. He was accusing them of discrimination! Although she remembered attending a lecture and small group on dealing with angry patients, her mind was a complete blank about how to respond. She watched to see how her attending physician, Dr. Zinsmeister, would handle this and hoped there might be some way to get out of this situation without making it worse.

Because behaving professionally is dependent on effective relationships and interactions among healthcare providers and their patients, much of the learning must be experiential in the complex, highly emotionally charged environment of care delivery. In this encounter, Suzanne realizes that it is one thing to talk abstractly about how one might interact with a challenging patient; it is an entirely different experience to actively participate in a difficult situation on the wards. As articulated by Knowles (1978), adults learn best when they feel they have an immediate need to know the information that is being taught and when they are engaged in solving problems. Suzanne is ready to learn and her attending must be prepared to deal both with the clinical needs of the patient as well as the educational needs of the learners.

Workplace, or experiential, learning is the home of the informal curriculum. Because it occurs in the setting of a patient's immediate (and sometimes lifesaving) needs, these informal interactions can be both highly unpredictable and highly impactful. In contrast to the hidden curriculum (also see Chapter 8, The Hidden Curriculum and Professionalism), the informal curriculum is explicit but usually unscripted and ad hoc. For example, in the formal curriculum, students may learn the textbook approach for how to deal with an ethical dilemma involving advance directives, including relevant rules, policies, and guidelines.

In the informal curriculum, they might also learn a variety of techniques and strategies for how to have end-of-life discussions.

Faculty who teach in the clinical environment must understand what was taught in the formal curriculum, allow students to apply those lessons in their clinical encounters with their patients, and help them explore and resolve any disorienting dilemmas (disconnects between past knowledge and new experiences) that arise (Mezirow, 2009; Kilminster & Jolly, 2000). They do so using effective techniques for role modeling, supervision, and critical reflection.

Role Modeling

The construct of role modeling in professionalism is often viewed with a negative lens. Students are more likely to remember dramatic examples when their role models behave in a manner counter to the professionalism lessons from the classroom, and fail to recall the many times when their role models exemplified professional behavior. One study found that up to 40% of students felt their teachers did not behave as humanistic caregivers and were not very good role models in teaching the doctor-patient relationship (Maheux et al, 2000). In another study, the majority of clinical clerks reported that their teachers appeared unconcerned about how their patients were coping with their illnesses (Beaudoin et al, 1998). Yet, when carried out effectively, role modeling is a wonderful introduction into the ways in which skilled professionals navigate challenging circumstances. Ideal role models are defined as "people we can identify with, who have qualities we would like to emulate, and are in positions we would like to reach" (Paice, Heard, & Moss, 2002). To realize the full potential of role modeling as an educational strategy requires planning, Althouse, Stritter, and Steiner (1999) have summarized the steps of education through role modeling as ***attention, retention, production, and motivation.*** To ensure that the student ***attends*** to the right behaviors, the teacher should make the goal of the role modeling experience explicit by priming the student for the encounter. As an example, the faculty member might say to a learner before entering the room, *"I am going to talk with Mrs. Jones about the results of her surgery. While I am talking to her, pay attention to how she responds to my words and we will talk about it after the encounter."* Alternatively, they might say, *"I am going to use a three step approach to delivering bad news. See if you can identify the steps that I use. I will be interested in hearing what you think worked well and what might need a new approach."* The goal of the priming conversation is to help direct the learner to pay attention to the most important aspects of the encounter. It can also be used to engage the student in active problem solving by encouraging them to analyze and prepare to discuss the physician's management of the encounter. The role model can help the student retain the lessons learned by debriefing the encounter after it has finished.

This is the opportunity for teachers to engage in a thoughtful dialogue with the learner about what they witnessed; specifically what aspects of the encounter they viewed as successful and what they thought was less effective. **Production** is the process by which the student learns to apply the lessons learned in one case to the next case. The faculty member can guide this process by working with the student to envision how they will apply new strategies to their next encounter with a patient and also by identifying a good "next patient" for that student. **Motivation** of the student to continuously learn and apply the lessons from the workplace can be facilitated by role models who easily demonstrate caring and concern for students, explicitly talk about the joy they get from being a physician, and openly discuss their strategies for managing professional challenges.

> *Suzanne watched as Dr. Zinsmeister stepped forward. She sat down next to the angry father and said, "I'm glad you are here and that you are so concerned about your daughter. It can be very frightening to see someone you love in the hospital with breathing problems. Let's talk about your concerns some more and we will make sure that your daughter gets the care she needs to stay healthy. Would that be ok with you?" The father grew visibly calmer and by the end of the encounter he thanked the team for all they had done for his daughter. When they left the room, Dr. Zinsmeister pulled them aside and said, "Let's debrief this encounter as a team and figure out how to help Anita and her family. I also want to make sure you all could handle a situation like this if I wasn't here. Who wants to make some observations about what went well in there and what could have gone better?"*

Dr. Zinsmeister is working to help her team attend to, retain, and reproduce the lessons learned in this encounter. While she wasn't able to prime the students before the unexpected event, she circled back with an open-ended question intended to encourage immediate reflection on a challenging encounter in which the professionalism values of respect, empathy, and altruism were demonstrated. Her openness to the father and the success of her approach will also serve as motivation for the learners to emulate her strategy in the future.

> *Dr. Green was feeling a bit rushed reviewing new patients on a post-call morning with his team. The last patient and her family were known to Dr. Green from a previous admission, which was for the same problem. Because he knew the issues and the family so well, he walked in ahead of the team and told the family he was aware of the admission and that there was a plan in place. He told them he'd be back later to follow up with them after some tests were done, and then he walked out. The residents were a bit taken aback, as*

Dr. Green usually spent so much time at the patient's bedside, including conducting an abbreviated physical exam. They wondered if maybe he didn't really like that patient, or wasn't sure what to do clinically.

Dr. Green was probably unaware that his team was making inferences about his behaviors that morning, and potentially interpreting them in a negative light—that he doesn't care, or isn't a good communicator. But Dr. Green actually had a longstanding relationship with this patient and her family, and they trusted him to treat the patient quickly and get her back home. In fact, the patient and family were often frustrated by having to tell their story over and over again to different teams, and were relieved that Dr. Green was there so that they didn't have to do that again. If Dr. Green had quickly explained the unique approach he took with this patient, the team would have made very different inferences about his behavior. Without that explanation, they might inappropriately model the approach Dr. Green used with this patient on subsequent patients who didn't share the same trust with the team.

The lesson from this case is that even when faculty and residents don't intend to be teaching, they are role models. Their behaviors can quickly impact the attitudes and behaviors of the students and residents who admire them. The good news is that this can work to our advantage as we strive to optimize the culture of professionalism. Burack and colleagues (1999) found that teams dramatically decreased their use of derogatory language in as little as 1 month of interactions with a senior resident who didn't use that type of language on rounds.

LEARNING EXERCISE 9-1

1. Think of a time that you witnessed a role model do something that appeared to be out of character.
2. What did you think of the behavior at the time? Did you inquire as to the reasoning behind the behavior?
3. Did the role model explain why he/she was doing things differently than expected?
4. What would you do differently if you saw something like this again?

Effective Supervision

Nicolas Guerra was in his third month of internship. Today was an unusual day. His new attending, Dr. Masters, told him that she wanted to make sure she gave him the coaching he needed to develop into the best doctor possible. She set aside time to watch him talk with and examine a patient who came in the night before. He had to admit, he was a bit wary about being observed—didn't she trust him to know how to do a history and physical? But his attitude changed when before the encounter, Dr. Masters asked him what areas of the clinical exam he wanted to work on. It did seem like she wanted to help! He asked her to help him get information effectively and efficiently. The entire encounter took less than 15 minutes but was tremendously helpful. Dr. Masters even pointed out some things that he hadn't been aware of—like that he tended to stand at the end of the bed with his arms folded. He definitely learned something and hoped this would happen again.

Authentic learning in the workplace requires that the learner not only observe others working but also engage in work themselves, with close supervision by a skilled clinical teaching faculty (Kilminster & Jolly, 2000). Experts in the supervision of learning in the clinical environment emphasize that the quality of the relationship between the learner and the faculty is paramount. Whenever possible, relationships between students and faculty should be of sufficient duration for the parties to develop a trusting relationship. Longitudinal continuity relationships between students, faculty, and care environments facilitate workplace learning because the clinical teacher develops confidence in their student's abilities and more readily assigns them authentic work (Hauer et al, 2012). In addition, these working relationships engender trust and increase the likelihood that students will be open to feedback and honest in expressing their learning needs. This is particularly important when dealing with subjects that may provoke strong emotions, such as whether a student is communicating effectively or demonstrating empathy with his or her patients. If a longitudinal relationship is not possible, the faculty member must take steps to convey their respect for the learner's own goals and interest in the success of the learner to engender trust more quickly, as Dr. Masters accomplished in the encounter described above.

A key element of supervision in the clinical environment is direct observation of the student while they are participating in authentic work experiences, but unfortunately this occurs far too infrequently (Kogan, Holmboe, & Hauer, 2009). Nicolas has been an intern for 3 months and each month the evaluations of him by attending physicians have rated him as above average on history and physical skills. Yet, this is the first time Nicolas remembers being observed! Too often faculty make inferences about the quality of a student's clinical skills by judging the quality of their clinical presentations. When assessing skills in relationship building and counseling, it is critically important that that faculty watch the students interact with the patients and provide them with immediate

Table 9-3 SUPERVISORS' BEHAVIORS IN THE CLINICAL SETTING	Helpful	Ineffective
Relationship with student	Supportive, encouraging	Aloof, judgmental
Drivers of lesson	Student- and patient-centric	Teacher-centric
Site of teaching	Patient bedside, with direct observation	Hallway or conference room, without direct observation of student
Method of teaching	Joint problem solving through dialogue	Lectures and questions
Content of teaching	Explicitly links theory to practice; teaches generalizable rules	Idiosyncratic approach to encounters
Feedback	Formative	Summative

Adapted from Kilminster S, Cottrell D, Grant J, Jolly B. AMEE Guide No. 27: Effective educational and clinical supervision. Med Teach. 2007 Feb;29(1):2–19.

coaching to enhance their existing skills. Observations can identify quirky or ineffective communication styles or body language habits, such as with Nicolas. Table 9-3 contrasts the helpful and ineffective supervisory behaviors in clinical supervision adapted from the work by Kilminster and colleagues (2007).

Reflection

Reflection on action and reflection in action have long been thought to be critical facets for developing professionalism. Reflecting on one's actions in the moment, or at some point afterwards, is an effective means to learn from one's successes and failures and promotes professional growth and development (Lingard et al, 2001). Reflection can take different forms, from simply thinking about one's actions during an event, talking to a peer or advisor, writing (either privately or publicly), and so on. What is important in reflection is not just the retelling (or thinking) about events, rather it should include some indication that learning has occurred. Many medical schools and residencies now include reflection as part of their curricula, for example, using portfolios, reflective writing, and peer discussion as a way to promote self-awareness. Reflective writing has been noted to improve learning and performance, including for professionalism. However, there is often confusion surrounding the word "reflection" and what it is meant to accomplish. Critics have raised concerns that mandatory reflection, especially when attached to grades, will be superficial and lack meaning. That is, students might go through the motions and use the right language without really learning or changing their way of thinking.

There has also been concern that when reflections are used for assessment they may reinforce certain accepted narratives while marginalizing others. For example, it might be hard for a student to turn in an honest reflection about an event that increased his or her cynicism or sense of helplessness versus a story that had a "better" outcome of positive learning and growth. Therefore, it is important to be clear about what the reflection is meant to achieve and for what purpose(s) it will be used, so that maximal benefit to learning will be achieved.

Aronson (2011) created a set of guidelines to use when introducing reflection into a curriculum in order to maximize its benefit and minimize potential downsides (Figure 9-4).

It is often considered useful to assess learners' reflective exercises in some way. Even if these exercises are done as part of formative assessment, some type of evaluation, along with feedback, can help students and residents learn how to become more reflective. In addition, assessments certainly may ensure that students take the exercise seriously. Some scoring rubrics have been developed to assess the depth and degree of reflection, such as the following, adapted from Learman, Autry, & O'Sullivan (2008) for use in obstetrics and gynecology (Figure 9-5).

One might be concerned that students' skills in writing or story-telling might confound the assessment if the exercise involves writing (i.e., good writers and story-tellers may get higher scores than students for whom writing

1. Define reflection for your learners in a way that they will understand what you intend.
2. Set learning goals for the exercise.
3. Choose an appropriate instructional method (where, how, paper or electronic, and so on).
4. Decide whether reflections will be structured or unstructured and create a prompt for them to respond to.
5. Have a plan for dealing with ethical and emotional concerns that may arise in a student's writing.
6. Create a mechanism to follow-up on learners' plans.
7. Create a conducive, supportive, nonjudgmental environment for reviewing reflections.
8. Teach learners about reflection before asking them to do it.
9. Provide timely feedback and follow-up on any concerns.
10. Assess the reflection.
11. Embed the exercise as part of a larger system/curriculum to encourage professional growth.
12. Reflect on your reflection!

Figure 9-4 ▪ Tips for teaching reflection in medical education.

Adapted from Aronson L. Twelve tips for teaching reflection at all levels of medical education. Med Teach. 2011;33(3):200–205.

1. Describes event but does not mention lessons learned.
2. States opinions about lessons learned but does not support opinions with examples.
3. Provides superficial justification of lessons learned.
4. Reasoned discussion well-supported with examples regarding challenges, techniques, and lessons learned.
5. Analyzes factors from experience that contribute to progress.
6. Includes justification for the strategies that were used and evidence for effectiveness.

Figure 9-5 ▪ Example of a scoring rubric on a 1 (worst) to 6 (best) scale.

Adapted from Learman LA, Autry AM, O'Sullivan P. Reliability and validity of reflection exercises for obstetrics and gynecology residents. Am J Obstet Gynecol. 2008 Apr;198(4):461.e1–8; discussion 461.e8–10.

is a struggle), but this myth has been essentially debunked—reflective ability, if assessed with an appropriate rubric, is not linked to writing ability (Aronson et al, 2010). However, there are other methods available to teach and assess reflection and promote professional awareness that don't involve writing at all. Some of these tools help students gain insight and self-awareness, which are important elements of professionalism. The scales identified in Table 9-4 have all been studied in medical students and purport to measure constructs such as attitudes toward reflection, insight, and self-efficacy. These are relatively new and it is not certain how widespread their use is, but they have all shown good internal consistency and some construct validity, and may be useful as a means to show students what we mean by reflection.

Table 9-4 **REFLECTION SCALES**			
Scale	Audience	Measures	Quality
Self-reflection and Insight Scale(Roberts & Stark, 2008; Grant, Franklin, & Langford, 2002)	Medical students, self-administered	Measures attitudes toward need for reflection, engagement in reflection, and insight	30 items, good internal reliability
Groningen Reflective Ability Scale (Aukes et al, 2007)	Medical students, self-administered	Self-reflection, empathetic reflection, reflective communication	23 items, good internal consistency
Scale of Reflection-in-Learning (Sobral, 2005)	Medical students, self-administered	Attitudes toward learning, self-efficacy	14 items, construct validity

Reflection as a Means to Understand One's Unconscious Biases

Dr. Matthews is a busy family doctor in a small city who sees patients from 9:00 am to 5:00 pm, 4 days per week, with a focus mostly on women's health issues. Her clinics are often over-booked, as she tries hard to make room to see any of her patients who may be in need. For the most part, her patients don't complain about the long waits in her office, as they know when it's their turn they will get Dr. Matthews' undivided attention. Recently, Dr. Matthews was asked to take on patients from the new weight loss center next door. These patients have no family doctor and require basic medical care during their weight loss efforts. Some of these patients are obese and many have mobility issues (e.g., some require scooters to get around, and many cannot get up onto the exam tables). Dr. Matthews worries that she may not have enough space or resources to adequately (and safely) look after these patients. But now she is starting to feel guilty, as she realizes these potential patients do need ongoing care. She never thought she had any biases against overweight or obese patients, although she now realizes on reflection that her own patients are all fairly healthy, active, and fit. This realization disturbs her and she is unsure of what to do.

We all have biases—they are part of being human. They come from our upbringing, our families, our education, and elsewhere. Biases in clinical decision making are well described, as are strategies to mitigate them (Elstein, 1999; Croskerry, 2013). Yet, biases may also affect other aspects of dealing with patients, such as ensuring equitable access to care, or in treating certain types of patients differently than others. These biases are often unconscious and it is important to be aware of them in ourselves and our colleagues. Thus, explicitly focusing on our biases can form an important component of reflection.

Through our language and actions we communicate how we feel—including the relative value, or worth, that we place on certain types of patients or other healthcare professionals. Several categories of patients are commonly described in more negative terms, including "frequent flyers" to the emergency room, drug addicts, nonadherent patients, those that are "defiant," and the elderly (Higashi et al, 2013). Doctors may treat obese patients differently than their normal weight counterparts (Gudzune et al, 2013). Emerging research from the American Board of Internal Medicine has found that physicians may treat patients differently based on more nuanced and even unconscious factors (Ginsburg et al, 2012). Patient-level factors that influence decision-making include existing relationships with patients, how long a physician has known them, how compliant a patient is with recommendations, whether or not they challenge the physician's expertise, and so on. These factors may make it more or less likely for physicians to accept new patients into their practice, order specific tests or treatments, or grant enhanced access to services. Physician-level factors include the doctor's own comfort level, knowledge of what others do in similar situations, time and efficiency issues, and fear of litigation. These factors often act in combination and can create situations where a physician may respond to two very similar situations in very different ways. Furthermore, physicians are often surprised to learn of their own "inconsistencies" in approaching professional dilemmas and they find such exercises illuminating.

What should Dr. Matthews in the preceding scenario do about her predicament? She has already started the process of self-reflection, by thinking about her current patients and by questioning her unconscious biases. One of her medical students tells her about a website where you can take a test, the "Implicit Assumption Test" (IAT), to determine your unconscious biases (Project Implicit, 2011). She decides to take the one related to obesity, and finds to her surprise that she has a moderate preference for thin people. This prompts reflection on her part and a concerted effort to be aware of her potential bias as it relates to weight. She initiates a discussion with her practice partners to determine if they can upgrade their equipment and resources in order to better deal with obese patients.

There are many tools available to assess one's own biases, which are contextually specific. For example, there are tools to assess one's attitudes toward mental illness, psychiatry careers, obesity, or dealing with the underserved. The purpose of these self-assessments is to reflect and to unearth one's own internal biases in an attempt to better understand them and hopefully counteract them. Although the focus here has been on negative biases, there also may be a problem with positive bias, that is, patients we treat differently because they are "nice" or "important" may actually receive worse care, by overdiagnosis and overtreatment (Detsky & Baerlocher, 2011).

LEARNING EXERCISE 9-2

1. Think of a time where you gave a patient (or student) a little bit "extra," for example, more time, preferential scheduling, or enhanced access.

2. What were your reasons?

3. Why this patient or student and not others?

4. At the time, were you aware that you were giving "extra"? Did it make you uncomfortable in any way?

5. How would you deal with a similar situation if it were to arise again?

CONCLUSION

In summary, education for professionalism requires preparing learners for authentic workplace learning experiences by introducing them to the multitude of skill sets that can help them live their professional values in practice. Learners must then be assigned to developmentally appropriate, but authentic roles, where they can contribute to the care delivery system while they are working to learn how to apply their new found knowledge in the clinical environment. Clinical supervisors need to prepare themselves to optimize the learning environment by planning to effectively role model ideal behaviors, supervising the educational work that learners engage in and coaching their learners to critically reflect as an essential strategy for life-long learning. Finally, educational programs must develop comprehensive assessment programs to accumulate meaningful and reliable data that can be used by the learner to improve their performance and used by the program to assess their readiness for independent practice.

KEY LEARNING POINTS

1. Professionalism can be taught and learned through a variety of effective strategies in both the informal and formal curricula.
2. Well-established educational theories exist that can help in the development of a curriculum, including theories of competency development, expertise, and workplace-based learning.
3. Teaching in the formal curriculum should be based on agreed-upon definitions and should be consistent throughout an institution (teachers, administration and leadership, all healthcare professionals).
4. Powerful informal teaching can occur by explicit role modeling, expert supervision, and self-reflection.

REFERENCES

1. Althouse LA, Stritter FT, Steiner BD. Attitudes and approaches of influential role models in clinical education. *Adv Health Sci Educ Theory Pract.* 1999;4(2):111–122.
2. Aronson L. Twelve tips for teaching reflection at all levels of medical education. *Med Teach.* 2011;33(3):200–205.
3. Aronson L, Niehaus B, DeVries CD, Siegel JR, O'Sullivan PS. Do writing and storytelling skill influence assessment of reflective ability in medical students' written reflections? *Acad Med.* 2010 Oct;85(10 Suppl):S29–S32.

4. Aukes LC, Geertsma J, Cohen-Schotanus J, Zwierstra RP, Slaets JP. The development of a scale to measure personal reflection in medical practice and education. *Med Teach.* 2007 Mar;29(2-3):177–182.

5. Baernstein A, Fryer-Edwards K. Promoting reflection on professionalism: a comparison trial of educational interventions for medical students. *Acad Med.* 2003 Jul;78(7):742–747.

6. Batalden P, Leach D, Swing S, Dreyfus H, Dreyfus S. General competencies and accreditation in graduate medical education. *Health Aff (Millwood).* 2002 Sep-Oct;21(5):103–111.

7. Beaudoin C, Maheux B, Côté L, Des Marchais JE, Jean P, Berkson L. Clinical teachers as humanistic caregivers and educators: perceptions of senior clerks and second-year residents. *CMAJ.* 1998 Oct 6;159(7):765–769.

8. Birden H, Glass N, Wilson I. Teaching professionalism in medical education: a Best Evidence Medical Education (BEME) systematic review. BEME Guide No. 25. *Med Teach.* 2013 Jul;35(7):e1252–e1266.

9. Burack JH, Irby DM, Carline JD, Root RK, Larson EB. Teaching compassion and respect. Attending physicians' responses to problematic behaviors. *J Gen Intern Med.* 1999 Jan;14(1):49–55.

10. Cooke M, O'Brien B, Irby DM. *Educating Physicians: A Call For Reform of Medical School and Residency.* San Francisco, CA: Jossey-Bass; 2011.

11. Coulehan J. The possible dream: a commentary on the Don Quixote effect. *Fam Syst Health.* 2004;22:453–456.

12. Croskerry P. From mindless to mindful practice—cognitive bias and clinical decision making. *N Engl J Med.* 2013 Jun 27;368(26):2445–2448.

13. Cruess RL, Cruess SR. Principles for designing a program for the teaching and learning of professionalism at the undergraduate level. In: Cruess RL, Cruess SR, Steinert Y, editors. *Teaching Medical Professionalism.* 1st ed. New York, NY: Cambridge University Press; 2009.

14. Detsky AS, Baerlocher MO. Do nice patients receive better care? *JAMA.* 2011 Jul 6; 306(1):94–95.

15. Dreyfus SE, Dreyfus HL. *A Five-Stage Model of the Mental Activities Involved in Directed Skill Acquisition.* Washington, DC: Storming Media; 1980.

16. Elstein AS. Heuristics and biases: selected errors in clinical reasoning. *Acad Med.* 1999 Jul;74(7):791–794.

17. Epstein RM. Mindful practice. *JAMA.* 1999 Sep 1;282(9):833–839.

18. Ericsson KA. Deliberate practice and the acquisition and maintenance of expert performance in medicine and related domains. *Acad Med.* 2004 Oct;79(10 Suppl):S70–S81.

19. Ginsburg S, Bernabeo E, Ross KM, Holmboe ES. "It depends": results of a qualitative study investigating how practicing internists approach professional dilemmas. *Acad Med.* 2012 Dec;87(12):1685–1693.

20. Goldie J, Dowie A, Cotton P, Morrison J. Teaching professionalism in the early years of a medical curriculum: a qualitative study. *Med Educ.* 2007 Jun;41(6):610–617.

21. Goldstein EA, Maestas RR, Fryer-Edwards K, Wenrich MD, Oelschlager AM, Baernstein A, Kimball HR. Professionalism in medical education: an institutional challenge. *Acad Med.* 2006 Oct;81(10):871–876.

22. Grant AM, Franklin J, Langford P. The self-reflection and insight scale: a new measure of private self-consciousness. *Soc Behav Pers.* 2002;30(8):821–835.

23. Gudzune KA, Beach MC, Roter DL, Cooper LA. Physicians build less rapport with obese patients. *Obesity* 2013;21(10):2146–52.

24. Hatem CJ. Teaching approaches that reflect and promote professionalism. *Acad Med.* 2003 Jul;78(7):709–13.

25. Hatem D, Ferrara E. Becoming a doctor: fostering humane caregivers through creative writing. *Patient Educ Couns.* 2001 Oct;45(1):13–22.

26. Hauer KE, Hirsh D, Ma I, Hansen L, Ogur B, Poncelet AN, Alexander EK, O'Brien BC. The role of role: learning in longitudinal integrated and traditional block clerkships. *Med Educ.* 2012 Jul;46(7):698–710.

27. Higashi RT, Tillack A, Steinman MA, Johnston CB, Harper GM. The "worthy" patient: rethinking the "hidden curriculum" in medical education. *Anthropol Med.* 2013 Apr;20(1):13–23.

28. Huddle TS; Accreditation Council for Graduate Medical Education (ACGME). Viewpoint: teaching professionalism: is medical morality a competency? *Acad Med.* 2005 Oct;80(10):885–891.

29. Kern DE, Thomas PA. *Curriculum Development for Medical Education: A Six Step Approach.* Baltimore, MD: Johns Hopkins University Press; 2009.

30. Kilminster S, Cottrell D, Grant J, Jolly B. AMEE Guide No. 27: effective educational and clinical supervision. *Med Teach.* 2007;29(1):2–19.

31. Kilminster SM, Jolly BC. Effective supervision in clinical practice settings: a literature review. *Med Educ.* 2000 Oct;34(10):827–840.

32. Knowles M. *The Adult Learner. A Neglected Species.* 2nd ed. Oxford, UK: Gulf Publishing; 1978.

33. Kogan JR, Holmboe ES, Hauer KE. Tools for direct observation and assessment of clinical skills of medical trainees: a systematic review. *JAMA.* 2009 Sep 23;302(12):1316–1326.

34. Kolb DA. *Experiential Learning: Experience as the Source of Learning and Development.* Englewood Cliffs, NJ: Prentice-Hall; 1984.

35. Kumagai AK. A conceptual framework for the use of illness narratives in medical education. *Acad Med.* 2008 Jul;83(7):653–658.

36. Lave J, Wenger E. *Situated Learning: Legitimate Peripheral Participation.* Cambridge, UK: Cambridge University Press; 1991.

37. Learman LA, Autry AM, O'Sullivan P. Reliability and validity of reflection exercises for obstetrics and gynecology residents. *Am J Obstet Gynecol.* 2008 Apr;198(4):461. e1-8; discussion 461.e8–10.

38. Lingard L, Garwood K, Szauter K, Stern D. The rhetoric of rationalization: how students grapple with professional dilemmas. *Acad Med.* 2001 Oct;76(10 Suppl):S45–S47.

39. Maheux B, Beaudoin C, Berkson L, Côté L, Des Marchais J, Jean P. Medical faculty as humanistic physicians and teachers: the perceptions of students at innovative and traditional medical schools. *Med Educ.* 2000 Aug;34(8):630–634.

40. Mezirow J. *Transformative Learning in Practice: Insights from Community, Workplace, and Higher Education.* 1st ed. San Francisco, CA: Jossey-Bass; 2009.

41. Monrouxe LV, Rees CE, Hu W. Differences in medical students' explicit discourses of professionalism: acting, representing, becoming. *Med Educ.* 2011 Jun;45(6):585–602.

42. Paice E, Heard S, Moss F. How important are role models in making good doctors? *BMJ*. 2002 Sep 28;325(7366):707–710.

43. Patterson K, Grenny J, McMillan R, Swizler A. *Crucial Conversations: Tools for Talking When Stakes Are High*. 1st ed. New York, NY: McGraw-Hill; 2002.

44. Piaget J. *The Equilibration of Cognitive Structures*. Chicago, IL: University of Chicago Press; 1985.

45. Project Implicit. 2011. Available at: https://implicit.harvard.edu/implicit/demo/takeatest.html

46. Roberts C, Stark P. Readiness for self-directed change in professional behaviours: factorial validation of the Self-Reflection and Insight Scale. *Med Educ*. 2008 Nov;42(11):1054–1063.

47. Senge P. *The Fifth Discipline: The Art and Practice of the Learning Organization*. New York, NY: Doubleday; 2006.

48. Smith AK, White DB, Arnold RM. Uncertainty—the other side of prognosis. *N Engl J Med*. 2013 Jun 27;368(26):2448–2450.

49. Sobral DT. Medical students' mindset for reflective learning: a revalidation study of the reflection-in-learning scale. *Adv Health Sci Educ Theory Pract*. 2005 Nov;10(4):303–314.

50. Stern DT, Cohen JJ, Bruder A, Packer B, Sole A. Teaching humanism. *Perspect Biol Med*. 2008 Autumn;51(4):495–507.

51. Vygotsky L. *Interaction Between Learning and Development. Mind in Society*. 1st ed. Cambridge, MA: Harvard University Press; 1978.

52. Wear D, Zarconi J. Can compassion be taught? Let's ask our students. *J Gen Intern Med*. 2008 Jul;23(7):948–953.

53. Wilkinson TJ, Wade WB, Knock LD. A blueprint to assess professionalism: results of a systematic review. *Acad Med*. 2009 May;84(5):551–558.

54. Yardley S, Teunissen PW, Dornan T. Experiential learning: AMEE Guide No. 63. *Med Teach*. 2012;34(2):e102–e115.

EVALUATING PROFESSIONALISM | 10

LEARNING OBJECTIVES

1. To articulate the importance of evaluating professionalism.
2. To describe the challenges involved when evaluating professionalism.
3. To review common instruments used for evaluating professionalism.

Lucy, a 4th-year medical student, is walking down the hall with her attending surgeon, Dr. Wong, at the end of their inpatient ward rounds. Lucy tells Dr. Wong that the patient they are about to see wants to know the results of her latest tests. The patient is a few days post-liver transplant, and on a postoperative film they discovered a large lung mass that was not noticed preoperatively, and no one has told the patient. Every day the patient asks about any new test results, and Lucy feels awkward not telling her. Dr. Wong tells Lucy that it is up to the medical team and not up to them, as they are just responsible for the surgery and postoperative care. Just then, Dr. Wong gets paged away to the operating room, and Lucy enters the patient's room on her own. The patient is in good spirits, and wants to go home soon. She asks Lucy, "What do my tests show?"
(Ginsburg, Regehr, & Lingard, 2003).

What should Lucy do? Her basic options are "tell" and "don't tell," but clearly it is more complicated than that. Let's assume Lucy has just been to a lecture on the importance of honesty and full disclosure with patients, and decides to "be honest" and tell the patient about the x-ray finding. What would happen next? The patient would be fully informed about her condition, which was the student's goal—but she would also likely be terribly distraught and would have many follow-up questions. Is Lucy equipped to deal with the patient's emotional reaction and answer all of her questions about diagnostic possibilities, prognosis, effect on her transplant recovery, and so on? How might the patient feel now, knowing that a mistake may have been made, potentially exposing her to unnecessary risk? And to make things worse, now she thinks that her other doctors were aware and hid it from her—how might that affect her trust in her doctors and the system in general?

Now let's assume that Lucy—for whatever reason—decides to obey Dr. Wong's directive to not tell the patient. What would happen next? Lucy would not get in trouble and eventually the patient would be told by one of the attending doctors. The patient might still be upset that people (including the student) knew and did not tell her. An attending doctor would likely be able to effectively manage the patient's emotional reaction and would be able to answer her questions about diagnostic and prognostic possibilities and create a mutually agreeable management plan.

What does this have to do with evaluation? What if you had to evaluate Lucy, and she had decided not to tell the patient about the x-ray result? If you feel that it is wrong to withhold the truth no matter what, this failure to disclose would be considered a lapse in professionalism. But if she happened to have an evaluator who felt that sometimes it is better to withhold the truth, at least temporarily until they can get someone more experienced to do so with them, the student might receive a very good evaluation of her professionalism, because she minimized the patient's anxiety overall. So the same behavior—essentially amounting to dishonesty—could be evaluated as either good or bad, depending on how the situation is construed by the person evaluating her (Ginsburg, Regehr, & Lingard, 2004).

This scenario is a good example of why evaluating professionalism can be so difficult. If we focus on the issue of honesty with patients, it is easy to say, "Always be honest," but it is clearly more complicated. Simply blurting out "the truth" without consideration of people's feelings and reactions can be just as damaging as lying. What this exemplifies is the importance of context in interpreting people's behaviors, a point that will be expanded on again later (Ginsburg et al, 2000).

WHY IS EVALUATING PROFESSIONALISM SO DIFFICULT?

In the past, professionalism was often treated (taught, discussed, and evaluated) in a different way than other knowledge and skills, and was often not taught at all. One reason is that professionalism has traditionally been tricky to define, and if it is not clearly defined it is hard to assess when it is done well or poorly. That is why the framework presented in this book is useful in terms of operationalizing professionalism as a set of behaviors that can be observed and evaluated. There is certainly no shortage of definitions of professionalism that one can find by doing a literature search and, in general, there is consensus around the major themes (Lynch, Surdyk, & Eiser, 2004). What often differs between definitions is the emphasis and priority given to various elements, as well as the boundaries drawn around them. For example, in Canada and some countries in Europe, the CanMEDS framework is used for student and resident evaluation and includes "professional" as one of seven essential roles required of physicians (Frank, 2005). Its definition, framed as "key" and "enabling" competencies is shown below in Figure 10-1. The Accreditation Council for Graduate Medical Education (ACGME) framework (Figure 10-2), used in the United States, includes professionalism as one of six competencies (Accreditation Council for Graduate Medical Education,

Key competencies followed by enabling competencies
Physicians are able to…

1. Demonstrate a commitment to their patients, profession and society through ethical practice
1.1. Exhibit appropriate professional behaviors in practice, including honesty, integrity, commitment, compassion, respect and altruism
1.2. Demonstrate a commitment to delivering the highest quality care and maintenance of competence
1.3. Recognize and appropriately respond to ethical issues encountered in practice
1.4. Appropriately manage conflicts of interest
1.5. Recognize the principles and limits of patient confidentiality as defined by professional practice standards and the law
1.6. Maintain appropriate relations with patients.

2. Demonstrate a commitment to their patients, profession and society through participation in profession-led regulation
2.1. Appreciate the professional, legal and ethical codes of practice
2.2. Fulfill the regulatory and legal obligations required of current practice
2.3. Demonstrate accountability to professional regulatory bodies
2.4. Recognize and respond to others' unprofessional behaviors in practice
2.5. Participate in peer review

3. Demonstrate a commitment to physician health and sustainable practice
3.1. Balance personal and professional priorities to ensure personal health and a sustainable practice
3.2. Strive to heighten personal and professional awareness and insight
3.3. Recognize other professionals in need and respond appropriately

Figure 10-1 ■ CanMEDS professional role.

Credit: Frank JR. The CanMEDS 2005 Physician Competency Framework. Better standards. Better physicians. Better Care; 2005. Available at: http://www.royalcollege.ca/portal/page/portal/rc/common/documents/canmeds/resources/publications/framework_full_e.pdf. Copyright © 2005 The Royal College of Physicians and Surgeons of Canada http://rcpsc.medical.org/canmeds. Reproduced with permission.

> The program must integrate the following ACGME competencies into the curriculum:
> i. Professionalism
> Residents must demonstrate a commitment to carrying out professional responsibilities
> and an adherence to ethical principles. Residents are expected to demonstrate:
>   1) compassion, integrity, and respect for others;
>   2) responsiveness to patient needs that supersedes self-interest;
>   3) respect for patient privacy and autonomy;
>   4) accountability to patients, society and the profession; and
>   5) sensitivity and responsiveness to a diverse patient population, including but not
>   limited to diversity in gender, age, culture, race, religion, disabilities, and sexual
>   orientation.

Figure 10-2 ▪ ACGME competencies.

Credit: Accreditation Council for Graduate Medical Education (ACGME). Program Director Guide to the
    Common Program Requirements September, 2012.

2012). These frameworks were developed to guide teaching and to enable evaluation in the postgraduate setting.

The CanMEDS definition is broader than the one from the ACGME, encompassing not only the usual behaviors we consider (honesty, ethical behavior, and so on) but also a duty to participate in self-regulation (including peer review) and to attend to one's own personal health and wellbeing. It is also evident that many of the behaviors listed involve effective communication, yet this word does not appear explicitly. That is not to imply that communication is unimportant to professionalism, only that explicit evaluation of communication is captured in other components of the CanMEDS and ACGME frameworks. Clarity about the definition of professionalism is critical before planning evaluation.

There are other reasons that evaluating professionalism can be difficult. One issue is that if one starts with abstract principles, such as "honesty," it can be difficult to operationalize exactly what that means and how to apply it in a given situation, like in the earlier example. Often we make it seem too black and white—the student told the truth or she lied; someone is "professional" or "unprofessional"—which leaves no room for gray, for interpretation in context (Ginsburg et al, 2000). Perhaps most importantly, issues of professionalism have often been considered to be issues of character, of a person's personality or traits—a student is "honest" or "a liar"—and not as issues of behavior. Nobody wants to judge someone else's character as good or bad and, hence, framing professionalism as a character trait has historically been a barrier to evaluating professionalism. In fact, we mostly find that lapses in professionalism occur in basically "good" (or well-intentioned) people who are acting in difficult situations; this framing makes it much easier to evaluate without judging (see Chapter 2, Resilience in Facing Professionalism Challenges).

RELATIONSHIP OF ATTITUDES TO BEHAVIORS AND IMPLICATIONS FOR EVALUATION

Dr. Reid, an attending on general surgery, is asked to complete an evaluation on Kevin, one of her residents, who she's been working with for the past 2 weeks. Between post-call days, clinics, and other events, she realizes she has not directly observed much of Kevin's performance. His patient assessments seem to be accurate and he is efficient in completing his work by the end of the day. He is quite good technically in the operating room (OR). She thinks he meets expectations for professionalism but is now feeling uneasy filling out this part of the form. On the one hand, she's heard no complaints about him, and has not witnessed anything egregious. On the other hand, there was that time he seemed a bit glib and insensitive when discussing an obese patient in the surgeon's lounge. She overheard him say it was the patient's fault that she now requires bariatric surgery. The other surgeons in the lounge did not react at all. Dr. Reid is now, in retrospect, concerned about this potentially negative attitude, although she has no evidence it altered his care of the patient.

Why is Dr. Reid feeling uneasy? Partly because she realizes (too late) that she did not spend sufficient time directly observing this resident's behavior, and the potential "red flag" has not been explored or addressed. But another reason is that she is not sure whether having a bad attitude toward something is really important, or whether it is the behavior that counts. She is not alone—in fact, an enormous body of research has confirmed that the link between attitudes and behaviors is tenuous. One meta-analysis of nearly 800 studies in psychology found that the relationship between a person's attitudes and their behaviors was only moderate (with a correlation of about 0.4) (Wallace et al, 2005). When the pressure to behave in a particular way is high, or the behavior is more difficult to enact, the correlation between attitudes and behaviors may be significantly lower (Rees & Knight, 2007). Overall, evidence suggests that if the attitude is not very strong, the behavior is difficult, and there is a lot of pressure involved, the attitudes themselves may not count for much. This is actually helpful when we try to understand why "good" people sometimes do "bad" things. Indeed, putting it into the context of medical education, this is exactly the situation we see in medical students, who likely have very good attitudes and intentions to behave in certain ways but face a great deal of pressure to act otherwise; some of these behaviors can be quite difficult (e.g., going against one's resident or attending's directive). Yet we neglect these important influences when we evaluate, focusing solely on the individual and neglecting the context—or, if not entirely neglecting it, believing that the student should be "strong enough" or mature enough to overcome these external factors (Ginsburg, Lingard, & Regehr, 2008).

The example of Kevin who comments negatively about the obese patient demonstrates the other side of this—a resident who may have a negative attitude but does not appear to have actually done anything wrong. Since nothing bad happened to a patient, should Dr. Reid ignore the attitude? The answer, of course, is no! This situation presents an excellent teachable moment to explore what lies behind Kevin's comment. For example, maybe Kevin was echoing what he heard from other surgeons and does not, in fact, have a negative attitude—maybe he was just trying to fit in. Alternatively, Kevin may have made a glib comment as a joke without understanding the negative impact of his comment on others, including students for whom he serves as a role model. Kevin may also have been using black humor as a cathartic way of dealing with a stressful situation, which Dr. Reid may be unaware of. To better understand Kevin's performance, Dr. Reid should attempt to gather information from other sources (e.g., other attendings, nurses, students, and so on) to see if this is an isolated issue or if patterns exist. Just because the behavior in this case did not appear to be a problem, we do not know if it will be in the future, so looking at patterns and consistencies in behaviors is much more important than evaluating any one point in time.

EVALUATION IN THE CONTEXT OF THE HEALTHCARE SYSTEM

An attending, Dr. Brown, is on the wards and sees that his resident, Dr. Kessler, is struggling to order a test on the computer. Dr. Kessler's password does not seem to be allowing her to log in and she does not have time to call information technology to get it reset. Last time it took over 20 minutes. She notices that another resident has walked away from one of the computer stations and forgot to log out, so she goes over and orders her patient's test on the other resident's account. She logs out and walks away.

What should Dr. Brown do? Dr. Kessler violated the hospital's policy, which clearly states that it is forbidden to use another healthcare provider's account for any reason. Her behavior could be considered a lapse. But Dr. Brown also realizes that the hospital's new computer system makes it difficult at times to get things done efficiently, and they have had lots of problems with passwords lately. How should he evaluate his resident's professionalism? If he decides to take the systems issue into account, how might that look on an evaluation form? The form only focuses on the individual.

Fortunately there is now a growing recognition of the importance of taking the bigger picture into account when evaluating professionalism. For example, an international working group on evaluating professionalism suggested that there are three main perspectives, or lenses, through which evaluation might be considered (Hodges et al, 2011).

1. The first perspective is that professionalism is an individual level characteristic, trait, or behavior.
2. The second considers professionalism as an interpersonal process (e.g., teacher-student, student-student, or student-patient).
3. The third, most often forgotten, is that professionalism is also a socially determined phenomenon associated with power, institutions, and society.

It is too easy to consider only one perspective (usually the individual level) and neglect the influence of the other two. It is equally important to not neglect individual responsibility when considering the effect of institutions and organizations. This is consistent with the framework used in this book that highlights the influences of teams, settings, and the external environment on professionalism in daily life.

For the preceding case, where the resident used another healthcare provider's computer access, we can see that although the resident did something incorrect, there were other issues involved: the challenging computer system, poor IT support, the other resident's failure to log out of his session, and perhaps a lack of other knowledge or resources that would have enabled her to behave more appropriately.

Despite recent advances, most of our evaluations of professionalism are still focused on individuals, largely for the practical reason that we need to ensure that individuals are able to behave professionally. In the past these evaluations would often involve an assessment of attitudes, but we have shifted significantly over the years to more of a focus on behaviors. As described earlier and elsewhere in this book, this is in part due to the recognition that attitudes are not very good predictors of behavior. It has also been argued that behaviors may be easier and more "objective" to evaluate, yet we have also seen (as in the first example of honesty with the patient) that a particular behavior may be judged differently by two different people, depending on what they think the underlying motivation was behind it (Ginsburg, Regehr, & Lingard, 2004). Some studies have found that the evaluator's opinion about the motivation may outweigh their opinion about the behavior itself. If we ascribe a behavior to what we think of as a "good" intention, we will think of the behavior as "good," and vice versa. But of course we usually don't know what the intention is, and instead we infer it.

You might think that if we knew people's intentions we would be much better positioned to judge their behavior. However, in reality it is difficult for people to decide what is more important—the behavior or the motivation behind it (Ginsburg, Regehr, & Mylopoulos, 2009). What is better—a student who does the wrong thing but for the right reason or a student who does the right thing for the wrong reason? As Hafferty (2006) asked, "Do we want physicians who *are* professional, or will we settle for physicians who can *act* in a professional manner?" A patient may greatly prefer the "right" behavior to be done, but from an education and development perspective it may be more important to focus on the students' reasons for action, as then we can form a basis for education (Rees & Knight, 2008).

It might seem strange to be critical of evaluating behaviors when our framework emphasizes them. Yet the two points of view are not contradictory—we advocate for assessing behaviors *in context*. Perhaps even more importantly, the patterns and consistencies in behavior are far more important than one-off events, however, good or bad they may be. In the case of Dr. Kessler, the resident who used someone else's computer password, the attending decided to have a conversation with her about this apparently common workaround. Dr. Brown had known Dr. Kessler for 3 weeks and had never witnessed problematic behavior, so this appeared to be a one-off event rather than part of a pattern. Although Dr. Kessler recognized that it was against the rules, it turns out that many others use the same strategy. Instead of recording a lapse in professionalism, Dr. Brown realized that what was more important in this situation was that Dr. Kessler learns better strategies for the future (e.g., being a bit more patient and waiting her turn, politely asking someone if she could use an occupied computer, using one on another nursing station, and so on). Together, they decided to approach the IT department and help come up with a solution to the problem so that the workarounds would no longer be necessary.

LEARNING EXERCISE 10-1

1. Think of an incident in which a student, resident, or physician displayed potentially unprofessional behavior.

2. Can you describe the responses, both verbal and nonverbal, of all who were present (including yourself)?

3. Do you think the responses were appropriate? Explain why or why not?

4. Was this behavior documented on an evaluation? Why or why not?

5. Would you do anything differently if it happened again?

INSTRUMENTS FOR MEASURING PROFESSIONALISM

A comprehensive analysis of all possible methods for evaluating professionalism is clearly beyond the scope of a single chapter. Luckily, several excellent resources exist for this purpose (Lynch, Surdyk, & Eiser, 2004; Stern, 2006; Goldie, 2013). No one instrument will be capable of evaluating every element of professionalism in all possible contexts and for multiple purposes. Thus a *system* of evaluation is critically important, one that includes multiple methods with varying strengths and weaknesses and importantly integrates them into a holistic assessment of an individual's competence (Schuwirth & van der Vleuten, 2012). If we remember that professionalism can be thought of as a multidimensional competency that evolves over the course of a persons' education, training, and professional career, we can start to imagine what good evaluations might look like along the way.

First, it is important to consider the purpose of assessment. There are many reasons to evaluate people, including:

- a need to ensure competence for practice (or for the next stage of learning);
- to plan remediation;
- to feedback to curriculum if systematic gaps are found; and
- for medical licensure.

But more recently there has been a recognition that assessment is not only *of* learning but *for* learning (Schuwirth & van der Vleuten, 2011). Assessment in and of itself is a learning experience. Usually we think of assessment as being either formative or summative (formative refers to assessment that does not "count" and is for feedback purposes only; summative counts for decision-making). Figure 10-3 depicts the components that evaluations should encompass.

Thus we should be thinking about systems of assessment rather than of individual tools (van der Vleuten & Schuwirth, 2005). Given the developmental nature of professionalism as a competency, it is also important to use different methods for different stages. Figure 10-4 provides one useful way of thinking of this by drawing our attention to "Miller's pyramid" and the developmental trajectory. Each level is important to assess and each requires different methods.

Specific Evaluation Methods

What are the most common methods for evaluating professionalism and what are the strengths and weaknesses of each? In addition to the caveats noted earlier, we should also mention that sometimes the same method may be appropriate for formative assessment (designed to provide feedback) in some situations and summative assessment in others. Table 10-1 summarizes a variety of evaluation, their advantages and disadvantages, and tips for their best use. The

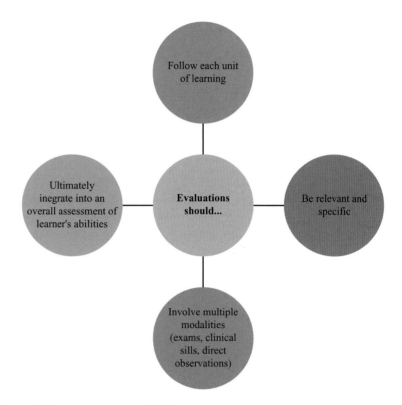

Figure 10-3 ▪ Components of effective evaluations.

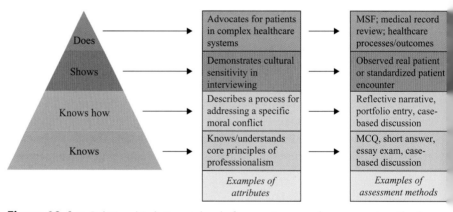

Figure 10-4 ▪ Relationship between level of competence and assessment methods.
From Hawkins RE, Katsufrakis PJ, Holtman MC, Clauser BE. Assessment of medical professionalism: who, what, when, where, how, and . . . why? *Med Teach.* 2009 Apr;31(4):348–361.

majority of evaluation methods are used for medical students and residents, but several are used frequently for practicing physicians or faculty members (these are indicated with an asterisk).

Table 10-1	EVALUATION METHODS – ADVANTAGES AND DISADVANTAGES		
Evaluation type and brief description	Advantages	Disadvantages	Tips for best use
In-training evaluation reports			
Usually used by faculty at end of rotation to evaluate residents/ students. Often has separate section for professionalism	Simple, familiar, evaluates what people actually "do" in practice, covers multiple competencies, may be reliable/valid if enough reports collected	Often not based on direct observation; recall bias; halo effect and other biases; thought to be too "subjective," which affects credibility; hard to know where to account for professionalism	Promote direct observations; use rating scales based on performance, not expectations; provide ample space for comments
Peer assessment*			
Evaluations from fellow students/residents, sometimes staff	Peers offer unique perspective, lots of observations in variety of contexts; peers are willing to participate if used appropriately; some good validity evidence	Concern about effects on relationships; often no link to reward or remediation	Consider whether open vs. anonymous; need good training and safe environment
Multi-source Feedback*			
Incorporates feedback from peers, self, patients, other healthcare professionals	Capitalizes on unique nature of others' observations; shown to be feasible and valid approach; credibility due to multiple sources	Need good infrastructure; lots of training needed for other healthcare professionals; need lots of ratings to be reliable (esp. from patients)	For formative feedback; best if well-structured teams with training; be clear on how they will be used and who will see them
Standardized patients (SPs) and OSCEs			
Can be used for teaching and evaluation, with structured evaluation instruments that often include elements of professionalism	Usually SPs are well trained and are able to assess empathy, humanism, and other elements of professionalism; often in use already and familiar	Lack authenticity and perhaps credibility for learners; SPs may attend to different types of behaviors than other evaluators; can encourage scripted responses that don't relate to how students act in practice; expensive to run	Consider which elements of professionalism are best to assess this way and don't try to do everything

(Continued)

Table 10-1 **EVALUATION METHODS – ADVANTAGES AND DISADVANTAGES (*Continued*)**			
Evaluation type and brief description	**Advantages**	**Disadvantages**	**Tips for best use**
Encounter cards			
Developed to be used at the end of a day or shift; like a small-scale ITER	Can include professional behaviors; simple to fill out; good research backing their use; usually part of a system of evaluation	Professionalism issues often not documented; issues that arise can get overlooked in the mass of data collected or dismissed as outliers	For planned or unplanned observations of professionalism behaviors
Critical incident reports			
To be used once a lapse has occurred	Written to reflect common lapses; easy to use and understand; allows for comparison across courses and detection of patterns	No role for most students; thresholds for reporting may differ between rotations; usually only capture lapses, not positive behavior	Should be embedded in a larger program of evaluation. Standardization between courses is useful.
P-MEX			
The Professionalism Mini-Evaluation Exercise was developed to parallel the mini-CEX (clinical evaluation exercise). Involves direct observation and feedback of trainees	Focused only on professionalism; mandates direct observation and written feedback; reliable with ~8; can use any time	Can be hard to find time to fit in with other evaluations; difficult to collect 8 or more	Planned observations of professionalism behaviors
Physician achievement review*			
A specific type of multisource feedback that is mandatory every 5 years in Alberta, Canada	Well-researched, specific forms relevant to various stakeholder groups; evidence of reliability and validity	Can be difficult for practicing physicians to accept 360-degree feedback; takes time and resources to provide feedback	Include trained professionals to give feedback and plan remediation; reward progress
Conscientiousness Index			
Type of evaluation that awards (or deducts) points for compliance with important administrative tasks	Objective as points awarded based on tasks done; correlates with future professionalism	Advantage can be lost if students know what's being measured; not all administrative staff may be happy playing this role	As part of a system of professionalism evaluation; also include potential for extra reward points for exemplary behavior.

*frequently used for practicing physicians of faculty members

SPECIFIC INSTRUMENTS

1. Assessment of trainees at the end of a rotation

Evaluations at the end of a rotation, or in-training evaluation reports (ITERs), are the most frequently used instruments for the evaluation of trainees' performance in general, and may have items that directly or indirectly relate to professionalism. They are usually filled out by faculty at the end of a rotation on the inpatient wards or in the clinic. Students and residents may work with multiple attending physicians and thus may receive many ITERs by the end of a rotation or year. They are very common, familiar to attending physicians, and have been studied extensively. The main benefit to using these evaluation forms for assessment of professionalism is that they are already incorporated into training programs and, hence, are part of normal routine. Both the CanMEDS and the ACGME framework form the basis for these common evaluation forms, and typically these have a section to evaluate each one of the competencies including professionalism. There is also an overall, or global rating, as well as space for comments.

Despite their widespread use, ITERs have often been criticized for not demonstrating good reliability or validity. However, if enough forms are gathered per learner (in the range of 8 or so, depending on the tool) the reliability can be acceptable. At least one specialty (internal medicine) has shown that these forms can be used to predict future professionalism issues in practice (Papadakis et al, 2008). The study demonstrated that trainees with lower professionalism scores on their evaluations during training were more likely to be disciplined by state medical boards in future practice.

One of the main drawbacks of these forms is that professionalism can be difficult to tease out and document. For example, poor communication with other team members might be considered poor professionalism—but may be captured on an evaluation form as difficulty in the competency of communication and interpersonal skills. So the tracking of professionalism issues, distinct from other competencies, might be difficult. For this reason some programs have used a separate form just for professionalism where these issues can be documented and tracked. The University of Toronto uses a separate rating form for professionalism of students on each course or rotation (Figure 10-5). It is framed in terms of behaviors, and the rating scale focuses on lapses (none, minor, or major). The items are based on behaviors relevant to students in that particular course.

2. Peer Assessment

There are advantages and disadvantages to asking students to evaluate each other (Norcini, 2003; Arnold et al, 2005). One clear advantage is that students are often in the best position to actually observe their peers' behaviors,

University of Toronto – Faculty of Medicine   81195

Clerkship Professionalism Evaluation Form - 2001–2002

Name: _____   Supervisor _____
                                          Please print

please use the following scale: W6

Meets professional expectations	Observed 1 or 2 minor lapses of professional behaviour	Observed 1 major lapse or 3 or more minor lapses of professional behaviour	Was not in a position to observe professional/ unprofessional behaviour	mark the box with dark ink ➡ ●
A	**B**	**C**	**N**	A B C N/O

A   Altruism

#		A	B	C	N/O
1	Demonstrates sensitivity to patients' needs	☐	☐	☐	☐
2	Takes time and effort to explain information to patients	☐	☐	☐	☐
3	Takes time and effort to comfort the sick patient	☐	☐	☐	☐
4	Listens sympathetically to patients' concerns	☐	☐	☐	☐
5	Puts patients' interests before his/her own	☐	☐	☐	☐
6	Shows respect for patients' confidentiality	☐	☐	☐	☐

B   Duty: Reliability and Responsibility

7	Completes assigned tasks timely and fully	☐	☐	☐	☐
8	Fulfills obligations undertaken	☐	☐	☐	☐
9	Takes on appropriate share of team work	☐	☐	☐	☐
10	Fulfills call duties	☐	☐	☐	☐
11	Reports accurately and fully on patient care activities	☐	☐	☐	☐
12	Always ensures transfer of responsibility for patient care	☐	☐	☐	☐
13	Informs supervisor/team when mistakes occur	☐	☐	☐	☐
14	Informs supervisor/team when faced with a conflict of interest	☐	☐	☐	☐

C   Excellence: Self Improvement and Adaptability

15	Accepts constructive feedback	☐	☐	☐	☐
16	Recognizes own limitations and seeks appropriate help	☐	☐	☐	☐
17	Incorporates feedback to make changes in behaviour	☐	☐	☐	☐
18	Adapts well to changing circumstances	☐	☐	☐	☐
19	Reads up on patient cases	☐	☐	☐	☐
20	Attends rounds, seminars, and other learning events	☐	☐	☐	☐

D   Respect for Others: Relationships with Students, Faculty & Staff

21	Establishes rapport with team members	☐	☐	☐	☐
22	Maintains appropriate boundaries in work and learning situations	☐	☐	☐	☐
23	Relates well to fellow students in a learning environment	☐	☐	☐	☐
24	Relates well to faculty in a learning environment	☐	☐	☐	☐
25	Relates well to other healthcare professionals in a learning environment	☐	☐	☐	☐

E   Honour and Integrity: Upholding Student and Professional Code of Conduct

26	Refers to self accurately with respect to qualifications	☐	☐	☐	☐
27	Uses appropriate language in discussion with patients and colleagues	☐	☐	☐	☐
28	Resolves conflicts in a manner that respects the dignity of those involved	☐	☐	☐	☐
29	Behaves honestly	☐	☐	☐	☐
30	Respects diversity of race, gender, religion, sexual orientation, age, disability, intelligence, and socio-economic status	☐	☐	☐	☐
31	Maintains appropriate boundaries with patients	☐	☐	☐	☐
32	Dresses in an appropriate professional manner (context specific)	☐	☐	☐	☐

F   Global Rating of Professionalism   6 = Excellent   1 = Poor   6☐ 5☐ 4☐ 3☐ 2☐ 1☐

If global rating is less than 4, please state reasons in critical comments section.

Critical Comments: *(note if there was a critical event, please document it here)*   **Critical Event:** ☐ Yes   ☐ No

This appraisal was completed by: ☐ a person   ☐ consensus of more than one person

Please sign below ONLY after the evaluation has been discussed with the student. Student signature does not necessarily imply agreement with the evaluation, only that it has been discussed.

Student's Signature: _____   Supervisor's Signature: _____
        Date: _____   Date: _____

Figure 10-5 ▪ University of Toronto clerkship evaluation form.
Reproduced with permission of Jay Rosenfeld, University of Toronto.

across varied settings and context and often over prolonged periods. It is important to note that they may be together in situations when no one else is present, so can offer a unique perspective on others' professionalism. On the other hand, students are often reluctant to evaluate one another because of concerns it may affect friendships or working relationships, or because they do not feel it is their responsibility. However, peer assessment is becoming more accepted in education and in some instances in clinical practice, so providing students with the opportunity to learn how to do it properly is an important goal.

There are two main types of peer assessment—ratings and nominations. Peer ratings are similar to ward assessments and ITERs in that they have multiple items tapping into different elements of competence, each rated on a Likert-type scale (e.g., from 1—5). They are designed to reflect what students can best assess in their peers (e.g., they might leave out assessment of knowledge base, but it would include items on collaboration, communication, and professionalism). There have been concerns that if students are able to choose who evaluates them that it may lead to bias—but in fact studies have shown that this is not the case. The method of evaluation can be reliable and valid, independent of whether students are assigned as raters or whether they are chosen by peers (Lurie et al, 2006). Centrally assigned peer evaluations allow for more anonymity if that is desired and may be easier to track.

The other main method of peer assessment is by nomination—that is, one can ask students to name or vote for classmates who they feel are highly professional, or who they would want to work with or send loved ones to one day. Similarly they can select peers who they feel the opposite way about. These systems have good reliability for picking up the very tops and bottoms of the class. One study showed that positive nominations were predictive of better clinical competence and empathy (Pohl, Hojat, & Arnold, 2011). Obviously most students will be somewhere in the middle and may never receive nominations at either end, so this system cannot be used for formative feedback on a day to day basis.

Some researchers have found that students may have strong preferences regarding the use of peer assessment of professionalism, especially concerning anonymity and confidentiality, and whether and how they might be used in a summative assessment. They also expressed a strong desire to see some results for their efforts; for example, if they went through the stress and effort to point out behavioral issues in a peer, that information should lead to remediation and improvement and not simply be filed away (Arnold et al, 2005).

3. Multisource Feedback

Dr. Verma is an accomplished surgeon who has been working in the same hospital for 15 years, and has never had any complaints.

Because of new accreditation standards, the hospital has recently instituted multisource feedback for all personnel. Dr. Verma just received his first round of evaluations from his team, which include the operating room (OR) nurses, anesthetists, respiratory therapists and other technologists, and booking clerks. They all comment on his excellent communication with patients, superb technical skills, and quality teaching. However, three evaluations noted that when things get stressful in the OR he "shuts down" and is difficult to communicate with. He has occasionally snapped at individuals who have interrupted him during these times. At first, Dr. Verma is shocked to read these somewhat negative comments, and initially tries to figure out who might have written them, as he wonders if they reflect "personality differences" and nothing more. But then he takes a moment to reflect, and considers that if three different people made the same observations that there may be some truth to them. He thinks back to some recent situations where this might have been an issue, and realizes that at those moments he is at tricky phases of the operation, concentrating intensely, and the background chatter distracts him. It never occurred to him that he might not only be offending his colleagues but may in fact be impeding good communication, which could affect patient safety. Dr. Verma decides that next time it happens he will tell the team he needs quiet in order to concentrate.

What is multisource feedback (MSF)? It is not a tool in itself but rather combines evaluations from multiple sources that "surround" the individual. Sometimes they are called 360-degree evaluations for that reason. The idea is that instead of having just one-way evaluations (faculty to learner), each learner might be evaluated by those above (supervisors, teachers), those at the same level (peer assessments), those below them (students), and those that surround them (nurses, administrators, pharmacists, social workers, and so on). The main advantages of MSF relate to the ability to combine assessments from multiple relevant sources, which adds to credibility and authenticity. As with Dr. Verma, it is harder to dismiss a criticism if it comes from multiple sources.

There are various methods for conducting MSF. Issues that require consideration include:

- whether to use the same form or different ones for the various groups;
- how to properly train individuals who are completing the forms; and
- whether to combine all the results or keep those from different groups separate (i.e., patient feedback separate from nurses, and so on).

Feedback from different groups often diverge, and when this occurs there is a tendency to believe the evaluations we like (i.e., that conform to our own self-images) and to discount the ones we disagree with or that we find threatening. Therefore, it takes skill and a safe environment to provide this feedback to the individual and to ensure that there are opportunities for questioning, learning, and setting goals for the future. It is also important to be aware of "evaluator fatigue" from having the same people fill out so many forms on each other on a recurrent basis. It helps to keep the forms brief and simple, and to stagger their administration so that they don't all come out at once. Having buy-in on the value of the assessments and their outcomes is also critical to the system's success.

4. Standardized Patients, OSCEs

Standardized patients (SPs) have been used for many years to both teach and evaluate clinical skills, especially involving patient interviewing and physical exam maneuvers. Whether in individual sessions or as part of Objective Structured Clinical Exams (OSCEs), standardized patients have been shown to be able to evaluate certain elements of professionalism. It is important to remember that different groups can have very different views of what it means to "be" or at least act professional—and SPs are no different (Zanetti et al, 2010). Just like real patients, SPs may value certain styles of communication or interaction, but if they are well trained they can assess learners with a fair degree of reliability. This makes them suitable for assessment of large groups of learners where standardization is critical. Indeed, they have been used extensively for licensing exams in the United States and Canada.

When it comes to assessment, the main downside to SPs and OSCEs is that they can feel forced and unrealistic, and these exams have been accused of promoting "checklist behaviors," in which the students learn to fire off questions to get points, at the expense of a more natural, holistic approach, which may be harder to standardize for assessment (Hodges et al, 1999). Good research has shown that a global rating on an OSCE station can actually be more reliable than checklist scores, but the trade-off is that the student may not receive sufficiently specific feedback to act on. Again, we struggle here with the difference between acting professionally for a test and behaving (or being) professional in real life with patients and colleagues. This issue may be particularly exacerbated by the artificiality of an OSCE. That said, SPs and OSCEs have proven to be useful for evaluating certain elements of professionalism, such as empathy, dealing with uncertainty, and conflict management. The key is to define the elements under study and to provide anchors to denote different levels of performance, and to train all raters so that they use the scale reliably. Overall, OSCEs are probably best used for formative feedback on professionalism rather than for any high-stakes assessment.

5. Encounter Cards

Encounter cards (Figure 10-6) can be thought of as "small-scale equivalents of ITERs" (Sherbino, Bandiera, & Frank, 2008) and are often used in disciplines such as emergency medicine or anesthesia, where a learner may spend a whole day or shift with a particular attending and then will receive an evaluation focused on that day. The advantages of encounter cards are that they are far less subject to recall bias as they are completed on the spot, and each day

Junior Resident Shift Feedback Card–Emergency Medicine (FRONT)

JUNIOR RESIDENT: ________ DATE ______ SUPERVISING PHYSICIAN: ________

1. Rate the Overall performance ON THIS SHIFT with a circle or 'x' on the line below.

AS EXPECTED

Performing > 1 yr Below PGY level	Somewhat behind for level	Somewhat ahead for level	Much better than Expected for level	Consultant Level

2. Using 2 or 3 of the following CanMEDS Roles, explain where the resident needs to improve to move up a level on the above scale. Provide specific examples for the assessments.

N = NEEDS ATTENTION; S = PARTICULAR STRENGTH

MEDICAL EXPERT:	Assessment		Example(s)
-Can APPROACH most presenting problems	N	S	________
-Safe basic procedural skills	N	S	________

JUNIOR Resident Shift Feedback Card–Emergency Medicine (BACK)

	Assessment		Example(s)
SCHOLAR: (Inquisitive, Evidence-based, uses IT well)	N	S	________
MANAGER: (Considers resource issues, efficient)	N	S	________
HEALTH ADVOCATE: (Knows determinants of health, advocates for patient)	N	S	________
COMMUNICATOR: (Patient interactions, case presentations, charting)	N	S	________
COLLABORATOR: (Collegial, understands roles)	N	S	________
PROFESSIONAL: (Punctual, responsible, has integrity, ethical)	N	S	________

3. GENERAL COMMENTS:

____

____

STAFF SIGNATURE: ________ RESIDENT SIGNATURE: ________

Figure 10-6 ▪ University of Toronto encounter card.
Reproduced with permission of Jay Rosenfeld, University of Toronto.

or shift has an evaluation, which translates into far more data collected per learner. This translates into more direct observation and feedback as well—indeed, the requirement for immediate feedback may be the greatest benefit. Encounter cards have been used for professionalism evaluation but there are challenges—even when professionalism issues arise they are not always documented; and because of the multitude of forms collected, any professionalism issues that are documented may get lost in the shuffle.

However, encounter cards also offer the distinct advantage, if used properly, of being able to illustrate patterns and consistencies in behavior that might otherwise go unnoticed. As discussed previously, these patterns may be far more important than single, one-off events.

6. Critical Incident Reports

Critical incident reports are instruments meant to be used for documentation when a lapse in professionalism has occurred. They are designed to be used as one part of a system of evaluation and clearly should not be the only method, because they just wouldn't apply to most learners. An exemplar program has been developed at the University of California, San Francisco, which has been widely published and adopted. Their instrument is called a Physicianship Evaluation Form (Figure 10-7) and is filled out and submitted

---

UCSF SCHOOL OF MEDICINE
PHYSICIANSHIP EVALUATION FORM

Student name (type or print legibly)_____

Course (Dept. & Course No.)_____

Site Director Quarter, Block and Year_____

Site Director's Signature Location_____

Date this form was discussed with the student _____

A student with a pattern of the following behavior has not sufficiently demonstrated professional and personal attributes for meeting the standards of professionalism inherent in being a physician:

Circle the appropriate category. Comments are required.

1. Unmet professional responsibility:

a. The student needs continual reminders in the fulfillment of responsibilities to patients or to other healthcare professionals.

b. The student cannot be relied upon to complete tasks.

c. The student misrepresents or falsifies actions and/or information.
_____
_____
_____
_____   *(Continued)*

2. Lack of effort toward self improvement and adaptability:

a. The student is resistant or defensive in accepting criticism.

b. The student remains unaware of his/her own inadequacies.

c. The student resists considering or making changes.

d. The student does not accept blame for failure, or responsibility for errors.

e. The student is abusive or critical during times of stress.

f. The student demonstrates arrogance.

_____
_____
_____
_____

3. Diminished relationships with patients and families:

a. The student inadequately establishes rapport with patients or families.

b. The student is often insensitive to the patients' or families' feelings, needs or wishes.

c. The student uses his/her professional position to engage in romantic or sexual relationships with patients or members of their families.

d. The student lacks empathy.

e. The student has inadequate personal commitment to honoring the wishes of the patients.

_____
_____
_____
_____
_____

4. Diminished relationships with members of the healthcare team:

a. The student does not function within a healthcare team.

b. The student is insensitive to the needs, feelings and wishes of the healthcare team members.

_____
_____
_____
_____
_____

5. Please comment on an appropriate plan of action to pursue when counseling the student.

_____
_____
_____
_____
_____

This section is to be completed by the student.

6. My comments are: (optional)

_____

_____

_____

_____

7. I have read this evaluation and discussed it with the clerkship director.

Student signature_____

Date_____

2/27/03

Figure 10-7 ▪ Physicianship evaluation form.

From University of California, San Francisco. Undergraduate Medical Education: Physicianship Evaluation Forms
    and Policies; 2013. Available at: http://meded.ucsf.edu/ume/physicianship-evaluation-forms-and-policies.

for any student with less than satisfactory professionalism performance during medical school. The domains on the form include reliability and responsibility; self-improvement and adaptability; relationships with students, faculty, self, or patients; and upholding the medical student statement of principles. Research has shown that some domains of unprofessional behavior (i.e., poor reliability and responsibility, lack of self-improvement and adaptability, and poor initiative and motivation) were especially associated with future disciplinary action once students were out in practice (Papadakis et al, 2005).

This system has allowed the school to track issues of professionalism and to act on them decisively, for example, by dismissing students with repeated lapses despite feedback (Papadakis et al, 1999).

7. Professionalism Mini-Evaluation Exercise (P-MEX)

The P-MEX (Figure 10-8) was developed jointly by McGill University and the ABIM Foundation, as a professionalism-focused mini-CEX (clinical evaluation exercise) (Cruess et al, 2006). Instead of including all elements of a patient interview, physical exam, clinical reasoning, and so on, it focuses on behaviors of professionalism. This 24-item form has demonstrated good reliability and some validity, and has been used in various settings. One advantage is the focus solely on concrete issues of professionalism (e.g., demonstrated awareness of limitations, accepted feedback, maintained appropriate boundaries, and so on).

Each P-MEX includes a section for written feedback that is given to the learner "on the spot." Students are able to select when they wish to be observed, or alternatively an attending may happen to observe an encounter

Evaluator:_____

Student/Resident:_____

Level: (please check) □ **3rd yr** □ **4th yr** □ **res 1** □ **res 2** □ **res 3** □ **res 4** □ **res 5**

Setting: <u>Patient Related</u>: □ **Patient Present** □ **Patient Not Present**

□ **Ward** □ **Clinic** □ **OR** □ **ER**

<u>Non Patient Related</u>: □ **i.e. – general teaching, small group teaching, etc.**

	N/A	UN	BEL	MET	EXC
Listened actively to patient					
Showed interest in patient as a person					
Recognized and met patient needs					
Extended his/herself to meet patient needs					
Ensured continuity of patient care					
Advocated on behalf of a patient					
Demonstrated awareness of limitations					
Admitted errors/omissions					
Solicited feedback					
Accepted feedback					
Maintained appropriate boundaries					
Maintained composure in a difficult situation					
Maintained appropriate appearance					
Was on time					
Completed tasks in a reliable fashion					
Addressed own gaps in knowledge and skills					
Was available to colleagues					
Demonstrated respect for colleagues					
Avoided derogatory language					
Maintained patient confidentiality					
Used health resources appropriately					

▶Please rate this student's/resident's overall professional performance during THIS encounter:

□ Unacceptable □ MET expectations □ Below expectations □ Exceeded expectations

▶Did you observe a critical event? □ no □ yes (comment required)

Comments:_____

_____

_____

Evaluator's signature: _____

Student's/Resident's signature:_____

Date & Time:_____

Figure 10-8 ▪ Professionalism Mini-Evaluation Exercise.

Cruess RL, McIlroy J, Cruess SR, Ginsburg S, Steinert Y. The Professionalism Mini-evaluation Exercise:
a preliminary investigation. Acad Med. 2006 Oct;81(10 Suppl):S74–78.

and wish to document it. The form is filled out, and feedback is handed directly to the student. Thus it promotes direct observation, a focus on professionalism, and formative feedback. However, there are downsides, including the extra work required on top of other evaluations that faculty must do, which has limited feasibility, and the system support required to track all the forms and feedback.

8. Physician Achievement Review (PAR)

The PAR is a specific sort of multisource feedback that was developed in Alberta, Canada, as a method to "provide doctors with information about their medical practice through the eyes of those they work with and serve" (Physician Achievement Review, 2011). It is now mandatory for all practicing physicians in the province, who have to undergo assessment every 5 years. Although not specific for professionalism, elements of professionalism are represented, such as respect and communication. Different questionnaires are given to the relevant assessors, for example, 25 forms are collected from patients, 8 from physician peers, and 8 from coworkers. Physicians also assess themselves. The data are collated by an independent agency that provides summaries and reports, which then go to members of a Physician Performance Committee. If a problem is noted, the committee works with individual physicians to help them improve. Research has shown acceptable reliability, validity, and feasibility, and a majority of physicians find the feedback helpful. A longitudinal study showed that improvement in ratings occurred over time when assessments were done by medical colleagues and coworkers but not when assessments were done by patients (Violato, Lockyer, & Fidler, 2008).

Disadvantages include the time taken from practice to participate in a PAR (which is actually very little), and the potential distress and embarrassment from receiving negative feedback from one's patients or peers. That said, the advantages far outweigh these issues, and the existence of such systems greatly enhance the integrity and accountability of our profession in the eyes of the public.

9. Conscientiousness Index

> Dr. Smith is the Preclerkship Director and has noticed that Jacob, one of her 1st-year students, often needs repeated reminders to respond to simple requests by email. For example, most students respond immediately to confirm their schedules, but the secretary had to send Jacob three emails before he replied. He is behind in handing in course evaluations and has still not provided a copy of his immunization records, required to begin on the wards. Dr. Smith is concerned about this pattern of behavior but isn't sure what to do. Jacob shows up in class and has passed his exams. When she talks to him he doesn't seem to think these issues have anything to do with his becoming a doctor. Should she be concerned?

Stern, Frohna, and Gruppen (2005) wanted to predict which medical students might have difficulties with professionalism during training. They looked at grades, evaluations, MCAT scores—nothing was predictive. However, they noted that students who had not complied with simple administrative requests, like handing in course evaluations, or showing proof of immunization, were more likely to have professionalism issues arise during their clinical training.

Other groups picked up on this and began to track these issues, eventually resulting in the development of a "conscientiousness index" (CI). This has been shown to have some reliability and validity, and has the advantage of being fairly objective (that is, it's easy for administrators to assess compliance with tasks and to track students). One report suggests that a student's CI correlates well with peer evaluations of professionalism, lending further validity (Finn et al, 2009).

One downside is that once students learn what is being tracked they can easily adapt their behaviors to comply, and then the tool's predictive validity might be lost. On the other hand, students can gain extra points by participating in extra activities, volunteering, and so on. So if they try to "game the system" they will at least be doing—and learning—good.

LEARNING EXERCISE 10-2

You recently became the program director in a large academic pediatric residency. In reviewing the evaluations of residents you notice that the "professionalism" category has very few comments written by faculty and that the numeric scores have little variation (almost everyone is scored an 8 or 9 on the (1 to 9) scale.

You would like to introduce a new system of evaluation of professionalism. You want to create a positive environment and you are clear that your goal is to foster skills, rather than punish outliers. You know that residents might be concerned that your goal is to look for lapses. How would you proceed with this goal?

1. How would you proceed with this goal?
2. Whose advice or input would you seek?
3. What would an ideal system of assessment look like? That is, what sorts of evaluations, by whom, at what points in time, and so on?
4. What specific assessment instruments would best meet your goals? Are these feasible in your system? Why or why not?
5. What faculty (or resident) development of education would you need to have in place for this to be successful?
6. How would you evaluate whether you are meeting your goals?

CONCLUSION

Evaluating professionalism is essential to maintaining the public's trust in their doctors. Although there are challenges involved in evaluating professionalism, there are now many tools and strategies available for all levels of training, with more being developed as time goes on.

Each relevant stakeholder group (e.g., patients, students, attending physicians) may also have different tools, as each views different aspects of professionalism and from different points of view. As far as possible, methods should be formative—meaning there should always be feedback provided, with specific steps for improvement if necessary. It is best to think of a system, or program of evaluation, with different tools and methods embedded within. Self-assessment and reflection are keys to professional growth and can be incorporated in the form of portfolios.

Finally, it is important to remember that isolated incidents and lapses in behavior happen to everybody, especially to learners as they navigate their new roles as professionals. We all make mistakes but, hopefully we can learn from them. That's why it is so important to avoid labeling a person as "being" unprofessional; instead we should direct attention to the behavior, and provide feedback so that the behavior doesn't recur. Patterns and consistencies in behaviors noted over time are far more telling than isolated lapses. For the most part, lapses in professionalism occur in "good" people who are in difficult circumstances, so it is critical to develop an environment that fosters professional behavior.

CHALLENGE CASE

Sarah, a final year medical student, is at the nursing station charting on her patients. Her senior resident is post-call and has his coat on, ready to sign out and go home. He realizes he forgot to order a repeat chest x-ray on a patient who is being discharged that day. Routine x-rays can take up to 4 hours to be done so he tells Sarah to order it "stat" so it gets done within an hour. There is no clinical indication to rush it, but Sarah remembers her lecture on stewardship of finite resources and realizes that having a patient occupy an acute care bed for an extra half-day is also problematic. Just then the attending appears and overhears Sarah tell radiology that the x-ray is a stat order and has to be done immediately. Radiology apparently disagrees and says they won't do it without a clinical indication. Sarah doesn't know what to do and decides to tell them the patient has coughed up blood so that the x-ray gets done.

If you were the attending on the service and saw the student lie to radiology, what would your response be? How would you evaluate this student's professionalism?

What are some of the ways Sarah might be evaluated in this situation? The attending has heard her lie to the radiologist and this would be considered a lapse in professionalism. On the evaluation form there is an item on integrity, about behaving honestly, so he can record the lapse there. It might then be noticed by the clerkship director and end up on her final transcript. However, the attending physician might decide to have a conversation with Sarah first and ask her why she lied. Now she is torn—between coming clean and perhaps looking better in her attending's eyes or saying nothing and protecting her senior resident who forgot to order the x-ray. The senior resident has some influence on her final evaluation but that's not what concerns her now—she's worried that he may be upset and take it out on her in more subtle ways, like not giving her prime learning opportunities.

What are the implications for the resident's evaluation? If it becomes known that he was the one who initiated this situation he would be considered to have lapsed—and not just for being dishonest when it came to the reason for the urgent test, but for putting his medical student in such a bad position. That might be considered poor leadership, teaching, and role-modeling around professionalism.

In this case, multisource or peer evaluations may have been able to provide a more complete picture of the situation. For example, a nurse or social worker may have witnessed the entire event and considered that this was not a significant lapse—as they appeared to be acting in what they believed was the patient's best interest (i.e, allowing the patient to be discharged in a timely manner). The student is inexperienced but has otherwise been very responsible and honest in her interactions with others. In fact, this behavior seemed out of keeping, and was not part of a pattern. The multidisciplinary team would be able to put the behavior in context and use this opportunity for formative feedback. They would likely have suggestions for what she might do differently if the situation were to arise again.

It may go without saying, but if this was a standardized patient scenario or an OSCE station, it would probably play out quite differently. The student would probably politely explain to radiology why the test needed to be done, and if it still had to wait up to 4 hours then the student would explain to the patient and her family why she couldn't go home just yet. If done skillfully she might get a really good score on professionalism. That is because in a scripted scenario there would be no consequences to the student for her behavior and she knows she is being watched. So it would not be so helpful in that situation.

The examples above serve to remind us that most of our evaluation methods involve judgments that someone (attending physician, nurse, medical student) makes about someone else (fellow student, teacher, resident). What we haven't yet discussed is individuals' assessment of themselves. Although self-assessment in general is usually thought to be unreliable, self-reflection can be very useful. Many schools have instituted portfolio programs that can variably include students' own reflections on their actions. These reflections are thought to promote self-awareness and self-regulation, both important to resilience. Here is what Sarah wrote in her portfolio that week:

I feel just awful about what happened on the ward on Thursday. Things had been going so well on this rotation and I really wanted my staff to have a good impression of me. I'm even thinking of applying to internal medicine! And then this happened. I know the resident was post-call and it had been a brutal night, with two code blues and so many new consults. I know there were good reasons that he just forgot to order the x-ray—but I wish it didn't then become my problem. If only he had just taken care of it himself. But actually I know that's not the point. When you're totally fatigued and sleep deprived you need to go home, and I'm sure there were lots of other things he signed out as well. In fact, I'll be glad that that's the system when I'm a resident. But I could have done things differently—there was really no need to lie, plus I'm a really honest person! I should have just explained the situation to radiology, and admitted I was in a bind—maybe they would have helped me out. Or I could have asked one of the nurses what to do, as I'm sure this is not the first time something like this has happened. If worse came to worst, I could have politely explained our mistake to the patient and his family, and let them know that it might be a few hours before they could leave. Maybe they would have understood. Yeah, that's what I would do next time. I'm going to ask Dr. Y if he has time to meet this week and discuss it, so he knows I'm not a bad person.

These sorts of reflections can be very powerful, especially for the person who writes them. The student has worked through her disappointment and anger, and has come to a good solution by the end. She hopes that she will continue to write and reflect when she begins her residency. That would be an excellent strategy for demonstrating growth and increasing competency as a professional. Although portfolios and self-reflections can be very important to developing as professionals, they are not without controversy. In an education setting they are often read and sometimes scored by others, so true, honest reflections may be inhibited.

KEY LEARNING POINTS

1. Professionalism must be evaluated as explicitly and rigorously as every other competency.
2. Information and assessments should be gathered from a variety of stakeholder groups including attending physicians, colleagues, students, and patients.
3. Evaluations should be as formative as possible; that is, they should all provide specific feedback so that learners and faculty can improve where needed.
4. Multiple methods must be used as no single instrument will be sufficient to capture all important elements.
5. A well-designed program or system of evaluation is required to integrate and synthesize evaluations from multiple sources, courses, and rotations.

REFERENCES

1. Accreditation Council for Graduate Medical Education (ACGME). Program Director Guide to the Common Program Requirements September, 2012. Available at: http://www.acgme.org/acgmeweb/Portals/0/PDFs/commonguide/CompleteGuide_v2%20.pdf
2. Arnold L, Shue CK, Kritt B, Ginsburg S, Stern DT. Medical students' views on peer assessment of professionalism. *J Gen Intern Med*. 2005 Sep;20(9):819–824.
3. Cruess RL, McIlroy J, Cruess SR, Ginsburg S, Steinert Y. The Professionalism Mini–Evaluation Exercise: a preliminary investigation. *Acad Med*. 2006 Oct;81(10 Suppl):S74–78.
4. Finn G, Sawdon M, Clipsham L, McLachlan J. Peer estimation of lack of professionalism correlates with low Conscientiousness Index scores. *Med Educ*. 2009 Oct;43(10):960–967.
5. Frank JR. *The CanMEDS 2005 Physician Competency Framework. Better standards. Better physicians. Better Care*; 2005. Available at: http://www.royalcollege.ca/portal/page/portal/rc/common/documents/canmeds/resources/publications/framework_full_e.pdf
6. Ginsburg S, Lingard L, Regehr G, Underwood K. Know when to rock the boat: how faculty rationalize students' behaviors. *J Gen Intern Med*. 2008 Jul;23(7):942–947.
7. Ginsburg S, Regehr G, Hatala R, McNaughton N, Frohna A, Hodges B, Lingard L, Stern D. Context, conflict, and resolution: a new conceptual framework for evaluating professionalism. *Acad Med*. 2000 Oct;75(10 Suppl):S6–S11.

8. Ginsburg S, Regehr G, Lingard L. The disavowed curriculum: understanding students' reasoning in professionally challenging situations. *J Gen Intern Med.* 2003 Dec;18(12):1015–1022.

9. Ginsburg S, Regehr G, Lingard L. Basing the evaluation of professionalism on observable behaviors: a cautionary tale. *Acad Med.* 2004 Oct;79(10 Suppl):S1–S4.

10. Ginsburg S, Regehr G, Mylopoulos M. From behaviors to attributions: further concerns regarding the evaluation of professionalism. *Med Educ.* 2009 May;43(5):414–425.

11. Goldie J. Assessment of professionalism: a consolidation of current thinking. *Med Teach.* 2013;35(2):e952–e956.

12. Hafferty FW. Measuring professionalism: a commentary. In: Stern DT, *Measuring Medical Professionalism.* 1st ed. New York, NY: Oxford University Press; 2006.

13. Hawkins RE, Katsufrakis PJ, Holtman MC, Clauser BE. Assessment of medical professionalism: who, what, when, where, how, and . . . why? *Med Teach.* 2009 Apr;31(4):348–361.

14. Hodges BD, Ginsburg S, Cruess R, Cruess S, Delport R, Hafferty F, Ho MJ, Holmboe E, Holtman M, Ohbu S, Rees C, Ten Cate O, Tsugawa Y, Van Mook W, Wass V, Wilkinson T, Wade W. Assessment of professionalism: recommendations from the Ottawa 2010 Conference. *Med Teach.* 2011;33(5):354–363.

15. Hodges BD, Regehr G, McNaughton N, Tiberius R, Hanson M. OSCE checklists do not capture increasing levels of expertise. *Acad Med.* 1999 Oct;74(10):1129–1134.

16. Lurie SJ, Nofziger AC, Meldrum S, Mooney C, Epstein RM. Effects of rater selection on peer assessment among medical students. *Med Educ.* 2006 Nov;40(11):1088–1097.

17. Lynch DC, Surdyk PM, Eiser AR. Assessing professionalism: a review of the literature. *Med Teach.* 2004 Jun;26(4):366–373.

18. Norcini J. Peer assessment of competence. *Med Educ.* 2003 Jun;37(6):539–543.

19. Papadakis MA, Arnold GK, Blank LL, Holmboe ES, Lipner RS. Performance during Internal Medicine Residency Training and Subsequent Disciplinary Action by State Licensing Boards. *Ann Intern Med.* 2008 Jun;148(11):869–876.

20. Papadakis MA, Osborn MC, Cooke M, Healy K. A strategy for the detection and evaluation of unprofessional behavior in medical students. *Acad Med.* 1999 Sep;74(9):980–990.

21. Papadakis MA, Teherani A, Banach MA, Knettler TR, Rattner SL, Stern DT, Veloski JJ, Hodgson CS. Disciplinary action by medical boards and prior behavior in medical school. *N Engl J Med.* 2005 Dec 22;353(25):2673–2682.

22. Physician Achievement Review (PAR). *Information About The PAR Program*; 2011. Available at: http://www.par–program.org/information/

23. Pohl CA, Hojat M, Arnold L. Peer nominations as related to academic attainment, empathy, personality, and specialty interest. *Acad Med.* 2011 Jun;86(6):747–751.

24. Rees CE, Knight LV. Viewpoint: the trouble with assessing students' professionalism: theoretical insights from sociocognitive psychology. *Acad Med.* 2007 Jan;82(1):46–50.

25. Rees CE, Knight LV. Banning, detection, attribution and reaction: the role of assessors in constructing students' unprofessional behaviors. *Med Educ.* 2008 Feb;42(2):125–127.

26. Schuwirth LW, van der Vleuten CPM. Programmatic assessment and Kane's validity perspective. *Med Educ*. 2012 Jan;46(1):38–48.

27. Schuwirth LW, van der Vleuten CP. Programmatic assessment: from assessment of learning to assessment for learning. *Med Teach*. 2011;33(6):478–485.

28. Sherbino J, Bandiera G, Frank JR. Assessing competence in emergency medicine trainees: an overview of effective methodologies. *CMEJ*. 2008 Jul;10(4):365–371.

29. Stern DT. *Measuring Medical Professionalism*. 1st ed. New York, NY: Oxford University Press; 2006.

30. Stern DT, Frohna A, Gruppen LD. The prediction of professional behavior. *Med Educ*. 2005 Jan;39(1):75–82.

31. University of California, San Francisco. *Undergraduate Medical Education: Physicianship Evaluation Forms and Policies*; 2013. Available at: http://meded.ucsf.edu/ume/physicianship-evaluation-forms-and-policies

32. van der Vleuten CP, Schuwirth LW. Assessing professional competence: from methods to programmes. *Med Educ*. 2005 Mar;39(3):309–317.

33. Violato C, Lockyer JM, Fidler H. Changes in performance: a 5-year longitudinal study of participants in a multi–source feedback programme. *Med Educ*. 2008 Oct;42(10):1007–1013.

34. Wallace DS, Paulson RM, Lord CG, Bond CF. Which behaviors do attitudes predict? Meta–analyzing the effects of social pressure and perceived difficulty. *Rev Gen Psychol*. 2005 Sep;9(3):214–227.

35. Zanetti M, Keller L, Mazor K, Carlin M, Alper E, Hatem D, Gammon W, Pugnaire M. Using standardized patients to assess professionalism: a generalizability study. *Teach Learn Med*. 2010 Oct;22(4):274–279.

WHEN THINGS GO WRONG: THE CHALLENGE OF SELF-REGULATION

11

LEARNING OBJECTIVES

1. To describe the nature and frequency of professionalism lapses.
2. To explain the impact of unprofessional behavior on patients, students, and the healthcare team.
3. To identify why professionalism lapses occur.
4. To illustrate how most individuals who witness lapses respond to them.
5. To outline strategies to respond to a spectrum of professionalism lapses.

In today's complex and often chaotic environment, physicians are often challenged as they strive to live their professional values. Physicians may struggle to maintain their equanimity in the face of suffering and dying patients, heightened productivity demands, work-related fatigue, and distressed colleagues. As humans, we may also be dealing with struggles outside of work. Physicians are not immune to personal illness, relationship troubles, or distractions related to dependent children or parents. Rather than be surprised that lapses in professionalism occur, we should anticipate that they will occur and prepare to handle them in a way that honors the trust that society places in both individual physicians and the collective profession when they grant us the privilege of self-regulation.

Unfortunately, individually or collectively we do not always live up to this commitment. Highly publicized incidents of physicians as the perpetrators

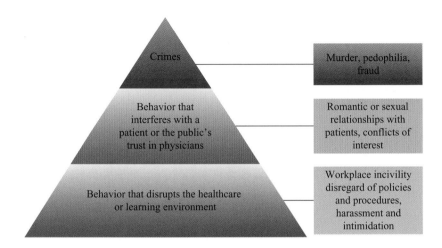

Figure 11-1 ▪ The iceberg of unprofessional behavior (with examples).

of crimes against society, ranging from financial fraud to sexual assault to even more egregious crimes are rare. When they occur, however, they raise questions about how the medical profession could have let someone with this flawed character enter or remain within the profession (Stewart, 2000). More common are examples of ethical transgressions, such as research- or practice-based conflicts of interest, where physicians have placed their financial or career success ahead of the best interests of their patients (Brownlee, 2008). Even more common are the type of professionalism lapses that don't make headlines, but that pervasively undermine the culture of respect that is essential to the effective functioning of our patient care and educational environments (Leape et al, 2012a; Walrath, Dang, & Nybert, 2013; Wear et al, 2009; Hickson et al, 2007; Samenow et al, 2013; Silverman et al, 2012). These include the daily incivilities that occur in the workplace and are characterized by disrespectful language, dysfunctional relationships, disregard of policies and procedures, and dismissive or destructive responses to clinical disagreement or uncertainty. Figure 11-1 describes these different types of breaches of professionalism.

WHAT DO PROFESSIONALISM LAPSES LOOK LIKE AND HOW COMMONLY DO THEY OCCUR?

Because unprofessional behavior covers a spectrum of actions that range from lapses to transgressions to crimes, it is difficult to pinpoint the frequency of professionalism lapses. The literature relevant to understanding these lapses can be found not only in articles that specifically address professionalism (Hickson et al, 2007; Teherani et al, 2005; Adams, Emmons, & Romm, 2008; Campbell et al, 2007; Buchanan et al, 2012; Humphrey et al, 2007; Arnold, 2006; Brater, 2007; Brainard & Brislen, 2007; Papadakis et al, 2005; Wasserstein, Brennan, & Rubenstein, 2007), but also in articles about the hidden curriculum (Hafferty, 1998; Testerman et al, 1996; Billings, 2011), moral distress (Wiggleton et al, 2010), disruptive people and behaviors (Walrath, Dang, & Nybert, 2013; Samenow et al, 2013; Silverman et al, 2012; Saxton, Heinz, & Enriquez, 2009; Reynolds, 2012; Leape et al, 2012a; McLaren, Lord, & Murray, 2011; Williams & Williams, 2008; Rosenstein & O'Daniel, 2008; Rosenstein & Naylor, 2012; Pronovost et al, 2003), problem residents (Wear et al, 2009; Adams, Emmons, & Romm, 2008; Brenner et al, 2010; Dupras et al, 2012; Sanfey et al, 2012; Zbieranowski et al, 2013), burnout (Billings et al, 2011; Dyrbye & Shanafelt, 2011; Dyrbye et al, 2010), and impaired physicians (Campbell et al, 2007) (Table 11-1).

Over the last decade, the profession's definition of what behaviors are unprofessional and disruptive has expanded. In the last century, a physician's professionalism was judged largely by how they interacted with patients, without regard to how they treated others in the healthcare environment. Comments like, "He is a fantastic doctor, just not very nice to the nurses," illustrated this belief. Previously unprofessional behaviors were viewed as limited to overt acts of verbal abuse and intimidation (yelling at or threatening the job

Table 11-1 **DEFINITIONS OF CONSTRUCTS LINKED TO PROFESSIONALISM PROBLEMS**		
Construct	**Definition**	**Comment**
Disruptive behavior	"Personal conduct, whether verbal or physical, that negatively affects or that potentially may negatively affect patient care" (Samenow et al, 2013).	Disruptive behaviors are unprofessional. When demonstrated by valued role models in the clinical environment, they create the hidden curriculum.
Hidden curriculum	Lessons learned that were not explicitly intended and that may be counter to the formal curriculum (Hafferty, 1998).	The hidden curriculum is often more powerful than the explicit curriculum because it is provided by role models who are successful in a role to which the students aspire.
Moral distress	Moral distress results when one knows the morally correct response to the situation but cannot act because of institutional or hierarchical constraints (Wiggleton et al, 2010).	As learners develop a professional identity based on classroom and workplace learning experiences, they may experience moral distress if they feel they are unable to act in the "right" way because of institutional barriers. *(Continued)*

Table 11-1 DEFINITIONS OF CONSTRUCTS LINKED TO PROFESSIONALISM PROBLEMS (*Cont.*)		
Construct	**Definition**	**Comment**
Burnout	Burnout is characterized by emotional exhaustion, depersonalization, and a decreased sense of personal accomplishment.	Moral distress and cynicism that comes from unresolved moral quandaries can contribute to burnout and further cynicism, depersonalization and more disruptive behaviors.
Impaired physicians	The Federation of State Medical Boards (FSMB) defines impairment as the inability of a licensee to practice medicine with reasonable skill and safety as result of a mental disorder, physical illness or condition or substance abuse (FSMB, 2011).	Illness does not equate to impairment. Impairment refers to the inability of the physician with the illness to meet standards.

or wellbeing of another healthcare professional) or physical violence (throwing a scalpel in the operating room). Presently, we hold a broader view of disruptive behaviors to include patterns of behavior that are passive-aggressive, including refusal to comply with evidence-based safety protocols or pathways, condescending or sarcastic responses to inquiries, failure to answer pages or complete documentation, hostile avoidance of or refusal to engage in collegial dialogue, disrespectful comments about patients or other professionals, and inappropriate humor (see Table 11-2) (Walrath, Dang, & Nyberg, 2013; Saxton, Hines, & Enriquez, 2009; Reynolds, 2012; Leape et al, 2012a).

Table 11-2 **THE SPECTRUM OF UNPROFESSIONAL BEHAVIORS**		
	Threatening	**Passive-aggressive**
Behavior that directly impacts patients	• Sexual misconduct • Refusal to provide care in emergency situations • Practicing beyond the scope of personal competence • Disclosing confidential patient information • Discrimination • Failure to respect patient's informed and autonomous decisions • Patient abandonment • Violence and threats toward patients • Failure to disclose serious medical errors	• Refusal to return calls or deliver on promised work • Research- or practice-based conflicts of interest • Disregard for stewardship of valuable resources • Refusal to demonstrate competence across the lifetime of practice

Table 11-2 **THE SPECTRUM OF UNPROFESSIONAL BEHAVIORS (*Continued*)**		
	Threatening	**Passive–aggressive**
Behavior that directly impacts other healthcare professionals and indirectly impacts patients	• Threatening or carrying out acts of physical violence • Physical intimidation • Hazing • Yelling • Use of profanity or abusive language • Racist, sexist, or discriminatory comments • Intimidation and humiliation • Public criticism or "dressing down" of other professionals • Sexual harassment	• Chronic lateness or unexplained absences • Condescension and sarcasm • Withholding of vital information • Humor about vulnerable people or populations • Active or passive refusal to comply with evidence-based safety practices • Specialty bashing or badmouthing of other professions • Gossiping about other healthcare professionals or trainees • Failure to answer pages, complete documentation, billing, or evaluations • Failure to address witnessed professionalism lapses in others

HOW COMMON IS UNPROFESSIONAL BEHAVIOR?

The percentage of physicians who exhibit behavior that is either sufficiently egregious or that persists enough to warrant intervention by an authoritative figure is fortunately small, estimated to be approximately 3% to 5% in any given institution (Hickson et al, 2007; Leape & Fromson, 2006). However, nearly everyone in the healthcare environment has had contact with or witnessed a physician who exhibited behavior they describe as unprofessional or disruptive at some time. More than 95% of physician executives attest that they are aware of problem physicians within their medical centers (Weber, 2004). The majority of nurses and physicians in operating rooms, emergency departments, and obstetrical units report incidences of unprofessional behavior (Rosenstein & Naylor, 2012; Saxton, 2012). More than 90% of pediatric nurses reported witnessing at least one disruptive behavior in the preceding 90 days (Saxton, 2012). In one survey of 102 hospitals, nurses were more likely to report witnessing disruptive behavior than were physicians, with 88% of nurses describing these behaviors in physicians and only 51% of physicians noting disruptive behavior in other doctors (Rosenstein & O'Daniel, 2008). These data raise questions about whether nurses and physicians agree on what constitutes disruptive behavior.

Residents and medical students observe, and also admit to, participating in unprofessional behavior including cheating, falsifying patient records, and engaging in disrespectful comments or humor about others. Between one fourth and one half of residents surveyed described witnessing multiple incidents (> 4 times) of disrespect of patients, residents, students, and nurses by other residents (Billings et al, 2011). Nearly all students responding to surveys describe witnessing unprofessional behavior on the part of faculty, residents, and peers (Wiggleton et al, 2010). Students themselves are the subjects of unprofessional behavior. The Association of American Medical Colleges (AAMC) monitors student mistreatment as a component of its Graduation Questionnaire (GQ), administered annually to all graduating medical students. In 2012, 33% of respondents reported that they had experienced public humiliation at least once in their medical school tenure and 15% noted that they had been subject to sexist remarks (Mann, 2012). Articles that describe specific anecdotes are profoundly disturbing (Brainard & Brislen, 2007).

WHAT IS THE IMPACT OF UNPROFESSIONAL BEHAVIOR?

Jeanette Smith-Johnson, a hospital pharmacist, was really upset. She had just received an order for an antibiotic dose that was too high, given the patient's age and renal function. When she went to the floor to talk with the prescribing resident, Dr. Estania chewed her out in the middle of the patient care unit, within earshot of multiple doctors, nurses, and patient families. Then Dr. Estania turned to her team and said, "All pharmacists are people who failed to get into medical school." Jeanette felt that it was too risky to say anything about the incident but it made her feel like the talk about interprofessional team work in the institution was just "lip service."

Physicians and nurses who display disruptive and unprofessional behaviors such as disrespectful comments, intimidation, harassment, physical threats, or violence negatively affect the culture of collaboration and respect that is so critical to the delivery of safe, high-quality care. Nurses, trainees, and students may hesitate to contact an attending physician about a change in a patient's status if they fear they will be subjected to verbal abuse. Members of an operating room team or intensive care unit may be reluctant to point out a break in sterile technique if they feel they may be the target of physical violence. These unacceptable behaviors are unfortunately common. In a study of personnel in more than 100 hospitals, almost three fourths of those responding felt that the presence of disruptive behavior contributed to poor quality and adverse events. Eighteen percent stated that they were aware of a disruptive event that directly compromised quality of care (Rosenstein & O'Daniel, 2008). Intimidation of a nurse or pharmacist was the cause of 7%

of medication errors in one hospital (Smetzer et al, 2005). Given our under-standing of how critical attention to detail is in today's dynamic medical envi-ronments, it is particularly worrisome that more than two thirds of nurses subjected to verbal abuse in pediatrics and perioperative units described a transient decrease in their concentration or ability to engage in critical think-ing as a consequence of the abuse (Saxton, 2012). Physicians who engage in disruptive or unprofessional behavior are bad for business as well. Verbal abuse on the part of physicians or other nurses toward nurses is described a significant cause of nursing turnover (Rosenstein, 2011). Physicians who refuse to comply with standards for documentation and billing also threaten the economic viability of their organization.

> *Dr. Stevens is a tenured faculty member in critical care who is on call for the intensive care unit (ICU). He is contacted by one of the senior surgical residents, Dr. Hussain, and asked to accept a transfer from one of the general surgical services. The patient in question was admitted today for revision of a dialysis shunt but had an episode of hypotension that was prolonged and took a long time to respond to treatment. Dr. Hussain felt that the patient needed intensive care. The faculty member refused to accept the patient and directed the resi-dent to admit the patient to the regular ward, stating that he didn't have room on his service for every dying dialysis patient.*

In the scenario above, Dr. Hussain is left feeling abandoned as he feels that his patient needs ICU monitoring but the staff physician is unwilling because of his views about dialysis patients. Dr. Hussain is in a difficult position that caused him moral distress and feelings of helplessness. In a study conducted at Vanderbilt University Medical School, students consistently described a greater degrees of moral distress when witnessing situations in which they felt that patients did not receive appropriate care than those in which members of their team made disrespectful comments about other services or patients who were not present (Wiggleton et al, 2010). Table 11-3 presents examples of situations that cause moral distress for students. It is notable that students sometimes witness disrespectful behavior directed at other physicians or ser-vices but do not find it particularly distressing, raising the possibility that they have accepted this type of behavior as normative.

> *Michael is a 3rd-year medical student. All students have been assigned to meet monthly with an elderly citizen as part of a program to introduce students to healthy elderly. After each monthly visit, the student is required to file a brief report. At the end of the winter quar-ter, Michael is doing surgery and submits his final report on his senior*

Table 11-3	**SITUATIONS THAT CAN LEAD TO MORAL DISTRESS IN MEDICAL STUDENTS**	
	Description
Situations Involving Patient Care	A patient presented with advanced disease because they had faced barriers to access to care.
	Optimal care was not provided to a patient because of insurance status.
	Poor communication between teams negatively impacted patient care.
	The team continued to provide aggressive care at the urging of patients or their family even when no potential benefit was evident.
	I felt that a patient was discriminated against by a member of my team.
	The attending physician or resident answered a patient's questions inadequately or simply ignored them.
	Our team withdrew care at the patient's or family's request, although I thought the patient could have survived with further treatment.
	A member of our team was rude or disrespectful to a patient or family member.
Situations Involving Self	One of my superiors behaved inappropriately but I did not report it, out of fear it would negatively impact my grade or because I felt pressured by the attending or resident.
	A member of my team was disrespectful to someone below him or herself in the team hierarchy.
	I performed a procedure that I did not feel qualified to do because I was afraid of being viewed as incompetent.

partner during the last week of the surgical clerkship. On the day following his report submission, his senior partner contacts the medical school to ask why he hasn't seen Michael for the past 2 months.

Uncorrected unprofessional behavior may have negative consequences for the individual as well. If Michael never gets feedback or does not correct these behaviors, he may be at risk of future difficulties. Studies consistently find a correlation between poor physician communication, patient dissatisfaction, and malpractice suits (Hickson et al, 2002). Students who were the recipient of more than one complaint about professional irresponsibility were 8.5 times as likely as their peers to be subjected to medical board sanctions in their subsequent career. In addition, students who demonstrated diminished capacity for self-improvement were 3.1 times as likely to be sanctioned (Papadakis et al, 2005). The presence of any negative descriptors about behavior in an individual's Medical Student Performance Evaluation showed a strong correlation with poor performance during residency (Brenner et al, 2010). In the case of Michael, the lapse needs to be dealt with even though the course is over.

1. Have you ever heard a colleague or trainee make a joke about a patient and his medical condition?
2. How did you feel?
3. Did you laugh with others? Did you say anything to the individual who made the joke? If so, what did you say? When did you say it?
4. If not, why didn't you? Were you planning on talking about it later, in private? If so, did later ever come?

WHY DOES UNPROFESSIONAL BEHAVIOR OCCUR?

Rafael was uncomfortable. His fellow intern, Delilah, was one of the smartest people in their residency group and he had been looking forward to working with her this month at the county hospital. They had a huge service of very sick patients, and overall they were providing very good care to them. But almost every day, Delilah made sarcastic or demeaning comments about patients—the hopeless guy with alcoholism, the woman who likes to turn tricks, and so on. Instead of anyone saying something about the importance of treating patients with respect, the rest of the team just laughed or ignored the comments. Rafael wasn't sure what he should do—perhaps he was overly sensitive. After all, what was important was what happened in the patient's room, not in the hallway, wasn't it?

Given that all physicians enter medicine to serve others, it is hard to understand why any physician or physician-in-training would engage in behaviors that interfere with their doctor-patient relationships, or with the effective delivery of high-quality healthcare. It is tempting to believe that if we simply sought out and removed the perpetrators of unprofessional behavior from the profession, the problem would be solved. This is certainly true for those who engage in truly egregious behavior and for those who, despite counseling, are unable to change the ways in which they are behaving. However, as we have discussed in other chapters, unprofessional behavior is often caused by good physicians and physicians-in-training who temporarily lack the knowledge skills or attitudes to manage the professionalism challenge in front of them (see Chapter 2, Resilience in Facing Professionalism Challenges, and Chapter 4, Fostering Patient-Centered Care). Some may also lapse because they have adopted a style of behavior that they fail to realize is unprofessional. In our modification of the Johns Hopkins Model for Disruptive Clinician Behavior (Walrath, Dang, & Nyberg, 2013) triggers for unprofessional behavior include personal issues, interpersonal issues, situational factors and organizational policies, procedures, and culture (Figure 11-2).

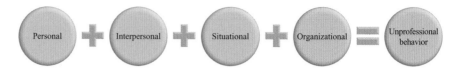

Figure 11-2 ▪ Triggers for unprofessional behaviors.

Examples in each of the categories listed earlier are presented in Table 11-4. Although any given healthcare provider may be able to manage a single issue without lapsing into unprofessional behavior, the presence of multiple issues may overwhelm the capacity of a given clinician to sustain their commitment to professionalism. Particularly vulnerable are physicians-in-training, who may lack the experience to recognize and respond to triggers before they lapse.

When educational and clinical leaders witness or hear reports about unprofessional behavior in the physicians for whom they are responsible, they may wonder if the person has a psychiatric illness or a substance abuse problem. Estimates vary about the extent to which professionalism problems are caused by unrecognized, unmanaged, or untreatable illness. Burnout appears to be a risk factor for unprofessional behavior that is modifiable if recognized (Dyrbye & Shanafelt, 2011; Dyrbye et al, 2010). In physicians whose behavior is sufficiently problematic to warrant formal evaluation, psychiatric disorders may be common (Williams, Williams, & Speicher, 2004). Psychiatric disorders identified include Axis I disorders such as depression, anxiety, bipolar illness, substance use, and dementia and Axis II disorders such as personality disorders (paranoid, narcissistic, passive aggressive, and borderline disorders) (Reynolds, 2012; Williams & Williams, 2008). Psychiatric disorders do not excuse unprofessional behavior, but their presence demands a comprehensive approach to preventing future lapses, involving medical therapy, counseling, and behavioral change.

HOW DO PEOPLE USUALLY RESPOND TO A WITNESSED PROFESSIONALISM LAPSE?

Dr. Sundera is a PGY-1 resident in surgery at a hospital different from where she had gone to medical school. She is appalled at the amount of joking that goes on in the operating room—mostly directed at the anesthetized patient but some at the medical students. All of the residents and the anesthesiology attending just laugh when they hear these comments. Was this the way her entire residency experience was going to play out?

When we observe a colleague or trainees behaving in ways that makes us feel uncomfortable we typically, and usually instinctively, respond in one of four ways: endorse, ignore, defer action or intervene to stop it (Figure 11-3).

Table 11-4	**EXAMPLES OF STRESSORS THAT MAY LEAD TO UNPROFESSIONAL BEHAVIOR**
Type of stressor	**Examples of stressors**
Personal	• Unmet deficit needs ○ Fatigue, hunger, safety concerns, isolation, sorrow, concern • Competency issues • Distractions ○ Family or relationship issues, high stakes exam • Physical illness • Psychological or psychiatric disorders ○ Burnout, affective disorders, bipolar illness, major depression • Substance abuse • Personality disorders
Interpersonal	• Prior relationship difficulties between individuals • Incongruent or unshared mental models • Clinical disagreement • Poor understanding of roles, responsibilities, and abilities • Infrequent, delayed, or inaccurate communication • Pattern of blaming rather than problem solving conversations • Language barriers • Unequal power relationships
Situational	• High workload • Clinical situations that evoke strong emotions ○ Death, trauma, sick children, obstetrical crises, surgical mishaps, violent patients, angry families, futile resuscitation efforts • Inadequate supervision • Unavailable backup
Organizational	• Inefficient workflows • Inadequate staffing • Poor staff training • Excessive bureaucracy • Conflicting policies and procedures • Financial pressures • New tools and technologies • Rigidly hierarchical culture • Unintentional reward of bad behavior by leaders • Culture that rewards bad behavior

Endorsing responses are behaviors that explicitly support, reinforce, or propagate the behavior in question. They may join in the laughter, respond with a similar anecdote or comment, gossip about the behaviors to others, or chide or marginalize others who attempt to interrupt the behavior. Inaction responses

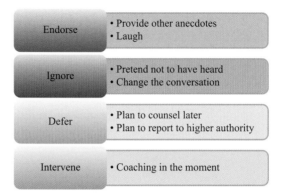

Figure 11-3 ▪ Options for immediate reaction to observed professionalism lapses.

are those that do not address the behavior as it is occurring. Examples include ignoring the questionable behavior or changing the subject without addressing the behavior. Deferral responses include those in which the observer plans to engage in counseling at a later time or to report the situation to a higher authority. Our intent in choosing one of these passive responses might be good. We might value unit cohesion in the midst of a busy call day; we might fear inducing more embarrassment in an otherwise good physician by calling attention to inappropriate comments or behavior; we might believe that we don't have sufficient authority to intervene; or we might want to just not get involved. But any response that ignores bad behavior, particularly in front of others, conveys tacit acceptance of the attitudes expressed. Planning to address this later with the colleague usually fails as a strategy because later almost never comes. The best approach when we witness a lapse is to accept our responsibility to self-regulate and skillfully intervene in the moment to stop the inappropriate comments or behaviors. In doing so, we teach important lessons about professionalism to both the offender (the one who lapsed) as well as to the bystanders who witnessed the lapse.

It turns out that this is more difficult than one might imagine. Learning to step in to help reinforce the values of professionalism requires a skill set that is robust enough to overcome the human instinct to let someone else handle a problem. Although our medical training prepares us to step in when a life is at risk (an infant who is choking, a teen motor vehicle accident victim who is bleeding, a middle aged man in cardiac arrest), rarely do we stop to think about how best to intervene when professional values are at risk.

Three sociological theories explain why we often do not take action when we see something amiss in the clinical environment:

1. The bystander apathy theory
2. Normalization of deviance
3. The law of invisible benefits

The bystander apathy theory resulted from a series of interesting experiments where people were observed reacting to a threat to someone else (an attack) or to themselves (smoke pouring into the room). The chance of any individual personally taking action in the face of the problem was inversely related to the number of people in the environment (Garcia et al, 2002). Translated into medicine, the likelihood that someone will speak up decreases when other members of the team are present. Many explanations exist for this observation. There appears to be a diffusion of responsibility. People think that it is someone else's job to speak up. This is particularly true when there is someone else present who is perceived to have more authority or experience, even if that authority or experience is self-declared, rather than defined by conventional hierarchy.

The second is a sociological theory related to how deviance is normalized. We take our cues from others when figuring out whether to respond. When hearing an intern make a tasteless joke, the resident and the other students might think that if no one else seems bothered by this comment, then maybe it isn't as problematic as they thought. If everyone in the environment accepts that disrespectful comments, even made in jest, as normal, the problematic comments become the new norm. The trainee learns that this joking is okay (this is the hidden curriculum).

The final theory is the law of invisible benefits. If I hear someone making a bad joke or a disrespectful comment and I attempt to intervene, the potential consequences to me of intervening are clear, immediate, and may be negative (e.g., I may lose my friend; I might be viewed by the team as a problem person myself). In contrast, the potential benefits of intervening may be less immediate and more indirect (e.g., how will I know if because of my comment Susan changed the way she approached patients and was happy because of it?). In addition to these sociological theories that pertain to everyone, for students and junior trainees who witness unprofessional behavior in someone with power over them, they may fear retaliation in the form of poor evaluations if they speak up about their concerns (Brainard & Brislen, 2007).

WHAT ARE STRATEGIES FOR GOOD RESPONSES TO PROFESSIONALISM LAPSES?

Given what we know about the impact of disruptive behavior on the culture of our workplace, the safety of our care delivery system, and the wellbeing of our trainees and peers, it is clear that all professionals need the attitudes and skills to embrace our responsibility for self-regulation (Papadakis et al, 2012). Living our responsibilities as professionals for self-regulation means that we need to prepare to deal with professionalism lapses, at all levels of severity, when they occur. Learning to address unprofessional behaviors in our colleagues and learners starts with embracing a series of assumptions about professionalism in physicians and physicians in training:

1. We all aspire to adhere to the highest standards of professionalism but sometimes fall short of the mark.
2. We all would want to know if our behavior is not meeting professional standards; if our reputation as a professional is suffering because of patterns of maladaptive behavior; and if we are role modeling anything other than excellent professionalism.
3. We all have the potential to improve our behavior and attitudes with the help of our colleagues.

With these assumptions in mind, we can turn to skills and strategies that can be used to address unprofessional behavior. Adapting Hickson's disruptive behavior pyramid, we can develop a stepped approach to dealing with the spectrum of professionalism lapses, in which the intensity and consequences of the intervention are proportionate to the severity and obstinacy of the unprofessional behavior observed (Figure 11-4) (Hickson et al, 2007).

When unprofessional behavior is at the low intensity end of the spectrum and appears to be an isolated problem, coaching in the moment (level I) is the right solution. For more serious but isolated situations, counseling after the moment (level II) is warranted. For persistent problems, correction and consequences conversations (level III) must be carried out. Lastly, physicians with

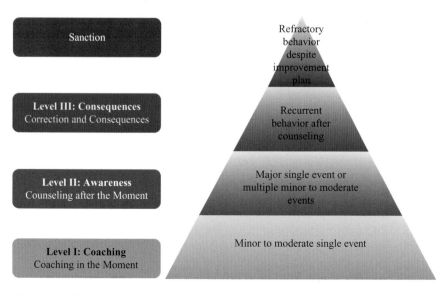

Figure 11-4 ▪ A stepped approach to intervention.

egregious professionalism lapses or those who persist in disruptive behavior despite coaching, counseling, or correction merit sanctions, up to and including dismissal from the profession (level IV).

LEVEL 1 INTERVENTION: COACHING IN THE MOMENT

Senior resident, Dr. Anderson, was helping Marta, his intern, insert an intravenous line in a patient with poor peripheral veins because of longstanding injection drug use. It was clear that Marta was increasingly frustrated, not only because she had to try repeatedly to get the IV in, but because the patient was crying loudly about the pain from the IV needle. After they left the room and rejoined their senior resident, the wound nurse assigned to the team and their students, Marta declared, "These whiny injection drug users really piss me off: they love their needles when they are full of heroin but not when they are full of antibiotics. I don't know why they even bother to come to the hospital."

Dr. Anderson finds himself in a common situation. He has just overheard an unprofessional comment made by another physician and now must decide how to react. Dr. Anderson knows Marta is a good physician; after all, she stayed up all night caring for this patient as well as several others. He understands how frustrating it was to put an intravenous line in someone without easily accessible veins. Many who resonate deeply with these feelings might choose to endorse her comment (intentionally or unintentionally) by laughing or joining in with an anecdote of their own, thus becoming co-conspirators of the undesired behavior. Alternatively, he might be worried that saying anything to Marta now would embarrass her in front of the students and damage their working relationship. He might imagine that Marta has already realized that she has said something uncharitable and will, upon reflection, correct herself. If these thoughts are dominant, Dr. Anderson might find himself in the group of people who say nothing and become bystanders. But inappropriate behaviors and comments that are reinforced or that are uncorrected are usually repeated. Clearly Dr. Anderson should intervene in a manner that is appropriate for the setting and proportionate to the seriousness of the event. For circumstances such as this, Dr. Anderson can engage in coaching in the moment.

Coaching in the moment (CIM) strategies should be thought of as coaching for improvement opportunities, not disciplinary events. The goal of a CIM intervention is to stop the lapse and to communicate the expected professional behavior to all involved. It is essential that the intervention occur in the presence of those who witnessed the lapse so that they understand that, while we can empathize with our peer who lapsed, we must stop unprofessional behavior before it becomes a pattern of disruption. The successful correction in the moment conversation allows the professional who hears a lapse (the coach) to recognize the cause of the lapse, express empathy for the one who lapses (the offender), reestablish the professionalism norm, and then redirect the conversation to appropriate care of the patient. The four steps of a CIM intervention are outlined below and literally take 90 seconds to complete (Table 11-5).

When a coach takes the time to engage in a coaching in the moment strategy, it makes it clear to the offender and the observers that he or she doesn't endorse the situation. It stops the group from engaging in similar activity. It provides the opportunity to simultaneously express empathy for both the offender and the subject of the disruptive comment.

Reactions to coaching in the moment vary widely but are generally positive. No one likes to have their mistakes acknowledged but if done gently and without labeling (no "that's so unprofessional!"), this correction can be tolerated and is sometimes very welcomed. In the ideal response, the offender acknowledges the lapse, apologizes for lapsing and asks the group to intervene again if they lapse another time. Of interest, a rapid recovery from a professionalism lapse makes malicious gossip about the lapse much less likely. Failure of the offender to acknowledge the coaching in the moment is less ideal but still represents a partial victory because the observers have witnessed others intervening in situations involving disruptive or unprofessional

Table 11-5	**COACHING IN THE MOMENT: FOUR STEPS IN 90 SECONDS**	
Step	**Example**	**Comment**
Recognize the underlying emotion	"I can see/hear how frustrated you are with this patient (or this nurse, or that service)."	"I" phrases are hard to argue with.
Relate to the offender	"I get frustrated with patients sometimes too." Or "I can relate to your frustration."	Showing understanding and empathy minimizes the risk of defensiveness or accusations of sounding "preachy."
Reestablish the professionalism norm	"We should try to remember that the patient is probably frustrated too—and possibly scared that we won't treat him well because of his habit."	Using "us" or "we" words implies that all of us need to remember or work on these issues. When possible, connect the behavior back to the patient or the subject of the inappropriate comment, creating a humanizing moment.
Redirect the conversation	"How can we (I) help you with this patient?"	Moving on reinforces the coaching nature of this conversation.

behavior. More challenging but fortunately much less common are responses that explicitly dismiss the concern ("don't be so uptight, what he doesn't know won't hurt him!") or attack the reactor ("who do you think you are? William Osler?") If this happens, it is best to simply state your disagreement ("I don't agree with what you are saying.") and, if needed, take a time out to allow tempers to cool.

LEARNING EXERCISE 11-2

Learning a new communication skill, like delivering bad news or coaching a peer through a professionalism lapse, takes practice. One needs to try on different words and phrases to see what feels most natural.

Try to identify specific phrases for the four CIM steps for each of the following situations.

1. Your intern is repeatedly badgering a medical student on rounds for not remembering to check on the computerized tomography (CT) results. You can see that the student is near tears.

2. While waiting for a conference to start, your fellow student is telling fat jokes about an obese patient that was on his surgical service.

3. You overhear another team joking and laughing in the cafeteria about a patient who was in a motor vehicle accident.

4. Your resident is badmouthing the nurses on unit 4D to the new interns, telling them never to pay attention to what they say, they are always wrong.

LEVEL II INTERVENTION: CORRECTION AFTER THE MOMENT (CAM)

Dr. Fahrabi was responsible for reviewing the incident reports for the emergency medicine department. She noticed that Dr. Rolando, the new emergency medicine physician, has received six complaints over the last 2 months from nurses who complain that he is condescending and impatient with them, and at times he refuses to answer their questions.

Dr. Fahrabi is faced with a slightly different challenge than in the prior case. Although she did not personally witness Dr. Rolando engaging in unprofessional behavior, she is expected to counsel him with a goal of improving his interactions with nurses. Assuming that these are the first negative reports that Dr. Fahrabi has received about Dr. Rolando, this circumstance merits a level II intervention, known as a Counseling After the Moment (CAM) conversation. Relying on the assumptions that all physicians aspire to behave professionally, want to know if others find them less than professional, and would be willing to work to improve recognized performance problems, the purpose of a CAM conversation is to make the subject of the complaints aware that negative reports have surfaced about them and to help them figure out how they might change their behavior. Hickson and colleagues (2007) have called these introductory conversations, "cup of coffee" conversations. This name reflects the belief that these are collegial conversations, carried out by a trusted peer or an authority figure with an intent to make the individual aware of how his or her behaviors are perceived, share available data, encourage reflection, and offer support so that the patterns of behavior that are viewed as objectionable do not continue. As truly formative feedback, they should not result in sanctions, and the counselor should assure the offender that these conversations would be kept confidential unless the behaviors are repeated.

Despite the intent to make CAM conversations low key and nonthreatening, talking about reports of unprofessional behavior is frequently difficult. One can imagine several potential responses when Dr. Fahrabi meets with Dr. Rolando to review the complaints about her from the nurses. Ideally, Dr. Rolando would thank Dr. Fahrabi, saying something like, "*I haven't handled my concerns about nursing very well. I wonder if you can help me think about a more effective way to deal with problems that I notice.*" This type of response would pave the way for a congenial conversation about how best to manage clinical disagreement and performance concerns. Unfortunately, Dr. Rolando is just as likely to respond with a conversation blocker, such as:

- "I don't have a clue what they are talking about."
- "I don't remember it like that. Are there any witnesses?"
- "I only get upset when patient care is jeopardized. Everyone agrees that someone has to get control over these nurses."
- "Why don't you talk with Federico, he gets a lot more complaints than I do?"

Responses such as these are frustrating but understandable. When people sense a threat to their wellbeing or to their reputation, their instinct is frequently flight or fight. Flight reactions can look like acquiescence: "*It won't happen again, you don't need to do anything else.*" While on the surface, this appears to be a good response, flight reactions often result in premature closure of a counseling conversation. This short-circuits a deeper exploration of issues that would truly help the offender avoid a repeat of the behavior in the future. Physicians who engage in fight reactions attempt to discount the validity or accuracy of the complaint, demand more proof, and justify their behavior because it supported high-quality patient care. The coach who is unprepared for this type of reaction may retreat from the conversation.

Counselor's Approach:	Coaching or Counseling	Discipline*
Preparation for encounter	**Understand perceptions:** Identify the behaviors that caused the individual to be perceived as unprofessional.	**Investigate facts:** Ascertain whether the observed behaviors occurred as described and whether extenuating circumstances were present.
Goals of encounter	**Formative:** Coach offender to better performance	**Summative:** Sanction offender for poor performance
Burden of proof needed to carry out encounter	Low	High

*Loss of or impact to reputation, privileges, benefits, position, license.

Figure 11-5 ▪ Contrasting the burden of proof required for different types of encounters.

The burden of proof required to engage in a counseling session about reported unprofessional behavior is proportionate to the possible outcomes of the session (Figure 11-5). If the physician is at risk of losing his or her position or license, then it is reasonable to expect that an extensive investigation into the accuracy of complaints has been undertaken. However, since the purpose of a CAM conversation is awareness and learning, rather than discipline and sanctions, the burden of proof for the "truth of the matter" is low. The job of the counselor in these conversations is not to conduct a detailed investigation but to help the involved physician understand the gap between what he or she intended to convey and how others perceived him or her. To do this effectively requires advance preparation and a strategy.

The counselor in a CAM conversation should take time to analyze the complaints and to prepare for the conversation. Communication skill workshops can be very helpful to people who are frequently responsible for difficult conversations like this (Saxton, 2012; Patterson et al, 2012; Sehgal et al, 2008). The CAM encounter has three goals:

1. To help the involved physicians understand and accept that regardless of their intent, others perceived their behaviors as inappropriate (empathy for others)

2. To engage in a structured exercise to uncover the root cause or causes of the behavior (personal learning and reflection)
3. To develop a plan for preventing similar complaints in the future (alternate strategy identification) and to identify whether new skills need to be developed (personal skill assessment)

If the institution has peer benchmark data, an additional goal may be to help the physician understand the frequency of complaints about them in comparison to complaints about others in the institution (Pichert, Hickson, & Moore, 2008).

A CAM conversation is typically carried out in three phases: framing, reflecting, and planning. In the framing phase of the conversation (Table 11-6), the counselor must establish the meeting as a safe place to discuss a serious issue, describe the complaint, allow the physician time to provide their insights into the situation, anticipate and deal with common and often defensive reactions, establish the goal of the encounter and reinforce their belief in the individual's ability to be an excellent professional.

In the reflecting phase of the CAM conversation (Table 11-7), the counselor guides the physician through a series of probing questions to help them understand what triggered the behavior in question, why others perceived them as unprofessional, and what they might do if they encounter a similar

Table 11-6 **FRAMING PHASE OF THE CAM**	
Objectives	**Examples**
Make it safe	"All great physicians want to be professional and I know you to be a great doctor."
Describe the objectionable behavior	"Three nurses have complained that you either mock them or speak to them in a condescending tone when they ask you for clarification of your orders."
Ask for a reaction	"Have you heard these concerns before? What is your reaction?"
Anticipate and manage reactions	"You might not agree with the way they characterized this encounter and I suspect you didn't meant to be condescending, but we have a responsibility to understand and manage the perceptions of others in the clinical environment. Nurses who are afraid of negative reactions will stop asking important questions and patient safety may be at risk." "I know you feel like this won't happen again but I would like to discuss this a bit more to make sure that we can prevent anything that damages your reputation in the future."
Set the goal	"Our goal today is to work through this case and see how you can be more effective next time."
Reinforce your belief in them.	"I know you want to have the reputation as someone who others can approach with their concerns."

Table 11-7	**REFLECTING PHASE OF THE COUNSELING AFTER THE MOMENT (CAM) CONVERSATION**

Sample questions:
1. What was happening when this encounter occurred? What else were you managing at the time?
2. What were you feeling at the time of the encounter?
3. What do you think (the other party) was feeling at the time?
4. Why do you think they interpreted your behavior in a negative way? What about your words or behavior led them to that conclusion?
5. If you had to do it over again, what changes would you make?

situation in the future. The following list of questions is derived from the emotional intelligence literature. Not all are relevant for every situation and they do not need to be followed in any particular order.

The answers the physician provides to these questions can provide insights into their self and social awareness and control. A physician who can describe that he was exhausted going into the encounter, who recognizes that it was a busy night and that the nurses were short staffed and stressed, who understands that he frequently uses sarcasm to deal with uncertainty, and who realizes that sarcasm can be misinterpreted when the people involved don't know each other well, is likely to be able to learn enough from this discussion to avoid repeating the same mistake in the future. Alternatively, a physician who rejects the notion that it is his responsibility to manage other's perceptions of him will likely continue to struggle.

The final phase of the CAM encounter is the planning phase. In the planning phase (Table 11-8), the physician is asked to make a specific commitment to try a new approach to similar interactions in the future. The counselor can help by asking if new skills are required, how the physician will learn them, who is able to help them with their goals, and how will they know if they are successful.

Table 11-8	**PLANNING PHASE OF THE COUNSELING AFTER THE MOMENT CONVERSATION**

Sample questions:
1. How will you approach situations like this in the future?
2. Who do you trust to help you with stressful circumstances?
3. Who will you be able to turn to if you need advice?
4. What will be the most difficult thing for you to do?
5. What kind of help or assistance or skills will you need for success?
6. How will you know if you are successful?
7. How can I help?

In a study by Pichert and colleagues (2008), 58% of those physicians with excessive patient complaints who were invited to participate in cup of coffee conversations reduced the frequency of patient complaints by at least 40%, with a median improvement of 79% over the period of observation. In 10 years of follow up, the recidivism rate of these responders was less than 3%. Of interest, one-fifth of high complaint physicians who received a cup of coffee encounter left the institution, perhaps because they realized that their personal styles were not compatible with the institution. While this is unfortunate for the physician, it preserves the desired culture of the institution.

LEVEL III INTERVENTION: CORRECTION AND CONSEQUENCES

Dr. Nanette Oscher, chair of the department of obstetrics and gynecology, was upset about a letter she had received. She had been thrilled to successfully recruit Jason Latcher, MD, away from a major competitor for the position of gynecologic oncology chief 2 years ago. Since then, although surgical volumes were up and Dr. Latcher's clinical outcomes were good, she had begun to rue that recruitment decision. Patients loved Dr. Latcher and raved about his compassion. But almost everyone else struggled with him. Nurses complained that he frequently yelled at them in front of patients. Residents routinely left the operating room in tears after being dressed down for perceived mistakes. The School of Medicine would no longer allow students to rotate on his service. Dr. Oscher had asked a seasoned senior surgeon to mentor Jason, but the cup of coffee conversations between them had not gone anywhere. Jason was charming in the encounters but he vigorously defended his actions by saying that he was simply holding people accountable to provide the highest quality care for patients. And each time he agreed to try and be more respectful in his interactions. Now Dr. Oscher was holding a letter signed by all of the interns saying that they could not work with Dr. Latcher because of the way he treated them in the operating room.

Although most physicians will not need counseling more than once, some physicians persist in engaging in unprofessional behavior even after an awareness intervention. In Pichert and colleagues' (2008) data, 21% of high complaint physicians failed to improve after the initial intervention. Dr. Latcher's case is not uncommon. He is kind and gentle with patients and his clinical outcomes are good, but he is disrespectful to the nurses, residents, and students. By engaging in such disruptive behavior, physicians such as Dr. Latcher engender fear and aversion in those who work with them. In doing so, they create a culture counter to the culture of respect and collegiality that is required to deliver safe, high-quality healthcare.

Why does someone as accomplished as Dr. Latcher repeatedly act in this manner? If this happened once or twice, it would be tempting to excuse this as just a bad day. Had that been the case, the coaching in the moment would have been successful. If Dr. Latcher was serious about fitting in to the culture of his new institution, the counseling after the moment conversation, where he was given data that demonstrated that he had four times the number of complaints compared with any other department physician, would have led to behavior change. Persistently disruptive behavior in a physician despite coaching and counseling interventions occurs for several reasons. The physician in question may be benefiting from the behavior that others find objectionable (Williams & Williams, 2008). The department, valuing his surgical skill and ability to attract patients, may have created work-arounds that benefit Dr. Latcher and thus unwittingly reinforce his disruptive behavior. Because of his response to the students, Dr. Latcher no longer has to have students on his surgical team. Because the residents have complained about him, he was assigned his own physician's assistant. Because the nurses are afraid to page him, other physicians manage his patients after-hours and on weekends. Alternatively, the physician with the disruptive behavior may not have the skills needed to function effectively in the environment. This may be an issue of professional competence, meaning that the individual is potentially capable of learning how to work in collegial manner but has not yet developed proficiency in those skills. A physical or mental illness, burnout, or substance abuse may also be present.

Dr. Latcher merits a level III intervention: a conversation about the need for behavior correction and the consequences if correction does not occur. In contrast to the counseling after the moment conversation, this needs to be carried out by an authority figure in a formal setting, and it must be documented. In planning for this encounter, Dr. Oscher may find it helpful to speak with a human resources or faculty affairs expert to develop an effective and legally supportable strategy. Because the stakes of this conversation are higher, it is expected that Dr. Oscher will have made sure that the reports she is receiving are accurate.

The purpose of a **Correction and Consequences** conversation is to make sure that the physician in question clearly understands what behavior is considered objectionable, what behavior is desirable, and what consequences will ensue if the objectionable behavior continues. It is critically important that Dr. Oscher identify how the department and institution might have inadvertently rewarded Dr. Latcher for disruptive behavior. She must develop a new set of strategies that reward good behavior and prevent gain from bad behavior.

A correction and consequences conversation includes a series of important steps. At the beginning of the meeting, the authority figure must describe this as a serious conversation. This is not the time to provide praise to the individual; doing so may minimize the impact of the subsequent corrective message. They should then describe the disruptive behavior and its impact on the environment. Following that, they must articulate the expected behavior. Next, they should outline the consequences of failing to behave in the expected manner and how the performance will be monitored. Finally, they should close with a show of support and a request for a reaction from the individual. Table 11-9 provides a sample conversation.

If Dr. Latcher attempts to interrupt this initial series of steps, Dr. Oscher should respectfully ask him to listen carefully to what she has to say and

Table 11-9 STEPS IN A CORRECTION AND CONSEQUENCES CONVERSATION	
Establish the seriousness of the conversation	"We need to have a serious conversation about your behavior. I know that this will be difficult to hear but I ask that you listen carefully to what I have to say without interrupting and then I will listen to you."
Describe the disruptive behavior	"Despite several counseling sessions about this, I continue to receive complaints that you use profanity in the operating room, raise your voice at the nurses, and use mocking and condescension in your dealings with the residents."
Outline its impact	"Your style of interaction is causing people to refuse to work with you or to be afraid of calling you about your patients. This is creating an unsafe culture in the patient care environment and a hostile learning environment. We have lost two experienced OR nurses this week and we were unable to recruit the Gyn-Onc fellow that you wanted."
Describe the desired behavior	"I want to make it perfectly clear that from this moment on, all complaints about your behavior must stop. I expect no reports of profanity or yelling in any clinical or learning environment, and I expect you to treat the residents and nurses with respect. When they point out an error in the operating room or call you on the phone about a patient, I expect you to thank them for their concern. If you disagree with them, I expect that you will express that disagreement in a civil manner, using language and tone that you would be willing to have me overhear."
Identify the consequences of failing to meet standards	"If I do not see improvement in your behavior within the next month, I will be forced to take correction action. First, I will assign one of our senior surgeons to proctor you in the operating room. You will not be allowed to post cases unless your proctor is available to participate. The proctor will guide you in positive interactions with operating room staff. If problems with trainees continue, I will be forced to close your gynecologic oncology fellowship, since I cannot, in good conscience, invite a trainee into a hostile work environment."

Table 11-9	STEPS IN A CORRECTION AND CONSEQUENCES CONVERSATION (*Continued*)
Outline how performance will be monitored	"We will monitor your performance using monthly 360 evaluations of your performance. Once it is clear that your behavior is improving, we will decrease the monitoring to every 3 months. Dr. X will be the recipient of these reports and will meet with you monthly to review them with you."
Support and ask for response	"Thank you for listening so carefully. I know that you are an excellent surgeon and care deeply about your patients. I'd like to hear your thoughts on how you will change the style of your work to create the culture of respect that we value here. I am committed to helping you as you work on this."

reassure him that he will have an opportunity to be heard when she is finished. She can anticipate and plan to respond to common but maladaptive reactions (Table 11-10), described by Mizrahi (1984) as denial, deflection, and distancing.

Dr. Oscher can select from a variety of leverage points to incentivize the desired behavior or discourage the disruptive behavior. She may choose to apply financial levers, such as modifying salary or bonus structures. She may change Dr. Latcher's access to operating room time or prime schedule slots.

Table 11-10	ANTICIPATING AND RESPONDING TO COMMON MALADAPTIVE RESPONSES TO CORRECTION AND CONSEQUENCES CONVERSATIONS	
Reaction	**Example**	**Response**
Denial	"I am not the one with the problem, you have hired a bunch of terrible residents. Did you see their in-service exam scores?"	"We are not here to talk about the resident's in-service scores, we are here to talk about your communication with them. Even if they are not meeting your standards, you must speak to them respectfully. Feel free to bring your concerns up with the program director."
Deflection	"Have you seen my latest billing? My most recent grant?"	"I appreciate your clinical and research skills, but your behaviors are interfering with your reputation and your effectiveness."
	"Wasn't that a great party last weekend? You've really built a great department."	"Thank you for your compliments, but I need you to listen to my serious concerns about your behavior."
Distancing	"All right, I admit that I am not the easiest person to get along with. I'll go apologize and promise to do better."	"I appreciate your willingness to apologize but that was your response the last time we had this conversation. I am afraid that we need to be more explicit about how you will avoid these complaints in the future."

She may consider altering support structures, such as access to physician's assistants or residents. She can modify Dr. Latcher's independence by mandating proctors in the operating room. Any of these levers for change may work; the best ones will be those that most closely relate to the disruptive behavior and to privileges viewed as important to Dr. Latcher.

LEVEL IV INTERVENTIONS: SANCTIONS AND DISCIPLINARY ACTIONS

Level IV interventions are reserved for the most recalcitrant disruptors and are generally conducted in accordance with institutional (academic medical center or university) bylaws. When permanent sanctions such as dismissal from medical school, nonrenewal of a resident's contract, loss of admitting privileges, removal of tenure, and loss of licensure are possible, the person in authority will work with institutional attorneys to ensure that due process is afforded to the individual accused of disruptive behavior that is either egregious enough or persistent enough to warrant these extreme responses. While important, these situations are less common and beyond the scope of this chapter.

THE ROLE OF SYSTEMS IN DEALING WITH UNPROFESSIONAL BEHAVIOR

Healthcare Institutions

As we have discussed in other chapters, the systems in which we work can unwittingly increase the risk of unprofessional behaviors or they can explicitly work to enhance the culture of professionalism. Swiggart and colleagues (2009) have summarized key institutional structures, policies, and procedures that can facilitate positive and constructive responses to unprofessional behavior. Wise healthcare leaders who intend to build a culture of safety and patient centeredness realize that they will need a multifaceted approach and that physicians must be involved in designing and co-leading any program that is aimed at improving professionalism (Humphrey et al, 2007; Leape et al, 2012b; Viggiano et al, 2007; Kitch et al, 2013; Smith et al, 2007). Strong approaches seek to optimize the culture and environment to support professionalism; provide educational programs and coaching resources to teach and sustain professional attitudes and behaviors; develop and consistently implement policies and procedures that address unprofessional behavior; and recognize and reward professionalism in all (Figure 11-6).

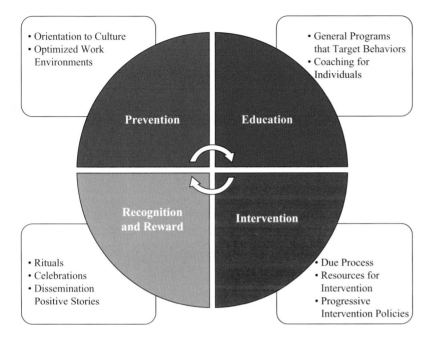

Figure 11-6 ▪ Components of institutional professionalism.

The healthcare environment should be constructed to support rest, reflection, and renewal for all professionals. Attention to appropriate staffing, shift length, and idealized workflow can mitigate some of the stressors inherent in caring for sick and dying patients. Quiet rooms for reflection and period rest breaks can also be helpful. Orientation to the desired culture of respect can help ensure that everyone who begins work at the institution understands what is expected of him or her. Education about the nature of unprofessional behavior, the impact of disruption on patient care and clinician wellbeing and the skills needed for coaching in the moment conversations must be provided to everyone, from medical students to practicing clinicians from all professions. All clinical, educational, and research leaders must be schooled in counseling after the moment and correction and consequences interventions. Resources must be invested in professional coaching and evaluation strategies for professionals who may benefit from them.

Policies and procedures that outline progressively more serious interventions and consequences must be developed and approved by institutional attorneys and should include guidelines for when reports to licensing boards or the national practitioner data bank are warranted. Many institutions have established covenants or compacts for behavior that are signed at the time of credentialing and include descriptions of ideal behavior for interacting with patients, students, trainees, and other healthcare professionals (Joint Commission, 2009). Due process for the professional accused of a serious transgression must be established to protect those who are wrongfully accused. However, the due process should not be so burdensome as to prevent an authority from taking corrective action when a professional will not adhere to the institution's or the profession's values. Service recovery strategies should be devised so that anyone who is the target of unprofessional behavior or retaliation for reporting unprofessional behavior receives an apology and any necessary support. Ideally, institutions will invest in data monitoring programs, such as the Patient Advocacy Reporting System (PARS) program (Pichert, Hickson, & Moore, 2008). Most importantly, all in the environment should understand that a culture of professionalism requires ongoing constant surveillance and reinforcement from all.

Finally, rituals that recognize and reward professionalism provide tangible evidence of the value the institution places on professional performance.

Accrediting and Professional Organizations

National professional organizations and accrediting bodies can provide important incentives for individuals and institutions to create and sustain a culture of professionalism. The Joint Commission requires organizations to have policies and procedures in place for dealing with disruptive behavior. Both the Accreditation Council for Graduate Medical Education (ACGME) and the Liaison Committee on Medical Education (LCME) mandate attention to and optimization of learner wellbeing and appropriate learning climate. Specialty societies like the American Board of Internal Medicine, the American Academy of Orthopaedic Surgeons, and the American College of Surgeons can provide educational materials to help members recognize and deal with unprofessional behaviors (American College of Physicians, 2009; Porucznik, 2013; Halverson, Neumayer, & Forcht Dagi, 2012).

| CONCLUSION

As we have learned from the medical errors literature, any endeavor that depends on humans to behave perfectly is bound to fail. Even the most committed physicians have days when they are not at their best, where they may be at risk for failing to live up to personal and professional standards. Our best safety net for these occasions is a group of dedicated peers who are committed to upholding the privilege and responsibility of self-regulation and who we can count on to intervene when we need a helping hand.

KEY LEARNING POINTS

1. Unprofessional behaviors range from those that disrupt the work and learning environment (like yelling or joking about patients) to crimes (like fraud). Most physicians and students witness disruptive behaviors, as they are frequent (3% to 5% of physicians in an institution warrant interventions due to more egregious lapses).

2. Unprofessional behaviors can compromise patient care by creating an environment where members of the team are afraid to speak up to correct gaps in quality. In an environment that allows unprofessional behaviors to go unchecked, students and others can experience moral distress and it can lead to poor morale and staff turnover.

3. A variety of triggers can contribute to unprofessional behaviors occurring, including ones that are personal, interpersonal, situational, and organizational.

4. Responses of individuals who witness unprofessional behaviors include endorsing, ignoring, deferring action, and intervening.

5. There is a step-wise approach to intervening in witnessed lapses ranging from coaching in the moment, to coaching after the moment, to consequences from recurrent lapses, to sanctions. Specific strategies can make these interventions more effective.

REFERENCES

1. Adams KE, Emmons S, Romm J. How resident unprofessional behavior is identified and managed: a program director survey. *Am J Obstet Gynecol*. 2008 Jun;198(6):692. e1–4; discussion 692.e4–5.

2. American College of Physicians Dealing with the Disruptive Physician Colleague. *ACP Ethics Case Studies*. 2009. Available at http://www.medscape.org/viewarticle/590319_2

3. Arnold L. Responding to the professionalism of learners and faculty in orthopaedic surgery. *Clin Orthop Relat Res*. 2006 Aug;449:205–213.

4. Billings ME, Lazarus ME, Wenrich M, Curtis JR, Engelberg RA. The effect of the hidden curriculum on resident burnout and cynicism. *J Grad Med Educ*. 2011 Dec;3(4):503–510.

5. Brainard AH, Brislen HC. Viewpoint: learning professionalism: a view from the trenches. *Acad Med*. 2007 Nov;82(11):1010–1014.

6. Brater DC. Viewpoint: infusing professionalism into a school of medicine: perspectives from the dean. *Acad Med*. 2007 Nov;82(11):1094–1097.

7. Brenner AM, Mathai S, Jain S, Mohl PC. Can we predict "problem residents"? *Acad Med*. 2010 Jul;85(7):1147–1151.

8. Brownlee S. *Overtreated: Why Too Much Medicine Is Making Us Sicker and Poorer*. 1st edition. New York (NY): Bloomsbury; 2008.

9. Buchanan AO, Stallworth J, Christy C, Garfunkel LC, Hanson JL. Professionalism in practice: strategies for assessment, remediation, and promotion. *Pediatrics*. 2012 Mar;129(3):407–409.

10. Campbell EG, Regan S, Gruen RL, Ferris TG, Rao SR, Cleary PD, Blumenthal D. Professionalism in medicine: results of a national survey of physicians. *Ann Intern Med*. 2007 Dec 4;147(11):795–802.

11. Dupras DM, Edson RS, Halvorsen AJ, Hopkins RH Jr, McDonald FS. "Problem residents": prevalence, problems and remediation in the era of core competencies. *Am J Med*. 2012 Apr;125(4):421–425.

12. Dyrbye LN, Massie FS Jr, Eacker A, Harper W, Power D, Durning SJ, Thomas MR, Moutier C, Satele D, Sloan J, Shanafelt TD. Relationship between burnout and professional conduct and attitudes among US medical students. *JAMA*. 2010 Sep 15; 304(11):1173–1180.

13. Dyrbye LN, Shanafelt TD. Physician burnout: a potential threat to successful health care reform. *JAMA*. 2011 May 18;305(19):2009–2010.

14. Federation of State Medical Boards (FSMB). *Policy on Physician Impairment*. 2011. Available at: http://www.fsmb.org/pdf/grpol_policy-on-physician-impairment.pdf

15. Garcia SM, Weaver K, Moskowitz GB, Darley JM. Crowded minds: the implicit bystander effect. *J Pers Soc Psychol*. 2002 Oct;83(4):843–853.

16. Hafferty FW. Beyond curriculum reform: confronting medicine's hidden curriculum. *Acad Med*. 1998 Apr;73(4):403–407.

17. Halverson AL, Neumayer L, Forcht Dagi, T. Leadership Skills in the OR. Part II: Recognizing disruptive behavior. *Bulletin of the American College of Surgeons*. 2012 Jun;97(6):17–23.

18. Hickson GB, Federspiel CF, Pichert JW, Miller CS, Gauld-Jaeger J, Bost P. Patient complaints and malpractice risk. *JAMA*. 2002 Jun 12;287(22):2951–2957.

19. Hickson GB, Pichert JW, Webb LE, Gabbe SG. A complementary approach to promoting professionalism: identifying, measuring, and addressing unprofessional behaviors. *Acad Med*. 2007 Nov;82(11):1040–1048.

20. Humphrey HJ, Smith K, Reddy S, Scott D, Madara JL, Arora VM. Promoting an environment of professionalism: the University of Chicago "Roadmap." *Acad Med*. 2007 Nov;82(11):1098–1107.

21. Joint Commission. Managing Disruptive Behavior. *The Joint Commission Perspectives on Patient Safety*. 2009 Jan; 29(1):8–10.

22. Kitch BT, Desroches C, Lesser C, Cunningham A, Campbell EG. Systems model of physician professionalism in practice. *J Eval Clin Pract*. 2013 Feb;19(1):1–10.

23. Leape LL, Fromson JA. Problem doctors: is there a system–level solution? *Ann Intern Med*. 2006 Jan 17;144(2):107–115.

24. Leape LL, Shore MF, Dienstag JL, Mayer RJ, Edgman-Levitan S, Meyer GS, Healy GB. Perspective: a culture of respect, part 1: the nature and causes of disrespectful behavior by physicians. *Acad Med*. 2012a Jul;87(7):845–852.

25. Leape LL, Shore MF, Dienstag JL, Mayer RJ, Edgman-Levitan S, Meyer GS, Healy GB. Perspective: a culture of respect, part 2: creating a culture of respect. *Acad Med.* 2012b Jul;87(7):853–858.

26. Mann S. *Efforts Increase to Eradicate Student Mistreatment, Improve Culture at Medical Schools.* AAMC Reporter; September 2012. Available at: https://www.aamc.org/newsroom/reporter/sept2012/303666/student-mistreatment.html

27. McLaren K, Lord J, Murray S. Perspective: delivering effective and engaging continuing medical education on physicians' disruptive behavior. *Acad Med.* 2011 May;86(5):612–617.

28. Mizrahi T. Managing medical mistakes: ideology, insularity and accountability among internists-in-training. *Soc Sci Med.* 1984;19(2):135–146.

29. Papadakis MA, Paauw DS, Hafferty FW, Shapiro J, Byyny RL; Alpha Omega Alpha Honor Medical Society Think Tank. Perspective: the education community must develop best practices informed by evidence-based research to remediate lapses of professionalism. *Acad Med.* 2012 Dec;87(12):1694–1698.

30. Papadakis MA, Teherani A, Banach MA, Knettler TR, Rattner SL, Stern DT, Veloski JJ, Hodgson CS. Disciplinary action by medical boards and prior behavior in medical school. *N Engl J Med.* 2005 Dec 22;353(25):2673–2682.

31. Patterson K, Grenny J, McMillan R, Switzler A. *Crucial Conversations: Tools for Talking When Stakes Are High.* 1st edition. New York, NY: McGraw-Hill; 2012.

32. Pichert JW, Hickson G, Moore I. Using Patient Complaints to Promote Patient Safety. In: Henriksen K, Battles JB, Keyes MA, Grady ML, eds. *Advances in Patient Safety: New Directions and Alternative Approaches* (Vol. 2: Culture and Redesign). Rockville, MD: Agency for Healthcare Research and Quality; 2008. Available at: http://www.ncbi.nlm.nih.gov/books/NBK43703/

33. Porucznik MA. How to Deal with the "Problem Physician." AAOS *Now.* January, 2013. Available at http://www.aaos.org/news/aaosnow/jan13/managing3.asp

34. Pronovost PJ, Weast B, Holzmueller CG, Rosenstein BJ, Kidwell RP, Haller KB, Feroli ER, Sexton JB, Rubin HR. Evaluation of the culture of safety: survey of clinicians and managers in an academic medical center. *Qual Saf Health Care.* 2003 Dec;12(6):405–410.

35. Reynolds N. Disruptive physician behavior: use and misuse of the label. *Journal of Medical Regulation.* 2012;98(1):8–19.

36. Rosenstein AH. The quality and economic impact of disruptive behaviors on clinical outcomes of patient care. *Am J Med Qual.* 2011 Sep-Oct;26(5):372–379.

37. Rosenstein AH, Naylor B. Incidence and impact of physician and nurse disruptive behaviors in the emergency department. *J Emerg Med.* 2012 Jul;43(1):139–148.

38. Rosenstein AH, O'Daniel M. A survey of the impact of disruptive behaviors and communication defects on patient safety. *Jt Comm J Qual Patient Saf.* 2008 Aug;34(8):464–471.

39. Samenow CP, Worley LL, Neufeld R, Fishel T, Swiggart WH. Transformative learning in a professional development course aimed at addressing disruptive physician behavior: a composite case study. *Acad Med.* 2013 Jan;88(1):117–123.

40. Sanfey H, Darosa DA, Hickson GB, Williams B, Sudan R, Boehler ML, Klingensmith ME, Klamen D, Mellinger JD, Hebert JC, Richard KM, Roberts NK, Schwind CJ, Williams RG, Sachdeva AK, Dunnington GL. Pursuing professional accountability: an evidence-based approach to addressing residents with behavioral problems. *Arch Surg*. 2012 Jul;147(7):642–647.

41. Saxton R. Communication skills training to address disruptive physician behavior. *AORN J*. 2012 May;95(5):602–611.

42. Saxton R, Hines T, Enriquez M. The negative impact of nurse-physician disruptive behavior on patient safety: a review of the literature. *J Patient Saf*. 2009 Sep;5(3): 180–183.

43. Sehgal NL, Fox M, Vidyarthi AR, Sharpe BA, Gearhart S, Bookwalter T, Barker J, Alldredge BK, Blegen MA, Wachter RM; Triad for Optimal Patient Safety Project. A multidisciplinary teamwork training program: the Triad for Optimal Patient Safety (TOPS) experience. *J Gen Intern Med*. 2008 Dec;23(12):2053–2057.

44. Silverman BC, Stern TW, Gross AF, Rosenstein DL, Stern TA. Lewd, crude, and rude behavior: the impact of manners and etiquette in the general hospital. *Psychosomatics*. 2012 Jan–Feb;53(1):13–20.

45. Smetzer JL, Cohen MR. Intimidation: practitioners speak up about this unresolved problem. *Jt Comm J Qual Patient Saf*. 2005 Oct;31(10):594–599.

46. Smith KL, Saavedra R, Raeke JL, O'Donell AA. The journey to creating a campus-wide culture of professionalism. *Acad Med*. 2007 Nov;82(11):1015–1021.

47. Stewart JB. *Blind Eye: The Terrifying Story Of A Doctor Who Got Away With Murder*. 1st edition. New York, NY: Simon & Schuster; 2000.

48. Swiggart WH, Dewey CM, Hickson GB, Finlayson AJ, Spickard WA Jr. A plan for identification, treatment, and remediation of disruptive behaviors in physicians. *Front Health Serv Manage*. 2009 Summer;25(4):3–11.

49. Teherani A, Hodgson CS, Banach M, Papadakis MA. Domains of unprofessional behavior during medical school associated with future disciplinary action by a state medical board. *Acad Med*. 2005 Oct;80(10 Suppl):S17–S20.

50. Testerman JK, Morton KR, Loo LK, Worthley JS, Lamberton HH. The natural history of cynicism in physicians. *Acad Med*. 1996 Oct;71(10 Suppl):S43–S45.

51. Viggiano TR, Pawlina W, Lindor KD, Olsen KD, Cortese DA. Putting the needs of the patient first: Mayo Clinic's core value, institutional culture, and professionalism covenant. *Acad Med*. 2007 Nov;82(11):1089–1093.

52. Walrath JM, Dang D, Nyberg D. An organizational assessment of disruptive clinician behavior: findings and implications. *J Nurs Care Qual*. 2013 Apr–Jun;28(2):110–121.

53. Wasserstein AG, Brennan PJ, Rubenstein AH. Institutional leadership and faculty response: fostering professionalism at the University of Pennsylvania School of Medicine. *Acad Med*. 2007 Nov;82(11):1049–1056.

54. Wear D, Aultman JM, Zarconi J, Varley JD. Derogatory and cynical humour directed towards patients: views of residents and attending doctors. *Med Educ*. 2009 Jan;43(1):34–41.

55. Weber DO. Poll results: doctors' disruptive behavior disturbs physician leaders. *Physician Exec*. 2004 Sep–Oct;30(5):6–14.

56. Wiggleton C, Petrusa E, Loomis K, Tarpley J, Tarpley M, O'Gorman ML, Miller B. Medical students' experiences of moral distress: development of a web–based survey. *Acad Med.* 2010 Jan;85(1):111–117.

57. Williams BW, Williams MV. The disruptive physician: a conceptual organization. *Journal of Medical Licensure and Discipline.* 2008;94(3):12–20.

58. Williams MV, William BM, Speicher M. A systems approach to disruptive behavior in physicians: a case study. *Journal of Medical Licensure and Discipline.* 2004;90(4): 18–24.

59. Zbieranowski I, Takahashi SG, Verma S, Spadafora SM. Remediation of residents in difficulty: a retrospective 10-year review of the experience of a postgraduate board of examiners. *Acad Med.* 2013 Jan;88(1):111–116.

ORGANIZATIONAL PROFESSIONALISM | 12

LEARNING OBJECTIVES

1. To explain how healthcare organizations influence professionalism.
2. To identify common themes in organizations that have successfully advanced professionalism in their institutions.
3. To identify the organizational "levers" for influencing professionalism.
4. To provide illustrative examples of how several specific organizations have advanced professionalism.

The framework for professionalism described in this book includes consideration of the role of organizations in building a culture of professionalism. Our premise is that systems in which physicians practice influence physicians' behaviors in positive or negative ways by shaping the practice environment. The chapters on patient-centered care, integrity and accountability, pursuit of excellence, and fair and ethical use of healthcare resources each included a section on the role of the healthcare system in contributing to professionalism. This chapter describes further the role of the healthcare system, including academic medical centers, ambulatory care centers, community hospitals, and integrated delivery systems, and provides some specific examples of organizations that have integrated some aspect of professionalism into their culture.

Egener and colleagues (2012) propose that healthcare organizations, particularly nonprofit ones, have a responsibility to uphold the values of professionalism because these organizations are perceived as the face of the profession by the public and because their tax exempt status requires them to serve the best interest of the public. We suggest that healthcare organizations should uphold the ethical values of beneficence, dignity, justice, honesty, and self-discipline, just as individual healthcare professionals should do. In order to live up to these values, they suggest that organizations need to develop competencies and demonstrate professionalism behaviors. For example, the value of beneficence means doing good and acting with generosity. For an organization, this may mean providing services not only to patients who come to the facility, but also proactively providing care for patients in the community who may not come in but need help to be healthy or to manage medical problems. Other organizational behaviors that demonstrate a commitment to this value could include caring for uninsured patients in the community or working to eliminate health risks in the community (e.g., environmental hazards, gun violence, and obesity). In other words, healthcare organizations can demonstrate professionalism by committing to a set of ethical values and acting to realize them. Table 12-1 presents a set of values, competencies, and behaviors to describe organizational professionalism. Organizations also set the internal culture that shapes the work of the physicians, nurses, and other members of the team. Healthcare organizations provide a powerful message about "how things are done around here" through formal policies and procedures, incentives, and informal and usually unwritten rules that are modeled by leaders.

> *A large multispecialty clinic made a commitment to engage patients in the organization to help improve their "patient-centered care." Furthermore, the clinic wanted to promote the message that relationships between patients and staff, and between staff members, were of the upmost importance. Patients were asked to participate in planning the new clinic space, and examination rooms were designed to allow patients and physicians to sit side by side using the computer chart together. Common work areas were designed for the physicians and staff to increase interaction and collaborative care. Several methods of obtaining patient feedback were implemented including regular surveys, focus groups, and advisory groups. Patient feedback was examined regularly and incorporated into quality improvement in a continuous fashion. To foster relationships between staff, the organization also implemented 360 degree evaluations for all physicians and key leaders in all disciplines.*

In this multispecialty group example, the clinic is seeking to provide "patient-centered care" and to build a "relationship-centered environment" for staff. Patient-centered care is a component of professionalism and the culture of the clinic supports this through engaging patients in decisions and through building both physical space and processes that foster relationships. Written rules are not necessary for patients or physicians to understand what is expected in this clinic. Over time, and with consistent leadership reinforcing the message, the unspoken rules become embedded in the processes of care and become the norm for all staff. Physicians who consider working at the clinic will choose

Table 12-1 ORGANIZATIONAL VALUES, PROFESSIONALISM COMPETENCIES, AND BEHAVIORS		
Value	Professionalism competency	Behavior
Beneficence (does good, acts with generosity and kindness)	• Service (to the patient, the community, and the profession)	• Promotes population health • Reduces harm • Promotes well-being • Aspires to improve the organization and the profession
Dignity (respects self, is worthy of esteem)	• Respect (for self, patients, and employees)	• Responds to regular assessments of the experiences of patients and employees • Provides access to care • Supports teamwork • Promotes cultural sensitivity • Rewards achievement
Justice (is impartial, upholds the laws)	• Fairness	• Practices and promotes ethical stewardship of resources • Incorporates voice of community • Advocates equitable payment policy • Reduces disparities
Honesty (is morally upright, truthful, and candid)	• Integrity • Accountability	• Practices transparency • Discloses meaningful performance information • Eliminates conflicts of interest
Self-discipline	• Mindfulness • Self-motivation	• Engages in collective self-reflection • Closes the gap between current performance and the ideal state • Utilizes supportive structures, e.g., ethics committees, quality improvement committees

From Egener B, McDonald W, Rosof B, Gullen D. Perspective: organizational professionalism: relevant competencies and behaviors. *Acad Med.* 2012 May;87(5):668–674.

to join the practice, or choose not to do so, based on whether the culture fits their values. Successful steps in changing the culture to one of patient-centered care are celebrated by leaders and staff, and this provides positive reinforcement for the change.

It is important to note that most organizations do not use the word "professionalism" to describe the behaviors they are trying to foster. This makes sense as the goal is to foster a set of values and behaviors that are well-accepted and enacted by all the professional staff. It is much easier to describe professionalism as a set of observable behaviors than to use the term "professionalism," which is interpreted in many different ways. Organizations may not even consider that they are working on professionalism when they develop efforts to foster these behaviors. Language used by the organizational leaders may be "plan for excellence" or "patient-centeredness." Hence, the language these organizations uses varies but we consider them examples of fostering professionalism, since they are working to uphold the values of the *Physician Charter*. (see Chapter 1, A Practical Approach to "Professionalism") and to foster the specific behaviors that demonstrate those values in action.

WHAT DO SUCCESSFUL ORGANIZATIONS COMMITTED TO VALUES OF PROFESSIONALISM DO TO ACHIEVE THEIR GOALS?

Cunningham et al (2011) conducted interviews with leaders of healthcare organizations about how they advance values consistent with the *Physician Charter*. Organizations selected were recognized by peers as successfully building cultures to support some aspect of professionalism. The common themes identified included:

1. articulating values clearly;
2. aligning organizational systems and structures to support the desired behaviors; and
3. cultivating strong interpersonal relationships within the organization.

A key commonality was that these leaders were very clear about the articulated goal and that this goal was communicated broadly through the organization. Second, the values were not only written and communicated but, more importantly, were reinforced through numerous mechanisms—hiring, training, evaluation, remediation, and so on. They described building structures like payment models, physical design of space, and technology to support the goals. Recognition of employees who exemplified the values was frequently reported by these leaders as a mechanism to reward and reinforce the values publically. Although financial incentives were used, it was rarely seen as the key motivator. Third, these organizations had a common theme related to the cultivation of strong relationships to realize professional behaviors. Some leaders cultivated these relationships by adopting frameworks such as "relationship-centered care" (see Indiana University example below), whereas others emphasized being accessible to providers and staff, engaging in ongoing conversations with all organizational stakeholders, soliciting and acting on workforce feedback to improve the organization, and encouraging provider and staff "champions" to role model desired behaviors . Table 12-2 provides an overview of the organizational themes.

In summary, there are a variety of levers that organizations can use to foster the values and behaviors of professionalism. For example, organizations' physical designs, hiring procedures, payment models, performance feedback efforts, training programs, policies on unprofessional behavior, and leadership engagement with providers and staff can all help to ensure that an organization's values are supported and sustained. The development of strong interpersonal relationships between leaders and healthcare providers and among team members appears to be a critically important element in all the examples. What follows are several detailed examples of how organizations have

Table 12-2 **COMMON THEMES OF ORGANIZATIONS ADVANCING PROFESSIONALISM**	
Theme	**Examples**
Clarity, and clear articulation, of values	• Well-developed organizational mission statements and goals • Mission and goals developed with input from organizational stakeholders • Values inform organizational systems and structures
Aligned systems and structures to support behavioral expectations	• Hiring and orientation procedures that emphasize behavioral expectations • Protected time for quality improvement activities • Strong policies for dealing with unprofessional behavior • Physical design that supports patient-centeredness, team-based care, or other core values • Regular performance feedback • Payment systems to incentivize desired behaviors
Cultivation of strong relationships	• Adopting model of relationship-centered care • Leadership that is accessible and is engaging in regular conversations with providers and staff • Leadership transparency about organizational initiatives • Cultivating peer relationships to encourage role models/champions of organizational values

From Cunningham AT, Bernabeo EC, Wolfson DB, Lesser CS. Organizational strategies to cultivate professional values and behaviors. *BMJ Qual Saf.* 2011 Apr;20(4):351–358.

LEARNING EXERCISE 12-1

1. Think about the organization in which you are working or learning.
2. What are the stated values of the organization?
3. How does the organization support these values?
4. What are some of the "unwritten rules" of the organization? How do they support or undermine its stated values?
5. What behaviors demonstrate the commitment to the values?

promoted a component of professionalism and the behaviors that demonstrate it in action. Each example includes a rationale for the approach taken, the key elements of the initiative, its outcomes, and lessons learned.

INDIANA UNIVERSITY SCHOOL OF MEDICINE STRIVES FOR THE PROFESSIONALISM VALUE OF RELATIONSHIP-CENTERED CULTURE

Rationale

Indiana University School of Medicine is the second largest allopathic medical school in the United States. In 1999, the school's leaders completed an 8-year self-study and redesign of the undergraduate medical curriculum. As a result of that process, the school instituted changes in both the formal and informal curriculum. The school implemented a new formal curriculum requiring students to demonstrate proficiency in nine core competencies. In addition, its leaders committed to changing the culture of the institution to one that promoted caring, respect, and collaboration. This initiative was spurred by survey data from medical students that showed that despite a formal professionalism curriculum, the informal or hidden curriculum did not support these same professionalism values (Cottingham et al, 2008).

How They Did It—Key Elements

As part of the formal curriculum, school leaders identified professionalism as a core competency for all students. Their primary goal was for students to translate the sometimes abstract principles of professionalism into everyday practice. Students participated in reflective writing and small group discussions on professionalism issues encountered during their education. They were also required to demonstrate specific professionalism competencies by the end of their second, third, and fourth years. Key competencies for the second year include an understanding of basic professionalism principles and demonstration of respectful interactions with peers and professors. Third-year competencies include professional interactions with patients, families, and members of the healthcare team, whereas fourth-year students are expected to better understand the challenges and conflicts they face as physicians. In addition, third- and fourth-year students received peer professionalism assessments (Litzelman & Cottingham, 2007).

To address the hidden curriculum, the school used the framework of relationship-centered care, which is characterized by respectful collaborative relationships between patients and clinicians, among members of interdisciplinary healthcare teams, and between a healthcare system and its community. In addition, relationship-centered care includes a commitment to self-reflection and self-care. The initiative's leaders advanced relationship-centered care by utilizing appreciative inquiry, a technique focused on discovering what is working well within an organization rather than identifying deficits. The initiative's leaders formed a task force comprising students and faculty, who conducted 80 appreciative inquiry interviews with students, residents, faculty, and staff about the school's informal curriculum. The task force then shared themes from these appreciative inquiry interviews at a school-wide meeting.

In addition, the initiative's leaders used a process of emergent design, by letting many of their projects emerge through conversations with community members. For example, the presentation of themes from the initial round of appreciative inquiry interviews inspired a group of medical students to conduct appreciative inquiry interviews with classmates. Results from these student interviews were compiled and shared at a white-coat ceremony for the incoming medical students.

Third, the leaders based their work on the view that small, local changes in behavior can lead to larger organizational change. Therefore, they instituted a number of "local" activities around the institution, such as redesigning the admissions process to select students with a "relational orientation"; implementing executive and leadership coaching on relationship-centered approaches to administrative activities such as faculty evaluations; and developing a Change Agent Program to train interested community members in relationship-centered care (Cottingham et al, 2008).

Outcomes They Measured

For the formal curriculum, course and clerkship directors assessed students' professionalism competencies based on their reflective writing, professional deportment, and other measures. The school tracks all students' progress and scores electronically. Focus groups with students have revealed that the competency-based curriculum was a significant factor in their decision to attend Indiana University School of Medicine (Litzelman & Cottingham, 2007). For the informal curriculum, quantitative measures included changes in medical students' survey responses to questions on the school's informal curriculum, and the number and types of individuals (e.g., students, faculty) engaged in the project. In addition, an external consultant gathered qualitative data through observations and key informant interviews. The initiative's leaders also tracked project events, shared their reflections in team meetings and recorded these events and reflections in project reports. Student ratings of their medical school experience increased dramatically, and the number of individuals engaged in relationship-centered care activities increased from 6 to over 900 in 3 years. Interviews, observations, and project reports showed lasting changes in meeting formats and practices, new admissions requirements, and communication about organizational culture (Cottingham et al, 2008).

Key Lessons

Indiana University School of Medicine's experience shows the importance of addressing both the formal and informal curricula of an institution. The organization's leaders felt that implementation of the competency-based curriculum, while challenging, led to, "A new sense of purpose and newfound energy for students and faculty who dream of more consistently aligning IUSM community members' behaviors with [its] institutional values" (Litzelman & Cottingham, 2007). Efforts to change the informal curriculum revealed that Appreciative Inquiry is a powerful tool for spurring organizational change. In addition, the emergent design format allowed activities to emerge naturally and encouraged individuals who were ready to be engaged, rather than forcing change on those who might not be ready. The use of complexity theory was also effective; the project demonstrated that small changes, such as the way meetings are conducted, can spread throughout an organization and promote lasting change (Cottingham et al, 2008).

ALASKA NATIVE MEDICAL CENTER ADVANCES THE PROFESSIONALISM VALUE OF PATIENT-CENTERED CARE

Rationale

In 1999, the Alaska Native Medical Center, an ambulatory care center and 170-bed hospital in Anchorage, came under Alaska Native ownership. Its new leaders wanted to infuse behaviors of patient-centered care at all levels of the organization, particularly in ambulatory care. When they began their work, the Center had long wait times for routine appointments and high no-show rates for appointments. Many local community members used the emergency room as their main source of care. The organization committed to improving the patient experience (Gottlieb, Sylvester, & Eby, 2008).

How They Did It—Key Elements

The new leaders developed a vision, mission, and operating principles to guide its strategic and annual plans. As part of their new vision, they stated that "our core product is relationships" and began referring to patients as "customer-owners." Their work was based on the following acronym (RELATIONSHIPS):

- **R**elationships between the customer/owner, family, and provider must be fostered and supported.
- **E**mphasis on wellness of the whole person, family, and community including: physical, mental, emotional, and spiritual wellness.
- **L**ocations that are convenient for the customer/owner and create minimal stops for the customer/owner to get all of their needs addressed.
- **A**ccess is optimized and waiting times are limited.
- **T**ogether with the costumer/owner as an active partner.
- **I**ntegration of services throughout all of Southcentral Foundation (SCF). No more islands.
- **O**ne seamless system.
- **N**o duplication of services or roles and responsibilities.
- **S**imple and easy to use systems and services.
- **H**ub of the system is the family.
- **I**nterests of the customer/owner are placed first, and the system is created around what works best for the customer/owner.
- **P**opulation-based systems and services.
- **S**ervices and systems are culturally appropriate and build on the strengths of Alaska Native cultures.

To develop and implement its new mission and plans, organizational leaders engaged in ongoing conversations with community members, and participated in quality improvement training (Gottlieb, Sylvester, & Eby, 2008).

Key elements of their patient-centered clinic include same-day appointments and several "talking rooms," which are rooms in which the patient and clinician sit side-by-side in a physical arrangement that allows the joint use of computers or materials. These rooms are well-suited for visits that are primarily focused on health education rather than clinical purposes. In addition, care is delivered by primary care teams of physicians, medical assistants, a nurse who focuses on care coordination, and an administrator. Social services, nutrition, and complementary and alternative medicine are integrated into primary care. Patients are seen by the same team each time they visit to cultivate long-term, trusting relationships (Cunningham et al, 2011). Many of the organization's employees are Alaska Natives, and the Center has strived to provide culturally sensitive care through efforts such as emphasizing the role of the extended family and spiritual issues in care (Institute for Healthcare Improvement, 2011).

Workforce recruitment and planning are also key to Alaska Native Medical Center's success. The organization reinforces its values through a group hiring process that assesses candidates' commitment to patient-centered care and teamwork and provides ongoing training to reinforce organizational culture. The organization encourages staff collaboration through regular "huddles" and open office designs that allow clinicians to easily discuss and plan patient care. Leaders also provide regular feedback to each team on their clinical and patient experience performance (Gottlieb, Sylvester, & Eby, 2008).

Outcomes They Measured

The organization has a variety of measures related to operations, quality assurance, quality improvement, and process improvement. Since 1999, they have seen a 40% decrease in urgent care and emergency department utilization, and has reduced the number of individuals on its behavioral health waiting list from 1300 to 0 (Gottlieb, Sylvester, & Eby, 2008).

Patient-centered outcomes that are measured include wait times for appointments and no-show rates. Patient experience surveys include questions about whether a patient feels they are listened to, had their questions and concerns answered, had their care coordinated effectively, and feel that their goals and values drive their care. The organization also gathers qualitative data on patient experience through focus groups, "mystery shoppers," and its patient advisory committee. Quantitative and qualitative results reflect high levels of quality and patient satisfaction (Cunningham et al, 2011).

Key Lessons

Alaska Native Medical Center exemplifies a commitment to professionalism through fostering the value of patient-centered care. To operationalize this goal they made organizational changes that set the conditions for professionalism to flourish and behaviors of patient-centered care to become the norm. These changes included physical design of exam rooms and office space, hiring and training processes, and gathering and acting on ongoing feedback from community members. Providing patient-centered care requires intensive effort by providers and staff at all levels of the organization, but can yield high-quality care and excellent patient experiences.

UNIVERSITY OF CALIFORNIA SAN FRANCISCO (UCSF) SCHOOL OF MEDICINE UNDERTAKE PROFESSIONALISM WITHIN ALL LEVELS OF MEDICAL EDUCATION

Rationale

Nearly 20 years ago, UCSF School of Medicine undertook a process to establish professionalism as a core element of the medical school curriculum, which included both teaching and evaluation. The goal at the time was to identify clerkship students' problematic behaviors early so that appropriate remediation could be instituted. Over time, the evaluation of professionalism was expanded to also include preclerkship students, and eventually faculty members.

How They Did It—Key Elements

Starting in the mid-1990s, the medical school developed evaluation forms for "physicianship" at the clerkship and ultimately preclerkship levels. It is important to note that these new evaluation forms were not isolated assessments; rather, they were developed as part of a system of evaluation, with the primary goal being remediation. The way it works is that a course director may submit a "Physicianship Evaluation Form" (Figure 12-1) for any student who is deemed to have displayed less than satisfactory behaviors with regard to professionalism. These forms are reviewed by the Associate Dean for Student Affairs at the school, who works with the student with the goal of remediation. If a student receives a form from more than one clerkship rotation, this may be documented on the Dean's letter, and the student may be

The student has exhibited one or more of the following behaviors that need improvement to meet expected standards of physicianship. This student needs further education or assistance with the following:

1. Reliability and responsibility
    a. Fulfilling responsibilities in a reliable manner
    b. Learning how to complete assigned tasks
2. Self-improvement and adaptability
    a. Accepting constructive feedback
    b. Recognizing limitations and seeking help
    c. Being respectful of colleagues and patients
    d. Incorporating feedback …

Figure 12-1 ▪ Examples from the "Physicianship Evaluation Form" for 1st- and 2nd-year students.

Credit: University of California, San Francisco. Undergraduate Medical Education: Physicianship Evaluation Forms and Policies; 2013. Available at: http://meded.ucsf.edu/ume/physicianship-evaluation-forms-and-policies.

placed on academic probation. Ultimately, a student may even be dismissed for poor professionalism, despite meeting all the other academic standards.

Embedded within this system of professionalism assessment were initiatives for faculty development to enhance the teaching and evaluation of professionalism, a transparent process for documentation and appeal, and supports for remediation. After this system was in place for a number of years, some outcomes were published indicating that the system had achieved its intended goals; the authors noted that their "faculty has embraced this evaluation system, and that within a year of its use it became part of the culture of the UCSF School of Medicine" (Papadakis, Loeser, & Healy, 2001).

As this system became well-established, it became apparent that students were not the only ones with professionalism issues. On review of the school's results on the Association of American Medical Colleges (AAMC) Graduation Questionnaire it was noted that a surprising proportion of students reported "mistreatment" by residents and staff (approximately 34% in 2004). Thus a concerted effort was made to address the issue, including the development of a system to monitor professionalism in faculty members. As one part of this initiative, two new items were added to faculty's current evaluation forms, both related to respect:

1. I was treated with respect by this attending physician; and
2. I observed others (students, residents, staff, patients) being treated with respect by this attending physician.

The response scale went from a score of 1 for "failed to treat me with respect and generally displayed an unprofessional or abusive manner in all interactions" to 5 for "consistently treated me with respect." If a student indicated that there was an issue of lack of respect, they were then given the option to select from the following (Figure 12-2).

All faculty were educated in advance of the new evaluation questions and reminded of behavioral expectations. Data were collected and monitored centrally.

Outcomes They Measured

Students' professionalism has been monitored centrally at UCSF since the development of the new form. The school keeps track of the numbers and types of lapses, as well as outcomes for each student. In addition, Papadakis et al (2004) have conducted important longitudinal studies and have reported that unprofessional behavior in medical school is associated with subsequent disciplinary action of physicians in practice. Students with comments indicating severe irresponsibility and severely diminished capacity for self-improvement were most likely to be disciplined in practice (Papadakis et al, 2005). These

	Belittled or humiliated me
	Spoke sarcastically or insultingly to me
	Intentionally neglected or left me out of the communications
	Subjected me to offensive sexist remarks or names
	Subjected me to racist or ethically offensive remarks or names
	Engaged in discomforting humor
	Denied me training opportunities because of my gender
	Required me to perform personal services (i.e., babysitting, shopping)
	Threw instruments/bandages, equipment etc.
	Threatened me with physical harm (e.g., hit, slapped, kicked)
	Created a hostile environment for learning
	Other

Figure 12-2 ▪ Sample graduation questionnaire items.

reports underscore the importance of identifying unprofessional behavior in medical school, although the authors themselves note that most students who have issues in medical school do not go on to face difficulties in practice.

In terms of faculty, the results were almost immediate—the year after the new system and evaluation were in place students' complaints about faculty dropped by half, to approximately 16% (personal communication, Maxine Papadakis, April, 2013). It isn't possible to state with certainty that the drop was because of the new form, and unfortunately further tracking was made difficult because the AAMC changed the relevant questions on the questionnaire. Still, this was an impressive effect and can be taken as evidence that changes at the level of the organization can have profound effects.

Key Lessons

An explicit system for evaluating and monitoring professionalism is not only feasible, it can help change the culture within a medical school. Including lots of education, resources, and faculty development were key to UCSF's success. Expanding the program to include faculty (and not just learners) helped reinforce the message that professionalism is a core competency expected by physicians at all levels.

BRONSON METHODIST HOSPITAL PURSUES THE PROFESSIONALISM VALUE OF HIGH-QUALITY CARE

Rationale

Bronson Methodist Hospital, a 404-bed facility in Kalamazoo, Michigan, moved to a new location in the 1999. The organization's leaders saw this move as an opportunity to redesign Bronson's culture and create a more focused mission that would inspire and engage organizational leaders, clinicians, front-line staff, patients and families, and community members as partners. Bronson's leaders were inspired by conversations with multiple organizational stakeholders, its history as a regional leader in quality outcomes, and national challenges to improve quality, including the Malcolm Baldrige Quality Award (National Institute of Standards and Technology, 2013) and declared their vision "to be a national leader in healthcare quality" (Harrelson et al, 2007).

How They Do It—Key Elements

The hospital constructed its new facility in collaboration with its staff and community members and using evidence-based healthcare design principles. These design principles included features such as private rooms with dedicated hand-washing sinks to minimize hospital-acquired infections (Van Enk, 2006). As they were moving into the new facility in 1999, Bronson leaders began developing their new vision. They used input from numerous, stakeholders, the Malcom Baldrige Quality Award criteria, a Presidential award for performance excellence in healthcare and other fields (National Institute of Standards and Technology, 2013) as well as the Institute of Medicine's six quality aims (Institute of Medicine, 2001) to develop its "Plan for Excellence." The Plan for Excellence outlines the organization's goals in the "3 Cs"—clinical excellence, customer and service excellence, and corporate effectiveness—as well as a philosophy of nursing excellence. Once completed, the Plan was distributed to all employees and redistributed regularly. To further inspire commitment to its vision, Bronson's leaders set the goal of receiving a Malcolm Baldrige award by 2010 (Harrelson et al, 2007).

Currently, the Plan guides the defining of quality goals in the hospital's annual strategic planning process and ongoing financial, capital, and human resources planning; the quality goals guide the development of quality scorecards, which contain measures in each of the "3 C" areas (Knapp, 2006). A number of multidisciplinary performance improvement committees throughout the organization implement the strategic plan goals, and leadership regularly monitors its progress (Harrelson et al, 2007).

Bronson Methodist maintains its commitment to quality through a hiring process that emphasizes organizational commitment to measurement and improvement (Cunningham et al, 2011). Employees also receive communications skills training and standardized processes of interacting with patients to assure patient satisfaction and high-quality care (Harrelson et al, 2007).The hospital also provides protected time for physicians and other staff to participate in quality improvement activities, and offers leadership training for staff interested in further quality improvement training. The organization also provides a number of educational incentives and recognition and reward programs for staff. In addition, the hospital's leaders model a commitment to quality improvement by conducting regular staff surveys on organizational climate and quality efforts. Leaders share survey results with all staff and commit to areas for improvement. The surveys also ask employees to rate the organizations' leaders, both collectively and individually, on the following: "competence, ethical, caring, fair, strategic, approachable, honest, and open." The organization's leaders examine the results both collectively and individually, and use it to develop individual leadership development plans (Harrelson et al, 2007). Bronson leaders also obtain regular patient and family feedback through a patient advisory council and focus groups (Cunningham et al, 2011).

Outcomes They Measured

The hospital measured the impact of its new design in a number of ways, including examining hospital-acquired infection rates. Bronson leaders compared the units in the new facilities with private rooms and dedicated hand washing stations to those with semiprivate rooms. They found that the majority of private room units had a statistically significant decline in hospital-acquired infections compared to other units (Van Enk, 2006). In addition, as part of ongoing quality improvement, all performance improvement committees have quality scorecards; their numerous quality measures include heart failure, pneumonia, and acute myocardial infarction process and outcome measures, skin breakdown rates, patient fall rates, and patient satisfaction measures. Recent quality measures include an 83% hand hygiene compliance rate, compared to 40% nationally, and a 91.4% survival rate for Medicare pneumonia patients, which exceeds the national average (Bronson Methodist Hospital, 2009). The organization applied for the Malcolm Baldrige Quality Award, the Presidential honor for quality and organizational performance, for five consecutive years, which involves an extensive application and site visits. Subsequently, in 2005 Bronson Methodist became the first healthcare organization to win the Baldrige Award (Bronson Methodist Hospital, 2005).

Staff surveys also reveal high satisfaction, and the organization reports turnover rates that are well below the national average. For example, Bronson has a 5% annual nursing turnover rate, which is one of the lowest in the country (Harrelson et al, 2007).

Key Lessons

A clear strategy, strong leadership support, engagement of all stakeholders, and ongoing measurement can help an organization achieve aggressive quality goals. Furthermore, a culture of high expectations, coupled with a strong interest in staff and patient feedback, can lead to high levels of staff and patient satisfaction and reduce staff turnover.

TULANE UNIVERSITY SCHOOL OF MEDICINE ADVANCES PROFESSIONALISM BY REDUCING DISPARITIES IN CARE

Rationale

Tulane University School of Medicine in New Orleans was hit hard by Hurricane Katrina in 2005. A number of the school's leaders remained in New Orleans to create urgent care sites. As New Orleans attempted to recover from the storm, these leaders observed that the already-existing health disparities in the city had worsened. Tulane's leadership, led by physician advocates, felt that it had an obligation to address these disparities. Immediately following the storm, their efforts consisted of setting up makeshift clinics around the city, often without power, drinkable water, or functioning sewage systems. Seeing an ongoing need for community-based care, Tulane's leaders saw an opportunity to reshape its mission (Niyogi et al, 2006).

How They Did It—Key Elements

Tulane University School of Medicine changed its mission to, "Education, Research, Patient Care: We Heal Communities." The School also created an Office of Community Affairs and Health Policy (OCAHP) with the vision that "OCAHP will be a leader in improving population health and building capacity through innovative and community engaged clinical care, education, research, and policy advancement" (Tulane University School of Medicine, 2013). While this was occurring, the Department of Health and Human Services (HHS) provided funding support for a network of clinics built on the principles of the patient-centered medical home through its Primary Care Access and Stabilization Grant, which provided funding for some of Tulane's community clinics along with nearly 90 other primary care clinics in the New Orleans region. Tulane also participated in the HHS-funded Louisiana Health Care Redesign Collaborative, a multistakeholder group committed to supporting evidence-based, high-quality care in Louisiana.

In 2006, the Collaborative developed four post-Hurricane Katrina redesign recommendations:

1. Expansion of access to affordable healthcare coverage
2. Implementation of medical home systems of care
3. The use of health information technology to support patients and providers
4. Establishment of shared quality standards and information (Tulane University School of Medicine, 2013)

Subsequently, the OCAHP instituted a number of new programs to implement the Health Care Redesign Collaborative's recommendations in consultation with community leaders. These programs include several community-based clinics, mobile children's health units that visit underserved areas, and depression treatment programs that incorporate music therapy and faith-based programs. In addition, Tulane has collaborated with local community groups on the REACH NOLA Mental Health Infrastructure and Training Project to integrate much-needed behavioral health services into community-based clinics (Association of American Medical Colleges, 2010).

Tulane's focus on community-based care has extended to its medical education and training programs. The School of Medicine offers a community health rotation that includes training in quality improvement, leadership, social justice, social determinants of health, and advocacy (Cunningham et al, 2011). Tulane has also created a nursing fellowship to train nurses in community-based healthcare; and a community health workers training institute to train community members in health outreach and promotion (Tulane University School of Medicine, 2013). Furthermore, Tulane's Internal Medicine Residency program also has a strong focus on primary care, and its residents complete their continuity clinics at the Tulane University Community Health Centers (Tulane University School of Medicine, 2010).

Outcomes They Measured

An evaluation of the Primary Care Access and Stabilization Grant (PCASG), which supported several Tulane clinics, found that PCASG-funded clinics provided critical access to primary care in underserved areas of New Orleans, and that the clinics made significant quality and safety gains during their funding period. Furthermore, "they provided primary and preventative care to twice as many African American residents as any other race helping to alleviate the long-standing disparity in access to care for the minority population"(Louisiana Department of Health and Hospitals, 2010). PCASG-funded clinics also made significant gains in quality and safety measures during their funding period (Rittenhouse et al, 2012).

Tulane's clinics also track a number of quality measures, and all of Tulane's clinics have achieved some level of patient-centered medical home recognition from the National Committee for Quality Assurance. Community-based clinic measures include community members' ratings of access to care, confidence in care quality and safety, and coordination of care; the clinics have received strong marks in these areas. In addition, the medical school saw significant increases in the number and quality of applicants after redefining its mission to focus on the community's needs (Cunningham et al, 2011). The Association of American Medical Colleges also recognized the school's efforts by awarding Tulane the 2010 Spencer Foreman Award for Outstanding Community Service (Association of American Medical Colleges, 2010).

Key Lessons

For Tulane, a tragedy provided an opportunity to redefine its mission. Their work since Hurricane Katrina also illustrates that academic medical centers can play a significant role in addressing local healthcare disparities by providing high-quality, community-based primary care. However, finding ongoing funding to provide care to underserved populations can be challenging and without that funding quality gains may be difficult to sustain (Rittenhouse et al, 2012). In addition, Tulane found that a focus on community-based care and healthcare disparities can be a significant attractor of medical students and residents and can improve the quality of its student body.

CONCLUSION

Healthcare organizations can influence professionalism through both formal and informal policies and procedures. Organizations that have successfully advanced professionalism have clearly articulated their values, aligned their organizational systems and structures to support desired behaviors, and cultivated strong relationships. Supporting professionalism requires sustained commitment from an organization's leaders. Table 12-3 provides further resources for organizations interested in fostering professionalism.

Table 12-3	**TOOLS FOR ORGANIZATIONS TO ADVANCE PROFESSIONALISM**
Organization	**Description**
ABIM Foundation (http://www.abimfoundation.org)	The ABIM Foundation is committed to advancing medical professionalism to improve healthcare. Its website contains information on the *Physician Charter,* profiles of organizations advancing professionalism, and a resource center with a medical professionalism bibliography, videos, and other tools.

Table 12-3 TOOLS FOR ORGANIZATIONS TO ADVANCE PROFESSIONALISM (*Continued*)	
Organization	Description
Institute for Healthcare Improvement (IHI) (http://www.ihi.org)	IHI has tools for implementing quality improvement and improving patient safety available, including: • IHI Open School is an interprofessional educational community that gives students the skills to become change agents in healthcare. Their resources section includes activities for IHI Open School Chapters, videos, case studies, and many other resources in topics such as quality improvement, patient safety, and error disclosure. The IHI Open School also offers online courses that are free to students, faculty, deans, and residents. • The IHI Triple Aim seeks to improve the health of the population, enhance the patient experience of care (including quality, access, and reliability) and reduce, or at least control, the per capita cost of care. Organizations can participate in a Triple Aim improvement community.
Institute for Patient and Family-Centered Care (http://www.ipfcc.org/advance/index.html)	IPFCC's website includes many profiles of organizations that have implemented patient and family-centered care. The IPFCC also makes a free download of specific tools available, including tools to foster collaboration with patients and families as advisors, and assessments for hospitals and ambulatory practices interested in advancing patient- and family-centered care.
Institute on Medicine as a Profession (IMAP) (http://imapny.org/)	The IMAP media library contains media presentations, videos, documents, citations and data related to IMAP's work. Visitors can search, filter, and download items from this library. • IMAP's Web-based curriculum "Promoting Change at AMCs and other healthcare organizations," offers a comprehensive guide to the issues surrounding conflicts of interest, medical professionalism, and best practices for the management of physicians' relationships with industry. • IMAP's research team has compiled the Conflicts of Interest Best Practices Toolkit, including case studies of healthcare organizations with innovative and effective policies for controlling conflicts of interest. These materials are relevant to a wide and varied audience with any interest in understanding and/or teaching conflicts of interest in medicine.
Malcolm Baldrige Quality Award (http://www.nist.gov/baldrige/)	Baldrige Award is a national program for performance excellence in a number of fields, including healthcare. The program offers self-assessments for leaders to assess an organization's current performance and opportunities for improvement. The Baldrige program also supports a network of state and local groups designed to support organizations that are new to the Baldrige program.
Relationship Centered Health Care (http://www.relationshipcenteredhc.com/)	Relationship Centered Health Care offers executive coaching and training for leaders interested in fostering relationship-centered care within their institutions. The website's Resources page features a relationship-centered care bibliography and links to related organizations.

KEY LEARNING POINTS

1. Healthcare organizations such as academic medical centers, ambulatory care centers, community hospitals, and integrated delivery systems play an important role in influencing physician professionalism.
2. Organizations can shape physician behavior through both written and unwritten rules and norms.
3. Organizations that have successfully advanced professionalism have used strategies such as clearly articulated values, alignment of systems and structures to support behavioral expectations, and the cultivation of strong, respectful relationships between individuals at all levels of the organization.
4. Organizational efforts to advance professionalism require sustained leadership commitment, hiring/admissions processes that support the organization's values, ongoing training, and soliciting and acting on feedback from staff, patients, and other stakeholders.

REFERENCES

1. Association of American Medical Colleges. *Spencer Foreman Award for Outstanding Community Service: Tulane University School of Medicine*; 2010. Available at: https://www.aamc.org/initiatives/awards/2010/155710/2010_ocsa_recipient_tulane.html
2. Bronson Methodist Hospital. *Malcolm Baldrige National Quality Award Application Summary*; 2005. Available at: http://www.baldrige.nist.gov/PDF_files/Bronson_Methodist_Hospital_Application_Summary.pdf
3. Bronson Methodist Hospital. *Report on Quality, Safety & Innovation*; 2009. Available at: http://www.bronsonhealth.com/system/media/steep-final/index.html
4. Cottingham AH, Suchman AL, Litzelman DK, Frankel RM, Mossbarger DL, Williamson PR, Baldwin DC Jr, Inui TS. Enhancing the informal curriculum of a medical school: a case study in organizational culture change. *J Gen Intern Med*. 2008 Jun;23(6):715–722.
5. Cunningham AT, Bernabeo EC, Wolfson DB, Lesser CS. Organisational strategies to cultivate professional values and behaviours. *BMJ Qual Saf*. 2011 Apr;20(4):351–358.
6. Egener B, McDonald W, Rosof B, Gullen D. Perspective: Organizational professionalism: relevant competencies and behaviors. *Acad Med*. 2012 May;87(5):668–674.
7. Gottlieb K, Sylvester I, Eby D. Transforming your practice: what matters most. *Fam Pract Manag*. 2008 Jan;15(1):32–38.
8. Harrelson K, McClurkan M, Reinoehl S, Sardone FJ, Serbenski M, Ulshafer SM. Bronson Methodist Hospital, 2005. Malcolm Baldrige National Quality Award Winner (Case Study). *J Innov Manage*. 2007;12(4):6–33.

9. Institute for Healthcare Improvement. *Alaska Native Medical Center: Values-Driven System Design*. 2011. Available at: http://www.ihi.org/knowledge/Pages/ImprovementStories/AlaskaNativeMedicalCenterValuesDrivenSystemDesign.aspx

10. Institute of Medicine. *Crossing the Quality Chasm: A New Health System for the 21st Century*. Washington, DC: National Academies Press; 2001.

11. Knapp C. Bronson Methodist Hospital: journey to excellence in quality and safety. *Jt Comm J Qual Patient Saf*. 2006 Oct;32(10):556–563.

12. Litzelman DK, Cottingham AH. The new formal competency-based curriculum and informal curriculum at Indiana University School of Medicine: overview and five-year analysis. *Acad Med*. 2007 Apr;82(4):410–421.

13. Louisiana Department of Health and Hospitals. *Louisiana's Vision for Access to Primary Care in the New Orleans Region*. 2010. Available at: http://new.dhh.louisiana.gov/assets/oph/pcrh/pcrh/LaVisionNORegionEmail.pdf

14. National Institute of Standards and Technology. *Baldrige Performance Excellence Program*; 2013. Available at: http://www.nist.gov/baldrige/

15. Niyogi A, Price E, Springgate B, Joplin C, Desalvo KB. Restoring and reforming ambulatory services and internal medicine training in the aftermath of hurricane Katrina. *Am J Med Sci*. 2006 Nov;332(5):289–291.

16. Papadakis MA, Hodgson CS, Teherani A, Kohatsu ND. Unprofessional behavior in medical school is associated with subsequent disciplinary action by a state medical board. *Acad Med*. 2004 Mar;79(3):244–249.

17. Papadakis MA, Loeser H, Healy K. Early detection and evaluation of professionalism deficiencies in medical students: one school's approach. *Acad Med*. 2001 Nov;76(11):1100–1106.

18. Papadakis MA, Teherani A, Banach MA, Knettler TR, Rattner SL, Stern DT, Veloski JJ, Hodgson CS. Disciplinary action by medical boards and prior behavior in medical school. *N Engl J Med*. 2005 Dec 22;353(25):2673–2682.

19. Rittenhouse DR, Schmidt LA, Wu KJ, Wiley J. The post-Katrina conversion of clinics in New Orleans to medical homes shows change is possible, but hard to sustain. *Health Aff (Millwood)*. 2012 Aug;31(8):1729–1738.

20. Tulane University School of Medicine. *The Tulane Internal Medicine Primary Care Track*; 2010. Available at: http://www.tulanemedicine.com/primary_care_career.html

21. Tulane University School of Medicine. *Office of Community Affairs and Health Policy*; 2013. Available at: http://tulane.edu/som/cahp/

22. Van Enk RA. Modern hospital design for infection control. *Health Des*. 2006;6(5):10–14. Available at: http://www.healthcaredesignmagazine.com/article/modern-hospital-design-infection-control

Index

Page numbers followed by *f* and *t* indicate figures and tables.